KT-480-598

Parkinson's
Disease Society

CLINICS IN DEVELOPMENTAL MEDICINE NO. 126

THE BIOLOGY OF THE AUTISTIC SYNDROMES
—2nd Edition

©1992 Mac Keith Press
5a Netherhall Gardens, London NW3 5RN

First published in this edition 1992

British Library Cataloguing in Publication Data

Gillberg, Christopher
  The Biology of the Autistic Syndromes.—
  2Rev.ed.—(Clinics in Developmental Medicine; No. 126)
  I. Title II. Coleman, Mary III. Series
  618.928982

ISSN: 0069-4835

ISBN   0 521 43228 6

Printed in Great Britain at The Lavenham Press Ltd., Lavenham, Suffolk
Mac Keith Press is supported by **The Spastics Society, London, England**

Clinics in Developmental Medicine No. 126

THE BIOLOGY OF THE AUTISTIC SYNDROMES—2nd Edition

CHRISTOPHER GILLBERG
Child Neuropsychiatry Clinic
University of Göteborg

MARY COLEMAN
Georgetown University School of Medicine
Washington, DC

1992
Mac Keith Press

Distributed by:
OXFORD: Blackwell Scientific Publications Ltd.
NEW YORK: Cambridge University Press.

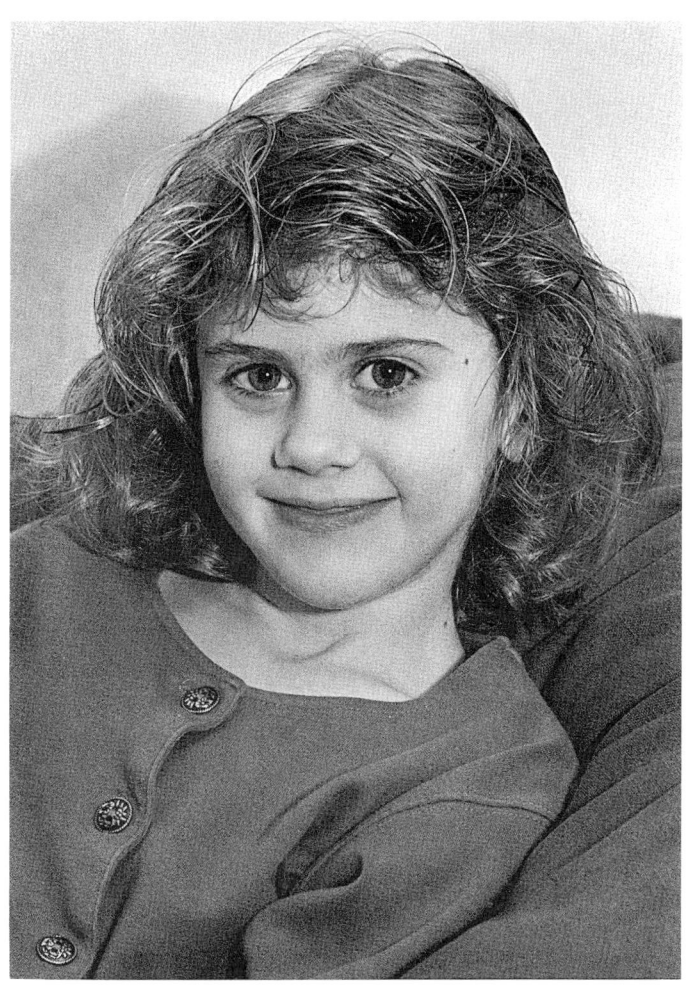

Frontispiece: 6-year-old girl with autism. (Photo by Michael Schmidt.)

AUTHORS' AFFILIATIONS

CHRISTOPHER GILLBERG,
M.D.

Professor of Child and Adolescent Psychiatry; Head, Child Neuropsychiatry Clinic, University of Göteborg

MARY COLEMAN, M.D.

Emeritus, Department of Pediatrics, Georgetown University School of Medicine, Washington, DC

CONTENTS

1
INTRODUCTION

In 1938, a small 5-year-old boy from Mississippi was brought to Baltimore, Maryland, to the Johns Hopkins University office of the child psychiatrist, Leo Kanner. According to Kanner:

I was struck by the uniqueness of the peculiarities which Donald exhibited. He could, since the age of 2½ years, tell the names of all presidents and vice-presidents, recite the letters of the alphabet forwards and backwards, and flawlessly, with good enunciation, rattle off the Twenty-Third Psalm. Yet he was unable to carry on an ordinary conversation. He was out of contact with people, while he could handle objects skillfully. His memory was phenomenal. The few times when he addressed someone—largely to satisfy his wants—he referred to himself as 'You' and to the person as 'I'. He did not respond to any intelligence tests but manipulated intricate formboards adroitly.

In the course of the next few years, Kanner observed ten more children who displayed similar behaviour patterns and noted that they had in common 'extreme aloneness from the beginning of life and an anxiously obsessive desire for the preservation of sameness.' He reported these 11 cases in a scientific journal (Kanner 1943), introducing to the world medical literature this group of children he labelled 'autistic'.

Once the syndrome was identified, several earlier accounts of children, probably autistic, were found (Darr and Warden 1951, Vaillant 1962, Wing 1976). In fact, strange, mysterious and enigmatic children have been part of our culture throughout history. Some of them were known as feral children, suckled and reared by wolves or other wild animals. In Roman history, Romulus and Remus were thought to have been cast into the Tiber River and somehow retrieved and reared by wolves until they could rejoin the human community in order to found Rome.

These legends are not confined to ancient history; such children have been a source of group fantasy in more recent centuries also. Victor, the wild boy of Aveyron, was first seen in 1797 running through the woods in the region of Lacaune, in south central France. He was captured, escaped twice, and recaptured when he was approximately 12 years old. The French physician Jean Marc Gaspard Itard devoted five years to teaching Victor, but eventually gave up his experiment (Lane 1976). The story of Victor has so caught our imaginations that it is the subject of many books and has been made into a movie.

The twentieth century has also had its feral children. The Reverend J.A.L. Singh discovered Kamala and her sister Amala in 1929 in Midnapore, India. The local inhabitants had been terrified by strange happenings and 'ghosts', and the Rev. Singh found that there were two wild children in the area. He reported that

1

the children were reared by wolves and found in a wolves' den. Dr Gesell of Yale University studied the reports on these children and in 'what now appears like a jarring suspension of rationality' (Schopler 1976) reconstructed, from his imagination, how the well-known Gesell norms manifested themselves in the wolves' den (Gesell 1941). He described Kamala's successful adjustment to the wolves' den, an adjustment which had admittedly been constructed purely from his imagination.

The Rev. Singh's diary of Kamala also interested the psychologist, Dr Bruno Bettelheim (1959). Bettelheim suggested that Kamala was not raised by wolves at all, but that she, like other feral children, behaved very much like children in his school who had autism. However, just as Gesell had done before him, he used the tools of his discipline to project fantasy medical history on Kamala. He argued that the so-called feral children were actually children with autism who had been neglected and emotionally deprived by their mothers. Without having any medical history to rely on regarding Kamala and her sister, he concluded that there were no feral children, only feral mothers.

According to Schopler (1973), Kamala's place in the history of autism is significant, not because of the theories widely-published experts claimed about her and her origin, but because of the myths that have evolved from these same theories, resulting in confused and misguided implications for the treatment of children with autism.

In a story published by the Russian author Gorky in 1921, there is a description of a boy who meets many autistic criteria. In this story, Gorky has the child fathered by a monk, and makes the child an attractive, enigmatic individual in spite of his mental deficiency. Thus, Gorky is describing the time-honoured notion that mentally deficient children may have a 'peculiarly close relationship to the almighty' (Gorky 1921).

In every culture, people as a group project their feelings onto unusual members of the group and target them for inappropriate fantasies and myths. This has been true, particularly, of mentally impaired children of all kinds, perhaps especially children with autism with their complex and unusual behaviour patterns. These cultural projections are not limited to the uninformed and poorly educated; the written history of children with autism and their parents is replete with examples of inappropriate interpretations. It is the purpose of this monograph to examine what hard data exist regarding these children so that the medical profession can move forward with appropriate diagnosis, treatment and care. They are not mystical, superhuman, subhuman, legendary, mysterious occult individuals in possession of non-human traits. They are simply children who are in trouble because their brains are not functioning as they should.

Since the syndrome was defined by Kanner in 1943, there have been a number of areas of major disagreement regarding this patient population. One is how the diagnosis is arrived at and which children are included or excluded from the term 'autistic'. Differing points of view on diagnosis are reviewed in the next chapter and a working solution is suggested by the authors of this monograph. In this chapter, the controversies regarding the multitude of aetiologies proposed as responsible for the symptoms in this patient group will be reviewed and discussed.

Controversies about the aetiology of the autistic syndromes

Kanner, who introduced the syndrome of autism, was a child psychiatrist deeply involved in the controversies in his field at the time. In the 1920s, theories of the parental causes of mental illness were being developed. Fromm-Reichmann's theory about schizophrenogenic mothers and Levy's theory about overprotective mothers are just two examples from that period. According to Victor (1983), Kanner, like many mental health professionals, was drawn into the conflict. His participation was said to be intense and he fought on both sides, foreshadowing the controversy about the role of parents of children with autism that was to follow. In 1941, during the period leading up to the publication of his paper on autism, Kanner published an article about mothers' destructiveness (Kanner 1941*a*). In the same year, he published *In Defense of Mothers*, a book in which he sought to relieve mothers of guilt in relation to their children (Kanner 1941*b*). This ambivalence toward mothers continued after he introduced the concept of autism.

In 1949, Kanner wrote:

The vast majority of the parents of autistic children have features in common which it would be impossible to disregard . . . Most of the parents declare outright that they are not comfortable in the company of people . . . They are polite and dignified people who are impressed by seriousness and disdainful of anything that smacks of frivolity. (Kanner 1949)

He also described them as perfectionists, and as obsessive, humourless individuals who used set rules as substitutes for life's enjoyment. His most extreme statement was made to *Time*, a popular magazine available to friends, families and neighbours of children with autism. He reported 'that children with early infantile autism were the offspring of highly organized, professional parents, cold and rational, who just happened to defrost long enough to produce a child' (*Time*, 25 July 1960). This was his view of the 'refrigerator' type of parent about whom he had been lecturing.

During this period, Kanner criticized the blindness of colleagues (*e.g.* van Krevelen 1952, Benda and Melchior 1959) who looked for physiological causes of autism rather than noting parental behaviour. He found the evidence for parental causes over physiological causes to be 'so obvious as to force itself on . . . an open-eyed observer' (Kanner 1948). Kanner also wrote that the condition usually could not be remedied because the parents sabotaged treatment. Therefore, unless the mothers could be helped by psychotherapy, the only hope for most children with autism lay in removal from the home and placement with foster mothers (Kanner 1952).

Yet this is the same Kanner who said:

Herewith I especially acquit you people as parents. I have been misquoted many times. From the very first publication to the last, I spoke of this condition in no uncertain terms as

3

innate. (Kanner 1969)

Kanner was ambivalent about the aetiology of autism, and here he was not alone.

Since his time there have been a great many aetiological theories developed, mostly psychodynamic, which assume that the infant was normal at birth and attribute its development of symptoms to poor nurturing, particularly poor mothering (as reviewed by Hingtgen and Bryson 1972). Many additional theories have been developed by Fraknoi and Ruttenberg (1971), Williams and Harper (1973), Szurek (1973), Ekstein and Friedman (1974), King (1975), Massie (1978) and Victor (1983). These various theories have postulated that the parents of children with autism were deficient either in touching, in feeding practices, in speech practices and/or in eye-to-eye contact with the child, or were thought to project dehumanizing fantasies onto their infant. They were viewed as extreme personality types: either very depressed, or cold, or full of rage, or without a sense of self, or actually psychopathic (as reviewed by DeMyer *et al.* 1981).

In addition to the theories of poor nurturing as a sole aetiological factor, DeMyer pointed out that there are also two varieties of a combined nature–nurture theory of autism. In one version, infants with autism were seen as biologically deficient and the parents viewed as failing to give proper emotional support to the vulnerable infant. In another version, some infants were viewed as organically damaged and others as biologically normal. In this latter version, the parents of the 'non-organic' infants were described as failing to a greater degree than the parents of 'organic' infants. Examples of these theories are those developed by Despert (1971), O'Moore (1972), Miller (1974) and Tinbergen and Tinbergen (1976).

One of the first authors to speak up prominently suggesting that the parents themselves may not be at fault and that there may be some other aetiology to autistic symptoms was Rimland, a parent/professional who wrote the book *Infantile Autism: the Syndrome and its Implications for a Neural Theory of Behavior* in 1964. Since then, in an attempt to address the large literature on parent deficits in child rearing, several investigators began studying parents of children with autism and comparing them to other control groups, using established scientific methodologies of obtaining data. Cox *et al.* (1975) investigated early stressful events and parental warmth, responsiveness and sociability in parents of children with autism compared to a matched group of parents of children with dysphasia. (Children with dysphasia have a delayed, usually aberrant, acquisition of language, but are not disabled in any other major area of functioning.) The two parent groups did not differ in interpersonal relationships or ratings of emotional warmth and sociability, except that parents of children with autism spent more time with friends than parents of children with dysphasia. This study suggested that parents of children with autism may be more, rather than less, sociable. Goldfarb *et al.* (1976) also failed to demonstrate parent group differences in psychopathology and functioning. McAdoo and DeMyer (1978a) decided to study the parents of children with autism

4

who had an organic diagnosis versus the parents of children who did not have an organic diagnosis. Using as a tool the Minnesota Multiphasic Personality Inventories, they found no difference between the two parent groups.

A study of infant care practices was also done comparing the parents of children with autism and a carefully matched group of parents of normal children. In this study there was no difference in infant acceptance, warmth, nurturing, feeding and tactile or general stimulation (DeMyer *et al.* 1972). Using the Ferreira and Winter unrevealed differences task, Byassee and Murrell (1975) found similar family interactions in both normal families and families with a child with autistim. Cantwell *et al.* (1978) compared families with children with autism to families with children with dysphasia and reported they were similar in quality and intensity, except that the children with autism received greater interaction. Using the Ittleson Center Scales, the authors found group similarities in spontaneity, decisiveness, anticipation, control, and meeting children's demands. Of interest because of earlier speculation regarding the use of language by the mothers of children with autism, the study by Cantwell *et al.* (1978) found the same linguistic clarity, complexity and grammaticality in the speech of the mothers. Other studies have also yielded no evidence that the speech of parents had any detrimental effect on their children (Frank *et al.* 1976, Cantwell and Baker 1978).

However, there were two studies which showed different results. Goldfarb *et al.* (1973) compared mothers of children with schizophrenia/autism with mothers of normal controls and described them as inferior in labelling and describing objects. King (1975), using a rating system on chart descriptions, compared mothers of children with autism with mothers of control children and reported more 'double bind' interactions in the mothers of children with autism.

The literature on parents was reviewed by McAdoo and DeMyer (1978*b*), who concluded that, as a group, parents of children with autism: (1) display no more signs of mental or emotional illness than parents whose children have 'organic' disorders, with or without psychosis; (2) do not have extreme personality traits such as coldness, obsessiveness, social anxiety or rage; and (3) do not possess specific deficits in infant and child care (see also Koegel *et al.* 1983, Schopler and Mesibov 1984).

DeMyer (1979) also wrote a sensitive piece acknowledging the difficulties of rearing a child with autism.

Although children with autism are some of the most difficult children to assess and evaluate, several studies have shown that parents can be trusted in the information they provide about their child (Schopler and Reichler 1972, Wing and Gould 1978). Schopler and Reichler (1972) pointed out:

Professionals, however, because of their distrust of parental judgment, frequently superficially reassure, or even worse, humiliate parents by labeling them overconcerned and overanxious, or blame the child's problems on parental management. Such criticism without appropriate evaluation and specific instructions in improved management can . . . leave parents on their own to cope with extremely difficult developmental problems, discouraging their seeking of further help, and harmfully delaying appropriate interventions.

To this day there are several myths in the field which tend to suggest that environmental factors cause autism. One is the myth that children with autism are from the upper social classes.

Kanner himself long believed that autism was a disease of the upper classes (Kanner 1943, 1949). When Lotter (1966) published the first epidemiological study of autism and found a small, but statistically significant, excess of parents from the highest social classes, this single result was at once incorporated into the Kanner theory as unequivocal proof. There are, however, several reasons why the social class theory cannot be regarded as proven or even plausible. First of all, Lotter's finding really was that the majority of children with autism do *not* belong to upper and upper-middle class families. Second, the calculated statistically significant difference rested on the shaky basis of a single child! If one child with autism had belonged to social class III instead of II the difference with regard to expected frequency would not be statistically significant. Third, Schopler *et al.* (1979) have provided evidence for a social class *referral* bias in studies of autism. Fourth and most importantly, there are at least six other epidemiological studies of autism (Brask 1970, Ritvo *et al.* 1971b, Wing 1980, Bohman *et al.* 1981, Andersson and Wadensjö 1981, Gillberg and Schaumann 1982) all of which have shown autism to be almost equally distributed over social strata. Thus, one can only conclude that the bulk of the data suggests beyond any reasonable doubt that autism is *not* associated with social class. The few authorities who still maintain that autism is correlated with high social class rely on the Lotter study and clinically referred samples for their argument, and do so in the face of a host of epidemiological data and other clinically referred samples not indicating a social class bias.

Another myth is the 'first or only child' theory. Several authors have reported an excess of first born children in series of children with autism (Despert 1951, Kanner 1954, Pitfield and Oppenheim 1964, Rimland 1964, Deykin and MacMahon 1980). This has been taken by some as firm evidence for psychogenetic theories. Two considerations are of major importance in this connection: (i) there is no study suggesting that *a majority* of children with autism are first-born, and (ii) there are several epidemiological studies that have not come up with results in support of the 'first-born notion' (Lotter 1966, Wing 1980, Gillberg 1984a). One study (Tsai and Stewart 1983) has suggested an increase among first and fourth or later-born children. This would be in line with biological hypotheses, as both first and fourth or later-born children are more at risk for pre- and perinatal hazards than second or third-born children. However, the results in this field are equivocal to say the least and cannot serve as a basis for any firm argument.

The notion that in a disproportionately large number of cases children with autism are only children has no scientific support that we are aware of. However, should this prove to be the case in a comparative study, the explanation that immediately presents itself is that the child's disabilities might deter the parents from trying to have more children, as has been confirmed by a number of parents.

More recently, the attempt to prove that autism does not have an organic basis has shifted. In 1981, a paper was written arguing that an organic origin is inconsistent with a review of the literature of the frequency of autism among Italian, Chinese, Hispanic, African and Israeli children (Sanua 1981). The author postulated that because of the family network available to various nationality groups and because of the isolation of mothers in nuclear families in the West, autism is seen more frequently in the West. He suggested that the Western family pattern prevents parental surrogates from compensating for the deficiencies of parents. However, this paper has several major weaknesses. For example, regarding the Israeli study, he quotes Kauffman (1972), who stated that he could identify eight out of 3000 children as having early childhood psychosis with autistic features. He did not want to count them as having autism if they had seizures, an inappropriate assumption (see Chapter 6). Since the incidence of autism elsewhere is somewhere around four to five per 10,000, what is being reported in this one paper is a much higher frequency than usual (25 per 10,000). However, we do not know what the incidence actually is, since no sound epidemiological studies are available from those countries. And, even if there are fewer cases of autism among Italian, Chinese, Hispanic, African and Israeli children, it still would not disprove an organic aetiology, since the prevalence of organic diseases can vary in different groups. An example is phenylketonuria, an established aetiology of the autistic syndromes (see Chapter 17), which is found more frequently in people of European extraction than of African extraction (Therrell *et al.* 1983). Gillberg (1984*b*) has suggested that divergent findings in epidemiology in autism might be due not only to different diagnostic criteria, but also to different aetiologies in different parts of the globe.

This present monograph is a review of the known information regarding the organic aetiology of the autistic syndromes. If we assume for the moment that the organic explanation appears to be the most reasonable explanation of the disease process in children with autism, the question then arises: why do highly intelligent, well-educated professionals continue to espouse the psychogenic theory of autism?

Several possible answers come to mind. The first is that the authority figure who first defined the syndrome—Kanner—himself wrote a number of medical papers suggesting that the parents were a major factor in their child's disability. As the innovative psychiatrist who established the syndrome and brought it to the attention of the world, his point of view would tend to be taken most seriously.

Secondly, perhaps the most compelling reason why the psychogenic/nurture/ environmental theory of autism persisted was that some reasonable parallels were drawn between behaviours observed in children with autism and in experimental animals. As summed up by Harlow and McKinney (1971), the theoretical linkages between the abnormal behaviour in Rhesus monkeys and human beings were elucidated by experiments with monkeys producing two prime behaviours: total social isolation, and disruption of affectionate bonds between mothers and infants or between peers. Harlow *et al.* (1955) were able to produce a syndrome in Rhesus monkeys that somewhat resembled autism by rearing infant monkeys from birth in a total isolation chamber where they had no contact with other monkeys or humans. The technique was effective in producing severe and long-lasting problems in monkeys, so that when they were removed from the chambers they spent most of their time huddled alone in a corner, rocking, self-clasping and refusing to enter into play or other normal social encounters with their peers. Some of them had self-abusive behaviours. It is not unreasonable to apply to children who share many of the characteristics of these monkeys the findings of the experiments.

For those who espouse an organic cause of autism, such a striking parallel in animal experiments and human behaviour must be explained. The answer probably lies in a similar lack of sensory input whether of an exogenous or endogenous nature at an early developmental state. If a small infant is in a normal environment, but has an endogenous central nervous system (CNS) impairment in the ability to process incoming sensory stimuli, the same effect might be achieved. Emotional nourishment, such as being hugged and kissed by a parent, is processed through the tactile sensory system, a system often impaired in children with autism who have tactile defensiveness. An infant's joy of visually exploring a mother's face depends upon a totally functional visual system, not a system relegated to avoidance of eye contact and fleeting glances. The pleasure of the parent's words and songs comes through the auditory processing system, a system so often impaired in children with autism that it has even been considered as a primary cause of autistic symptoms (Churchill 1978). But the baby with autism is not able to benefit from the environment and is often unable to send feedback messages through meaningful glances and smiles to further parent/child interaction. The nurturing environmental stimuli, just as essential for the organizational growth of a human brain as food is for the physical growth of the human body, are improperly processed by these children, thereby depriving them of much of the emotional and cognitive nutrients that they need in the first years of life.

A few individuals who suffered from autism as children have as adults been able to discuss their earlier experiences. The word common to all these accounts is 'confusion': as one boy put it, 'I did not know what was wanted from me.'

Where we stand today
The enigma of the beautiful child tip-toeing into your waiting room, gaze averted, is beginning to yield to the diagnostic techniques of contemporary science. The field of autism research has now moved beyond the outmoded concepts of parental culpability and of autism as a single disease entity (Fig. 1.1). There is a new understanding of the biological underpinnings of an infant's capacity for personal relatedness. This information is coming from the young field of developmental neuropsychiatry. Yes, there are those still clinging to the psychoanalytic point of view about autism (*e.g.* Haag 1984, Cecchi 1990), but they are fast becoming rare.

Developmental neuropsychiatry is a blend of once separate disciplines that

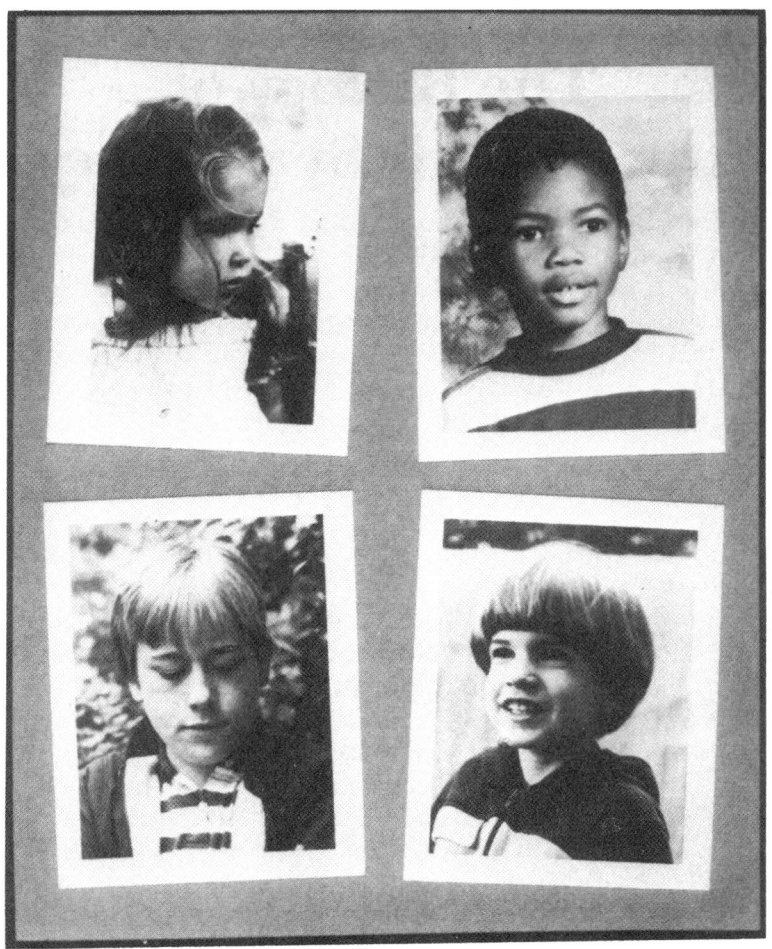

Fig. 1.1. Four children diagnosed with autism, each with a different diagnosis (*clockwise, from top left:* Rett syndrome, idiopathic autism, purine autism, neurofibromatosis).

have come to understand that major disorders of cognition and behaviour can coexist in the same child caused by the same aetiological agent. The many different disorders of maturation that affect temperament and behaviour also often affect areas of language and cognition in general. The autistic syndromes are a prime example of this developmental delay unevenly affecting the different spheres of maturation in each autistic child.

This book attempts to review the medical studies performed on autistic children to date. By summarizing currently available studies in the fields of neurophysiology, neuroradiology, biochemistry, genetics, immunology, neuro-pharmacology and neuropathology, the authors hope to pinpoint limitations, suggest some relevant new questions and stimulate further research. Because of the diagnostic confusion in many older studies, it is not always possible to sort out exactly who was being studied or if every child would meet our current definition of having an autistic syndrome. The authors did the best they could regarding this problem.

The old terms commonly used in the field of autism research are being redefined. Today, papers being published about 'parents of autistic children' now discuss the stress upon them of living full-time with a child with autism (Wolf *et al.* 1989) and their need for regular respite care (Factor *et al.* 1990). When the term 'environmental influences' is used, it is likely to concern the relationship of autism to a toxic factor such as lead poisoning (Accardo *et al.* 1988). There is finally a consensus about diagnostic criteria defining a child with autism (see Chapter 2). That autism is a disorder of multiple aetiologies is no longer in doubt (see Chapters 16 to 21).

Yet, this book has few final answers. Some patients with an autistic syndrome do not have a well-defined disease entity. There are many more research questions than medical answers.

However, enough knowledge now exists to recommend that every child with autism should have a thorough neuropsychiatric work-up (see Chapter 25). Each person with an autistic syndrome is entitled to a state-of-the-art work-up, for diagnostic, genetic and therapeutic purposes. A very few rational biomedical therapies are beginning to be available; as further understanding of the basis of the condition develops, more are anticipated. There is now a considerable body of experience and know-how about special educational techniques designed for children with autism.

Each person with autism who undergoes a thorough evaluation is a teacher as well as a patient: the physician, the family and the child are all learning together. This textbook is a framework to help that process.

REFERENCES

Accardo, P., Whitman, B., Caul, J., Rolfe, U. (1988) 'Autism and plumbism.' *Clinical Pediatrics*, **27**, 41–44.
Andersson, L., Wadensjö, K. (1981) *Early Childhood Psychosis in Malmöhus län.* Lund: Socialavdelningen. *(In Swedish.)*
Benda, C.E., Melchior, J.C. (1959) 'Childhood schizophrenia, childhood autism and Heller's disease.' *International Record of Medicine*, **172**, 137–154.
Bettelheim, B. (1959) 'Feral children and autistic children.' *American Journal of Sociology*, **64**, 455–467.
Bohman, M., Björck, P.O., Bohman, I.L., Sjöholm, E. (1981) 'Barndomspsykoserna-forsummade handikapp? Epidemiologi och habilitering i ett glasbygdslän.' *Lakartidningen*, **78**, 2361–2364. *(In Swedish, summary in English.)*
Brask, B.H. (1970) 'A prevalence investigation of childhood psychosis.' *Paper presented at the 16th Scandinavian Congress of Psychiatry.*
Byassee, J.E., Murrell, S.A. (1975) 'Interaction patterns in families of autistic, disturbed and normal children.' *American Journal of Orthopsychiatry*, **45**, 473–478.
Cantwell, D.P., Baker, L. (1978) 'The language environment of autistic and dysphasic children.' *Journal of the American Academy of Child Psychiatry*, **17**, 604–613.

———— Rutter, M. (1978) 'Family factors.' *In:* Rutter, M., Schopler, E. (Eds) *Autism: a Reappraisal of Concepts and Treatments.* New York: Plenum, pp. 269–296.

Cecchi, V. (1990) 'Analysis of a little girl with an autistic syndrome.' *International Journal of Psychoanalysis*, **71**, 403–410.

Churchill, D.W. (1978) *Language of Autistic Childen.* New York: V.H. Winston.

Cox, A., Rutter, M., Newman, S., Bartak, L. (1975) 'A comparative study of infantile autism and specific developmental receptive language disorder. II: Parental characteristics.' *British Journal of Psychiatry*, **126**, 146–159.

Darr, G.C., Warden, F.G. (1951) 'Case report 28 years after infantile autistic disorder.' *American Journal of Orthopsychiatry*, **21**, 559–570.

DeMyer, M.K. (1979) *Parents and Children in Autism.* New York: V.H. Winston.

———— Pontius, W., Norton, J.A., Baron, S., Allen, J., Steele, R. (1972) 'Parental practices and innate activity in normal, autistic and brain damaged infants.' *Journal of Autism and Childhood Schizophrenia*, **2**, 49–66.

———— Hingtgen, J.N., Jackson, R.K. (1981) 'Infantile autism reviewed: a decade of research.' *Schizophrenia Bulletin*, **7**, 388–451.

Despert, J.L. (1951) 'Some considerations relating to the genesis of autistic behavior in children.' *American Journal of Orthopsychiatry*, **21**, 335–350.

———— (1971) 'Reflections on early infantile autism.' *Journal of Autism and Childhood Schizophrenia*, **1**, 363–367.

Deykin, E., MacMahon, G. (1980) 'Pregnancy, delivery and neonatal complications among autistic children.' *American Journal of Diseases of Children*, **134**, 860–864.

Ekstein, R., Friedman, S.W. (1974) 'Infantile autism: from entity to process.' *Reiss-Davis Clinic Bulletin*, **11**, 70–85.

Factor, D.C., Perry, A., Freeman, N. (1990) 'Brief report: stress, social support, and respite care use in families with autistic children.' *Journal of Autism and Developmental Disorders*, **20**, 139–146.

Fraknoi, J., Ruttenberg, B.A. (1971) 'Formulation of the dynamic economic factors underlying infantile autism.' *Journal of the American Academy of Child Psychiatry*, **10**, 713–738.

Frank, S.M., Allen, D.A., Stein, L., Myers, B. (1976) 'Linguistic performance in vulnerable and autistic children and their mothers.' *American Journal of Psychiatry*, **133**, 909–915.

Gesell, A. (1941) *Wolf Child and Human Child.* New York: Harper.

Gillberg, C. (1984*a*) 'Infantile autism and other childhood psychoses in a Swedish urban region. Epidemiological aspects.' *Journal of Child Psychology and Psychiatry*, **25**, 35–43.

———— (1984*b*) 'On the relationship between epidemiological and clinical samples.' *Journal of Autism and Developmental Disorders*, **14**, 214–217.

———— Schaumann, H. (1982) 'Social class and infantile autism.' *Journal of Autism and Developmental Disorders*, **12**, 223–228.

Goldfarb, W., Yudkovitz, E., Goldfarb, N. (1973) 'Verbal symbols to designate objects: an experimental study of communication in mothers of schizophrenic children.' *Journal of Autism and Childhood Schizophrenia*, **3**, 281–298.

———— Spitzer, R.L., Endicott, J.A. (1976) 'A study of psychopathology of parents of psychotic children by structured interview.' *Journal of Autism and Childhood Schizophrenia*, **6**, 327–338.

Gorky, M. (1921) 'Nilushka.' *In: Through Russia: A Book of Stories.* (Translated by Hogarth, C.J.) London: Everyman's, Dent.

Haag, G. (1984) 'Autisme infantile précoce et phénomènes autistiques. Réflexions psychanalytiques.' *Psychiatrie de l'Enfant*, **27**, 293–354.

Harlow, H.F., McKinney, W.T. (1971) 'Nonhuman primates and psychoses.' *Journal of Autism and Childhood Schizophrenia*, **1**, 368–375.

———— Dodsworth, R.O., Harlow, J.K. (1955) 'Total social isolation in monkeys.' *Proceedings of the National Academy of Sciences of the USA*, **54**, 90–97.

Hingtgen, J.N., Bryson, C.Q. (1972) 'Recent developments in the study of early childhood psychoses: infantile autism, childhood schizophrenia, and related disorders.' *Schizophrenia Bulletin*, (5), 8–54.

Kanner, L. (1941*a*) 'Cultural implications of children's behavior problems.' *Mental Hygiene*, **25**, 353–362.

———— (1941*b*) *In Defense of Mothers.* Toronto: Dodd.

———— (1943) 'Autistic disturbances of affective contact.' *Nervous Child*, **2**, 217–250.

—— (1948) *Child Psychiatry. 2nd Edn.* Springfield: Charles C. Thomas.

—— (1949) 'Problems of nosology and psychodynamics in early infantile autism.' *American Journal of Orthopsychiatry*, **19**, 416–426.

—— (1952) 'Emotional interference with intellectual functioning.' *American Journal of Mental Deficiency*, **56**, 701–707.

—— (1954) 'To what extent is early childhood autism determined by constitutional inadequacies?' *In:* Hooker, D., Hope, C.C. (Eds) *Genetics and the Inheritance of Neurological and Psychiatric Patterns.* Baltimore: Williams & Wilkins.

—— (1969) *Keynote Address Given at the Annual Meeting of the National Society of Autistic Children, Washington, D.C.*

Kauffman, M. (1972) 'Characteristics of the emotional pathology of the kibbutz child.' *American Journal of Orthopsychiatry*, **42**, 692–709.

King, P.D. (1975) 'Early infantile autism: relation to schizophrenia.' *Journal of the American Academy of Child Psychiatry*, **14**, 666–682.

Koegel, R.L., Schreibman, L., O'Neill, R.E., Burke, J.C. (1983) 'The personality and family interaction characteristics of parents of autistic children.' *Journal of Consulting and Clinical Psychology*, **51**, 683–692.

Lane, H. (1976) *The Wild Boy of Aveyron.* Cambridge, MA: Harvard University Press.

Lotter, V. (1966) 'Epidemiology of autistic conditions in young children. I. Prevalence.' *Social Psychiatry*, **1**, 124–137.

Massie, H.N. (1978) 'Blind ratings of mother–infant interaction in home movies of pre-psychotic and normal infants.' *American Journal of Psychiatry*, **135**, 1371–1374.

McAdoo, W.G., DeMyer, M. (1978*a*) 'Personality characteristics of parents.' *In:* Rutter, M., Schopler, E. (Eds) *Autism: A Reappraisal of Concepts and Treatment.* New York: Plenum, pp. 251–268.

—— —— (1978*b*) 'Research related to family factors in autism.' *Journal of Pediatric Psychology*, **2**, 162–166.

Miller, R.T. (1974) 'Childhood schizophrenia: a review of selected literature.' *International Journal of Mental Health*, **3**, 3–46.

O'Moore, M. (1972) 'A study of the aetiology of autism from a study of birth and family characteristics.' *Journal of the Irish Medical Association*, **65**, 114–120.

Pitfield, M., Oppenheim, A. (1964) 'Child rearing attitudes of mothers of psychotic children.' *Journal of Child Psychology and Psychiatry*, **5**, 52–57.

Rimland, B. (1964) *Infantile Autism.* New York: Appleton-Century-Crofts.

Sanua, V.D. (1981) 'Cultural changes and psychopathology in children: with special reference to infantile autism.' *Acta Paedopsychiatrica*, **47**, 133–142.

Schopler, E. (1973) 'Current approaches to the autistic child.' *Pediatric Annals*, **2**, 60–74.

—— (1976) 'Toward reducing behavior problems in autistic children.' *Journal of Autism and Childhood Schizophrenia*, **6**, 1–13.

—— Mesibov, G. (Eds.) (1984) *The Effect of Autism on the Family.* New York: Plenum.

—— Reichler, R.J. (1972) 'How well do parents understand their own psychotic child?' *Journal of Autism and Childhood Schizophrenia*, **2**, 387–400.

—— Andrews, C-E., Strupp, K. (1979) 'Do autistic children come from upper-middle-class parents?' *Journal of Autism and Developmental Disorders*, **9**, 139–152.

Szurek, S.A. (1973) 'Playfulness, creativity and schisis.' *In:* Szurek, S.A., Berlin, I.N. *Clinical Studies of Childhood Psychoses.* New York: Brunner/Mazel, pp. 10–28.

Therrell, B.I., Brown, L.O., Dziuk, P.E., Peter, W.P. (1983) 'The Texas newborn screening program.' *Infant Screening*, **5**, 1–3.

Tinbergen, E.A., Tinbergen, N. (1976) 'The etiology of childhood autism: a criticism of the Tinbergens' theory: a rejoinder.' *Psychological Medicine*, **6**, 545–549.

Tsai, L.Y., Stewart, M.A. (1983) 'Etiological implication of maternal age and birth order in infantile autism.' *Journal of Autism and Developmental Disorders*, **13**, 57–65.

Vaillant, G.E. (1962) 'Historical notes: John Haslam on early infantile autism.' *American Journal of Psychiatry*, **119**, 376.

van Krevelen, A.v.D. (1971) 'Early infantile autism.' *Zeitschrift für Kinderpsychiatrie*, **19**, 91.

Victor, G. (1983) *The Riddle of Autism.* Toronto: D.C. Heath.

Williams, S., Harper, J. (1973) 'A study of aetiological factors at critical periods of development in autistic children.' *Australian and New Zealand Journal of Psychiatry*, **7**, 163–168.

Wing, L. (1976) 'Epidemiology and theories of etiology.' *In:* Wing, L. (Ed.) *Early Childhood Autism: Clinical, Educational and Social Aspects.* Elmsford, NY: Pergamon, pp. 65–92.

—— (1980) 'Childhood autism and social class: a question of selection.' *British Journal of Psychiatry*, **137**, 410–417.

—— Gould, J. (1978) 'Systematic recording of behavior and skills of retarded and psychotic children.' *Journal of Autism and Childhood Schizophrenia*, **8**, 79–97.

Wolf, L.C., Noh, S., Fisman, S.N., Speechley, M. (1989) 'Psychological effects of parenting stress on parents of autistic children.' *Journal of Autism and Developmental Disorders*, **19**, 157–166.

PART I

CLINICAL CONSIDERATIONS

2
CLINICAL DIAGNOSIS

Autism is not a single disease entity in the sense that, for instance, phenylketonuria is. Rather, the concept of infantile autism (autistic disorder, childhood autism) represents a comprehensive diagnosis, along the same lines as cerebral palsy, epilepsy or mental retardation. Hundreds of papers and books have already been written under the impression that autism will one day turn out to be a disorder with a single aetiology, be it psychogenic or biological. However, there is overwhelming evidence that the behavioural syndrome of autism represents the final expression of various aetiological factors. Furthermore, even within a purely behavioural/ phenomenological framework of autism, one is struck by the complexity of the symptomatology and the difficulty of fitting all individual cases into one operational diagnostic model. Hence the plural form (autistic syndromes) in the title of this book.

The term autism was coined by Bleuler (1911) to designate a category of the thought disorder that is present in schizophrenic syndromes. When Kanner (1943) described infantile autism (or rather, autistic disturbances of affective contact in young children) he used the term differently, although with special reference to schizophrenia which he at first thought was related to infantile autism but later tried to distinguish clearly from the 'Kanner syndrome'. The use of the word autism in connection with this latter syndrome is somewhat misleading, implying as it does a (spurious or perhaps even non-existent) link with schizophrenia and also that 'extreme aloneness' (synonymous with 'autism' according to Kanner) is at the aetiological root of the syndrome. In later years, some authors have argued for the use of terms other than autism, but so far without much success. Autism will probably be used as a descriptive term for years to come in connection with children and adults who at one time in their life showed the marks of the 'Kanner syndrome'.

Kanner's description of children with autism was accurate enough, and even though substantial progress has been made since 1943 as regards the pathogenetic mechanisms in autism, few later authors, with the exception of Wing (1980) and Frith (1989), have given a more vivid or clear presentation of them. Certainly, some development in diagnostic criteria has been made since Kanner's time, but for a classic presentation of a typical case of autism, one is well advised to study Kanner's 1943 paper.

The person with autism
The autistic syndromes (Coleman 1976, Coleman and Gillberg 1985) are variously

referred to as childhood autism (Wing 1980, World Health Organization [WHO] 1990), infantile autism (Rutter 1978, American Psychiatric Association [APA] 1980), autistic disorder (APA 1987), pervasive developmental disorders (APA 1980, 1987; WHO 1990) and childhood psychosis (Fish and Ritvo 1979). Of these latter categories, infantile autism is the concept that has received the most attention and about which there has been some consensus with regard to diagnostic criteria. Several of the criteria considered necessary for this diagnosis have also been listed among the crucial features of so-called childhood psychosis. The label of childhood psychosis has been considered a comprehensive diagnostic term, with infantile autism constituting one of the subgroups. For the last ten years, at least, many leading authorities have argued for the abolition of the term 'psychosis' in connection with the autistic syndromes and suggested the substitution of 'developmental disorder' or 'pervasive developmental disorder'. The move away from the psychosis/schizophrenia branch was clearly evidenced in the late 1970s when the leading scientific journal in the field changed its name from *Journal of Autism and Childhood Schizophrenia* to *Journal of Autism and Developmental Disorders*. Neither the DSM-III-R (APA 1987), nor the ICD-10 (WHO 1990) mention the term childhood psychosis. Both diagnostic systems now refer to pervasive developmental disorders instead. The removal of the psychosis label seems to indicate a step forward in the understanding of the autistic syndromes. However, the term pervasive developmental disorder is not the final answer. For one thing, it is unclear why mental retardation is not included as a 'pervasive' developmental disorder. Also, it would seem more appropriate to regard autism as a 'specific' rather than a 'pervasive' disorder.

In recent years, there has been concern that Kanner's concepts have been stretched too much and that the 'autistic-like conditions' have come to be lumped with the Kanner syndrome in an all-inclusive group of disorders of social relatedness (Rutter and Schopler 1987). Conversely, others have argued for a broadening of the concept of autism (Wing and Gould 1979, Waterhouse and Fein 1989, Wing 1989, Gillberg 1992a). Even though most authors agree that it is possible to 'branch off' Kanner's form of autism in the broader group now receiving diagnoses of autism and autistic-like conditions, there is no good clinical or scientific support for the notion that Kanner autism is a more 'specific' kind of autism than are other forms (Gillberg 1992a). For instance, the evidence of stronger validity for Kanner syndrome than for so-called Asperger syndrome (Gillberg and Gillberg 1989) just is not there. Kanner, among his original criteria, included both good intellectual potential and lack of neurological dysfunction. Given today's methods of examination, these two criteria would exclude virtually all children diagnosed by Kanner himself as 'autistic' from that category. The best validated category appears to be a rather broader concept as advocated by Wing (1989). Her 'triad of social, communication and imagination impairments' does have some better validity (Wing and Gould 1979, Steffenburg 1991). The authors of the present volume no longer feel confident that parents and children with autism have benefited at all from Kanner's original publications, implying as they did the uniqueness of a syndrome which is probably not so unique after all.

The criteria for autism (autistic disorder, childhood autism, autistic syndromes) currently agreed upon by most authorities are: (1) early onset (before age 3 to 5 years); (2) severe abnormality of reciprocal social relatedness; (3) severe abnormality of communication development (including language); and (4) restricted, repetitive and stereotyped patterns of behaviour, interests, activities and imagination.

These four criteria agree well with those set out for infantile autism by Rutter (1978) and the DSM-III (APA 1980). They are also very similar to those for childhood autism proposed in the draft versions of the ICD-10 (*e.g.* WHO 1990). The DSM-III-R (APA 1987) also agrees that criteria (2), (3) and (4) in the above definition are essential for a diagnosis of autistic disorder to be made. However, specific subcriteria are set out and a specified age of onset is not required (only that onset shall be in childhood and that age shall be specified) (Table 2.1). A recent statistical analysis of a series of autism spectrum cases found criteria 1 and 13 (see table) to have the strongest discriminating capacity of the 16 in differentiating autistic disorder from other conditions (Siegel *et al.* 1989). These two criteria are very similar to those considered essential by Kanner and Eisenberg (1956), *viz.* autistic aloneness and elaborate repetitive routines.

Many American authors (*e.g.* Coleman 1976, Ornitz 1983) would require that a fifth criterion be met for a definite diagnosis to be made, namely abnormal responses to sensory stimuli. This criterion is supported by a number of studies on early symptoms in autism (Dahlgren and Gillberg 1989, Ornitz 1989, Gillberg *et al.* 1990) and we included it among the autism criteria in the original edition of this book (Coleman and Gillberg 1985). However, in order to achieve consensus in the field, at the present stage we have refrained from including it as a necessary criterion, because we consider that criteria (2), (3) and (4) are necessary *and sufficient* and that the 'purity' of autism would not be enhanced by demanding the inclusion of the abnormal sensory response criterion.

Before discussing specific criteria, we need to be aware that a majority of children with autism are also mentally retarded (Fig. 2.1). We need to bear this in mind in order that distinctions between autism and mental retardation 'symptoms' are kept as clear as possible. A minority of children with classic autism function in the normal or near normal IQ range. The behaviour patterns unique to autism are often most clearly evident in such children.

Also, we need to keep in mind that 'Kanner autism' is possibly on a spectrum with 'Asperger syndrome' (Wing 1981*a*) and autistic-type problems in so-called DAMP (deficits in attention, motor control and perception) (Gillberg and Gillberg 1989) on the one hand and the 'triad of social impairments' (Wing and Gould 1979) on the other. There appears to be a spectrum—or continuum—of autistic syndromes or autistic disorders. Any cut-off between the various subcategories on this spectrum at the moment appears to be relatively arbitrary. The overlap of

TABLE 2.1

Diagnostic criteria for autism according to DSM-III-R (APA 1987)

Qualitative impairment in reciprocal social interaction as manifested by at least two of the following:

    (1) marked lack of awareness of the existence of feelings of others
    (2) no or abnormal seeking of comfort at times of distress
    (3) no or impaired imitation
    (4) no or abnormal social play
    (5) gross impairment in ability to make peer friendships

Qualitative impairment in verbal and non-verbal communication, and in imaginative activity, as manifested by at least one of the following:

    (6) no mode of communication, such as communicative babbling, facial expression, gesture, mime or spoken language
    (7) markedly abnormal non-verbal communication, as in the use of eye-to-eye gaze, facial expression, body posture or gestures to initiate or modulate social interaction
    (8) absence of imaginative activity, such as playacting of adult roles, fantasy characters, or animals: lack of interest in stories about imaginary events
    (9) marked abnormalities in the production of speech including volume, pitch, stress, rate, rhythm, and intonation
   (10) marked abnormalities in the production of speech including stereotyped and repetitive use of speech
   (11) marked impairment in the ability to initiate or sustain a conversation with others, despite adequate speech

Markedly restricted repertoire of activities and interests, as manifested by at least one of the following:

   (12) stereotyped body movements, *e.g.* hand-flicking, twisting, spinning, head-banging, complex whole-body movements
   (13) persistent preoccupation with parts of objects
   (14) marked distress over changes in trivial aspects of environments, *e.g.* when a vase is moved from its usual position
   (15) unreasonable insistence on following routines in precise detail, *e.g.* insisting that exactly the same route always be followed when shopping
   (16) markedly restricted range of interests and a preoccupation with one narrow interest, *e.g.* interested only in lining up objects, in amassing facts about meteorology, or in pretending to be a fantasy character

Onset during infancy or childhood

At least 8 of the 16 specified items above must be fulfilled

autism and the aforementioned syndromes plus the fact that in certain individuals with other diagnoses (obsessive–compulsive disorder, anorexia nervosa, paranoia) there may be a history—or even persistent symptoms—of autism, have led some authors to speculate that underlying all the phenomenological syndromes might be a common psychological denominator. In the chapter on neuropsychology (Chapter 15) we shall see that one recent hypothesis is that autism spectrum disorders share a common lack (or failure of normal development) of a 'theory of mind' (the ability to conceive of other people as having mental states). Having a well-developed theory of mind might be seen as synonymous with having

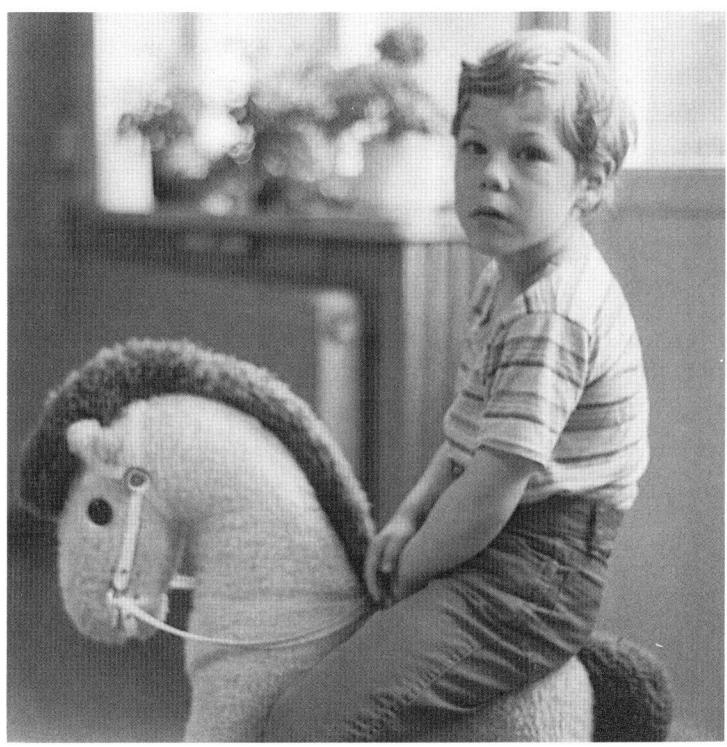

Fig. 2.1. 6-year-old boy with autism and high CSF levels of HVA. He has severe mental retardation, hyperactivity syndrome, cow's milk intolerance and abnormal brainstem auditory evoked potentials.

'empathy'. This, in turn, has led to the suggestion that autism might be but one of several subclasses among 'disorders of empathy' (Gillberg 1992*a*).

Early onset

With regard to the age of onset, most clinicians and researchers seem to agree that the behavioural disorder—or some major indication of abnormal development —must have been apparent before age 30 to 36 months (Rutter 1978, APA 1980, Coleman and Gillberg 1985, WHO 1990). However, some would require an even earlier age of onset, while others (Lotter 1966, Wing and Gould 1979) would allow the appearance of first symptoms to be delayed until the child's fifth birthday. Some authors have gone further still (Bohman *et al.* 1983) and have accepted cases with onset up to the age of 7 years. Nevertheless, the age limit of 2½ to 3 years is widely accepted.

Evans-Jones and Rosenbloom (1978), while arguing that disintegrative psychosis (childhood disintegrative disorder in the ICD-10) forms a separate diagnostic category from autism, maintain that sometimes the symptoms (which are often symptoms compatible with a diagnosis of autism) may begin before 2½ years of age, and yet not qualify the child for a diagnosis of autism but rather for disintegrative psychosis (see Table 2.2, p. 38).

Even though the criterion of early onset rarely causes much dispute in controversies over diagnostic symptoms in autism, the description of typical autistic syndromes beginning in previously normal people between the ages of 4 and 31 years in connection with herpes encephalitis (DeLong *et al.* 1981, Gillberg 1986, Gillberg, I.C. 1991) shows clearly that the matter cannot be regarded as settled. As has already been noted, the DSM-III-R does not include specified early onset among the diagnostic criteria.

In the great majority of cases with autistic syndromes, however, onset is quite clearly during the first few years and often even in the first six months of life. Wing (1989) has suggested that 'infantile autism' is congenital in approximately 80 per cent of cases. In the remaining 20 per cent there is either too scanty evidence from the medical history, or there are definite clues that the typical symptoms began sometime between the age of 6 and 20 months. Only rarely are there cases that commence around age 30 months or later. Cases with documented set-back after a period of clearly normal development are rare, but their relative frequency within the whole group is not known.

Many authors have assumed that the early onset of the disorder is one of the reasons for symptoms taking on such a stereotyped and primitive appearance. While this seems reasonable in a developmental–theoretical perspective, the whole notion is contradicted by the clear documentation of Kanner-type autism with onset as late as 14 years of age.

Conversely, it should be made clear that symptom onset after, for instance, 18 months of age does not mean that the disorder may not be congenital. One possibility in such cases is that there may be a brain abnormality allowing normal development up to a specific age but that later, the available neural circuitries can no longer match the requirements for further development and only then will symptoms begin to appear.

Abnormality of social relatedness
The disturbance of social relatedness—as all other symptoms—has to be out of proportion in comparison with the often concomitant mental retardation. The central features of this abnormality seem to be a lack of reciprocity in social interaction with other humans and a failure to recognize the uniqueness of other human beings (Wing 1980, Rutter 1983).

Frith (1989) has suggested that the basic failure in autism is the lack of early development of a 'theory of mind', such that a child with autism cannot conceive that other people think and feel and certainly cannot intuit *what* they think and feel (see Chapter 15). This 'underdeveloped' theory of mind will inevitably lead to extreme deficits in empathy, showing in all interactions with people. The empathy deficits, however, will not affect the ability to observe the world or to reason logically about visible and audible realities. Neither will basic emotions such as anger, fear or happiness necessarily be affected.

Some children with autism already during the first three years of life (and to a lesser extent later also) display, in Kanner's words (1943), an 'extreme autistic aloneness'. Others are described as 'easy so long as they are left to themselves in their bed or in their room'. Still others are difficult, 'terrible', or scream at all hours and need little sleep. Imitation and imitation play are deficient or lacking (personal observations). Feeding and sucking difficulties are very common (Wing 1980).

The 'typical' child with autism avoids eye contact, stares into thin air or is observed to have an abnormal gaze contact from before the end of the first year of life (Mirenda *et al.* 1983). Many gaze out of the corner of the eye and only very briefly. Quite a number do not show anticipatory movements when about to picked up, may resist being held or touched, and will not 'adjust' to 'fit' in a hug or something similar. However, contrary to popular belief, many children with autism enjoy body contact, which may constitute their only mode of 'communication' with other people. Infants who later receive a diagnosis of autism have often seemed to lack initiative, and the interested curiosity and exploratory behaviour seen in normal babies is often completely lacking.

Frequent responses include: 'He was so happy if we left him all to himself, but started to scream as soon as someone picked him up'; 'She was so stiff to hold'; or 'I don't know what it was, but he just wasn't "there".' There is an impression that humans, animals and soft and hard objects are treated alike. People are often treated by the child as if they were technical tools, there only for the benefit of the child to reach certain objects (exemplified by the child who leads their mother's hand, not only by the hand but by the wrist, to their spoon, and then directs the spoon via the mother's hand/wrist to their own mouth). The child does not usually come to parents, brothers or sisters—or anybody else for that matter—for help or comfort.

However, not all children with autism show these typical features and, to be sure, even in those who do, there is often a gradual decrease in the severity of symptoms.

Typical of all in the early preschool years is a failure to develop normal relationships with age-peers. This inability usually persists throughout childhood, adolescence and often into adult life.

As the child grows older, the abnormalities of social relatedness become less immediately obvious, particularly if the child is seen in familiar surroundings. The resistance to being touched and held often decreases with age, even though rough-and-tumble play is sometimes preferred to gentle stroking. The gaze avoidance behaviour may decrease. There is evidence (Rutter 1978, Mirenda *et al.* 1983) to suggest that it is not the amount of gaze contact that is abnormal in autism, but rather that—at least after infancy—there is a qualitative difference, the gaze of people with autism being stiffer and lasting longer on an individual basis. In some instances, *e.g.* autism associated with the fragile X chromosome abnormality, there is clear gaze avoidance (Hagerman 1989), and it seems likely that with the emergence of more and more aetiological subgroups, a multifaceted view of gaze abnormalities in autism will emerge. What is already quite clear at this stage is that gaze avoidance is definitely not a *necessary* feature of autism at any age.

Symptoms pertaining to the avoidance of visual or physical contact are often classified in the category of social abnormalities. However, several authors including Wing (1980) and the present authors (Coleman and Gillberg 1985, Gillberg *et al.* 1990) would argue that these abnormalities are best dealt with in the context of abnormal sensory responses. Be that as it may, the result of the changes in the child in these respects is that the child becomes somewhat more cooperative and easy to *relate* to. Unfortunately, the inability to play reciprocally with age peers remains sadly unchanged throughout the years in most cases, although this characteristic may not be as conspicuously apparent in the school-age child with autism as it was in that same child during the preschool years.

In some cases, and at some stages of development, the abnormality of social relatedness takes on the form of a lack of selectivity and distance. However, even in children with autism who show seemingly attention-seeking, distance-lacking behaviour, the inability to reciprocate and the failure to treat humans as anything but objects are clearly evident. These hallmarks differentiate them from superficially similar behaviour seen in emotionally deprived children.

Abnormalities of communication development including language
Usually from a very early age, the child with autism shows major problems in the comprehension of human mime, gesture and speech, and, accordingly, shows little social use of communication skills. Social imitation is lacking or deficient, and common early imitation play such as waving bye-bye or doing pat-a-cake is not elicitable. Some—though by no means all, perhaps not even the majority (Gillberg *et al.* 1990)—do not babble, and some yield strange monotonous sounds instead of the varied babble patterns heard in normal children.

Abnormal babbling is often inferred to be a crucial symptom of abnormal language development in autism. Actually there is little scientific evidence to uphold such a view, and some children with autism have indeed babbled in what appears to be a normal fashion. The few studies which have examined early language development (according to parental interview data) of children with autism do not suggest clear-cut abnormalities of babble (Dahlgren and Gillberg 1989, Gillberg *et al.* 1990). In fact, language and babbling may be more discrete functions and not as intrinsically interwoven as hitherto believed (Zetterström 1983).

Almost without exception, children with autism are delayed in their development of spoken language. This delay runs parallel with an impairment in the understanding of spoken language, which may vary from an almost total lack of understanding to more subtle deviances leading to literal interpretation. An example of this kind of literal interpretation is provided by the 10-year-old girl with autism with a full-scale WISC IQ of 100 who appeared panic stricken when the nurse, about to do a simple blood test said: 'Give me your hand: it won't hurt.' The girl calmed down immediately when another person, who knew her well, said: 'Stretch our your index finger.' The girl had understood, at the first instruction, that she was required to cut off her hand and give it to the nurse. Comprehension is usually severely impaired in such high-functioning persons with autism who excel in the use of vocabulary.

Many children with autism learn to follow simple instructions if given in a particular social context, but appear to fail to grasp the meaning of these instructions when given out of that context. Quite unlike deaf children, children with autism make little, if any, use of mime or gesture. Often they seem totally to misinterpret human facial expressions and begin to laugh when somebody cries or vice versa.

Approximately one in two children with autism fail to develop useful spoken language. The vast majority of these are also mentally retarded (usually severely or profoundly so). Of those who do develop speech, all show major abnormalities of speech development, such as sustained phases of seemingly non-communicative immediate and/or delayed echolalia (present only during short phases and integrated with the development of communicative speech in normal children), avoidance or confusion of personal pronouns (such as the substitution of 'you', 'he' or the child's first name for 'I', 'he' for 'she' and 'you' for 'we', thought to be a consequence of the echolalia), confusion of prepositions, and repetitive speech without talking *with* so much as *to* someone. The echolalia encountered in autism is often so well-developed that the casual listener/observer will have difficulty in recognizing the severity of the abnormality of language. Some may parrot whole conversations and go on talking as if at a cocktail party or ask endless questions. Those who constantly ask questions often become very irritating for people around them. It is sometimes difficult to understand why they should want to ask all these questions when everybody knows that they know all the answers. If a theory of mind deficit underlies autism it becomes easier to accept that in autism you can only ask questions that already have an answer which is well known to the person asking. If you cannot conceive that other people have mental states or, as it were 'inner worlds', how can you ask them about matters unknown to you?

We have come across quite a number of people with autism who eventually develop some communicative language, but who, nevertheless, retain some of their echolalia in that they whisper in an echolalic fashion every question directed at them. This may be particularly common in autism associated with the fragile X chromosome abnormality (Gillberg 1992b).

A minority of people with autism not only parrot conversations in an echolalic fashion, but imitate one's every movement and gesture. This phenomenon is sometimes referred to as echopraxia.

Some talking children with autism have very good rote memory skills and can repeat whole conversations word by word. However, these same children may have great difficulty or may not be at all able to extract meaning from sentences based on the order and the meaning of the words (Hermelin and O'Connor 1970).

Some non-speaking people with autism may be able to imitate and sing songs with baffling accuracy and some may even know the words of the song without being able to repeat them without singing.

In speaking children with autism it has been commonly noted that they can relate a series of real events if allowed to do that according to their own rigid structure of telling about the events, but cannot do so if interrupted by questions or remarks. Especially in brighter children with autism, there may be quite a lot of spontaneous speech. Rarely, if ever, do they communicate to others about their feelings and needs. They may hold lengthy and detailed disquisitions on the subject of a given, concrete experience, such as a dinner, or travelling on a bus, but will usually be unable to answer even simple questions about this same topic, in spite of having no difficulty al all 'recreating' the whole journey from start to finish in their own very concrete, descriptive words.

It is important to make note of the fact that comprehension of spoken language is always seriously compromised in autism. Even in high-functioning individuals who have well developed expressive speech there are usually severe comprehension problems. They may be able to understand most single words such as substantives and verbs (and even adjectives referring to visible or audible phenomena) and yet have enormous difficulty comprehending what these words mean if sequenced together and particularly if set in a social context. In other words, their pragmatic comprehension skills are very limited. Some high-functioning people with autism may have better skills with regard to language comprehension if they are allowed to read a text than if they hear the same text spoken by somebody. It appears that spoken language produces few if any 'mental states/pictures' in people suffering from the syndrome of autism.

There are often grammatical immaturities consistent with the overall developmental level of the child's speech (Bartak *et al.* 1975).

Typically there are peculiarities in respect to vocal volume and pitch, with a tendency to use staccato-like or scanning speech. Problems of pronunciation arise when using spontaneous, but not echo phrases (Wing 1966, Howlin 1982). Phrased differently, this sometimes implies that when language spoken by people with autism sounds stiff or monotonous it is more likely to be communicative than when it sounds 'perfect' or 'just as though it had been spoken by somebody else'.

Judging from the, so far limited, study of high-functioning people with autism, it appears that a flat prosody may be more characteristic than any other problems in the language domain. Also it is important to note the abnormalities of mime and gesture which usually prevail throughout the life of people on the autism spectrum. Little facial mimicry (including stiff and stereotyped smiles on the one hand and 'depressed' appearance on the other) and an extreme poverty, or indeed lack, of gestures are typical of almost all cases.

Restricted, repetitive and stereotyped behaviour, activities and interests
Children with autism often form bizarre attachments to certain objects or parts of objects, such as stones, curls of hair, pins, pieces of plastic toys or metals. They may also be fascinated by any object that glitters (glasses, earrings, necklaces, etc.). The objects are usually selected because of some particular quality (*e.g.* colour, surface texture) and are carried or followed around by the child, who becomes distressed or even frantic if anybody tries to remove them. Other children line up toys or household equipment for hours on end. Round and spinning objects, such as wheels of toy cars, coins, gramophone records and tape recorders often hold a distinct fascination for children with autism (Fig. 2.2).

Many children, adolescents and adults with autism demand that certain routines be adhered to in a pathologically rigid fashion. One 6-year-old boy insisted that his mother had to put the frying pan on the stove and heat some butter in it before he would have his breakfast. This 'show', as it were, had to be put on every morning or he would scream for hours, refusing to eat altogether. Another boy of 7 would eat only if one of the legs of his father's chair was one inch away from one leg of the dinner table and his mother had one elbow on the table. A girl of 4 would scream in rage if her mother did not always walk on the same pavement on her way to the post office. A child of 1 year would scream for hours if his mother, when taking him out in his pram, did not always take him twice around the block going to the right (as she had done the very first time she took him out in the pram).

It is often impossible to predict what environmental change will cause the emotional outbursts. On the whole, it appears that minor changes tend to be more upsetting and to cause more severe temper tantrums than do major changes. For instance, a 5-year-old boy cried desperately for almost an hour until his mother realized that she had removed a book from one of the shelves of the bookcase. When she put it back, he stopped crying within seconds. This boy, who was considered by his parents and professionals as unable to cope with even the smallest kind of environmental change, accepted going abroad without any outward reaction at all.

The 'insistence on sameness' may also affect the verbal skills of the child, who may demand that only certain words or phrases be used or that things be talked about or repeated in exactly the same fashion. As noted above, standard questions with demands for standard answers are common.

Especially during the school years and after, some relatively brighter persons with autism show unusual preoccupations with, for example, weather reports, birthdays or train schedules.

Various other ritualistic and obsessive–compulsive phenomena are common. Some people with obsessive–compulsive disorders are very much aware that their rituals are unhelpful and limit their capacity for doing other things. People with autism are usually not as well aware of the handicapping nature of their own rituals, but their obsessive–compulsive behaviours may be very similar to those of people who are diagnosed as suffering from obsessive–compulsive disorder. Also among

27

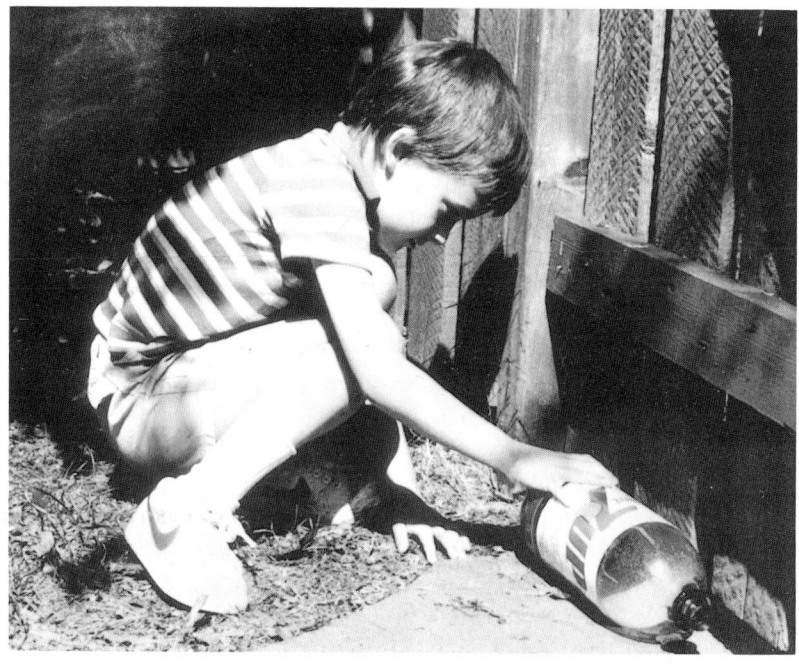

Fig. 2.2. *(Above)* Children with autism often prefer to play with shiny or mobile trash rather than toys. *(Below)* Even a flickering birthday candle can be a source of visual self-stimulation.

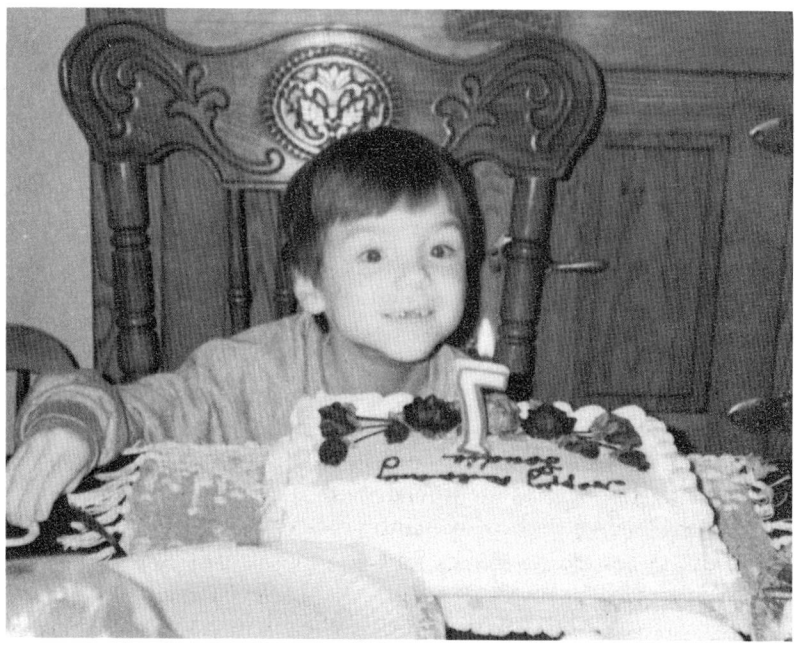

children with the latter diagnosis, there are many who are not aware that their rituals are 'negative'. It has been our experience that some children receive a diagnosis of obsessive–compulsive disorder when, in fact, they show all the hallmarks of autism. Conversely, many children with classical autism would also qualify for a diagnosis of obsessive–compulsive disorder.

Some authors include less complex stereotypic behaviour—such as simple stereotypies or toe-walking—among the elaborate repetitive routines. Even though some stereotypies, especially hand-flapping with flexion of the elbows and extremely 'high' tip-toeing, appear to be rather typical of autism, most authors do not include these kinds of stereotypic behaviours as *necessary* criteria for a diagnosis of autism. Nevertheless, in low-functioning individuals with autism, elaborate motor routines (stereotypies) may be the only way of 'expressing' the repetitive behaviour pattern considered essential for a diagnosis of autism to be made.

One way of looking at the 'behavioural criterion' of the autism diagnosis would be to say that the restricted pattern reflects the fact that you can only do what you know how to do. People with autism, because of their inability to communicate with the 'inner worlds' of other people, have to learn through copying what they see, hear or sense in other ways. This will necessarily mean a severe restriction of the behavioural repertoire even in high-functioning cases. In low-functioning cases, repetitive motor patterns may be the only behaviours individuals with autism may know how to do, whereas in higher functioning cases, more elaborate patterns of behaviour may be possible.

Symptoms which are almost universal but not among the diagnostic criteria
Perhaps the most characteristic symptom of autism which is not currently included as a necessary diagnostic criterion is the abnormal response to sensory stimuli.

Of these symptoms, an abnormal response to sound may be thought of as the most characteristic of all. In our experience all children with typical autism have shown abnormal responses to sensory stimuli when very young. The child who 'acts deaf' and does not react at all when an explosion is suddenly heard near by may moments later turn at the sound of a paper being removed from a chocolate. Many children with autism cover their ears to shut out even 'ordinary' noise levels. There may also be strange reactions, such as the covering of ears or eyes at a special sound. There is often an extreme variability in the reaction to sound and light from one second to another.

Reduced or in other ways abnormal sensitivity to pain, heat or cold is often encountered in autism. A typical example is that of a boy who seemingly derives pleasure by biting the back of his hand. Some children withdraw or squeal if touched or stroked lightly, but enjoy being handled roughly. Other kinds of tactile stimuli may give pleasure to a child who can stand for half-hours just feeling and scratching differently textured surfaces.

One boy of 7 years was 'helping' his mother by the stove. He put his hand down and did not remove it until the smell of burnt flesh attracted his interest. He had to undergo several operations after this, but his hand function was never totally recovered. He did not seem to experience pain or heat from the burn wound. Another Swedish boy of 9 years got up early on one extremely cold morning and went out, naked, to play in the snow for what must have been more than an hour without feeling the need for warm clothes (and, incidentally, without any untoward consequences).

Abnormal responses to visual stimuli are probably present in a large majority of young children with autism, who often give the impression of having difficulty recognizing the things they see. People may ask the parents if the child is blind; in fact, every now and then autism is mistaken for blindness. Some children with delayed visual maturation show many or all of the symptoms of autism (Goodman and Ashby 1990). The peculiarities of gaze reported in the section on abnormality of social relatedness (p. 23) could also be taken as evidence of abnormal perceptual responses, as could the extreme fascination with contrasts of light (including that produced by shadows in the sunshine).

Children with autism often want to smell people and objects. This is a characteristic not usually encountered in normal development or in mental retardation without major autistic features.

By and large, clinical experience suggests that perceptions relating to auditory and tactile stimuli may be more impaired in autism than are perceptions of visual and, especially, olfactory stimuli. The two latter functions make their first intracranial nerve connections at a higher level in the nervous system than do the two former. A preference for proximal stimuli has also been experimentally evidenced in autism (Hermelin and O'Connor 1970). Masterton and Biederman (1983) have argued that proprioceptive input dominates over visual input in children with autism. They see this dominance as the effect of an alternative strategy to compensate for a lack of visual control over fine motor performance. In this context, it is of some interest that certain children, who otherwise yield good gaze contact, can talk coherently only when avoiding gaze contact.

Although abnormal sensory responses in autism are regarded by many as 'primary' and in their view should therefore be included among the diagnostic criteria, the most influential diagnostic manuals do not do this. Nevertheless, most authorities agree that for instance 'undue sensitivity to sound' is an extremely common feature in autism and that it differentiates autism from, for instance, dysphasia (Rutter 1978, 1983). In a prospective study of children with autism seen before their third birthday, 'abnormal responses to sensory stimuli' was the class of symptoms which most clearly distinguished autism from mental retardation (Gillberg *et al.* 1990). Similar findings were reported by Ornitz (1989).

Other common symptoms
Hyperactivity is a very common symptom, especially in young children with autism. Sleep problems are most often apparent in infancy, when the child may keep the

whole family awake by crying, but may sometimes continue right through to adulthood. Many people with autism are awake for long periods each night. An almost total lack of initiative is a dominating problem in certain children with autism.

Food fads are the rule rather than the exception. Many children with autism have great problems chewing. Hard objects are sometimes orally preferred to soft ones.

Self-injurious behaviour (head banging, wrist or knuckle biting, chin knocking, cheek smacking, eye poking, hair tearing, clawing, etc.) is seen in many children with autism. It has been proposed as being concomitant to the mental retardation, but in fact could not be, since such behaviour is often seen even in children with autism of normal intelligence.

Cognitive profile
Many children with autism are mentally retarded. However, it appears that there are certain characteristics in the cognitive patterns of a majority that differentiate them from children without autism regardless of whether they are mentally retarded or not.

First, it is well established (Shah and Frith 1983), that some, though not all, show 'islets' of special abilities, particularly in the fields of rote memory (*e.g.* numerical skills), music, art and visuospatial skills (such as is sometimes demonstrated in a particular aptitude with jigsaw puzzles).

Second, many seem to have an impaired memory for recent events (Boucher 1981). Specifically, their memory difficulties impair their ability to recall past activities in response to 'open' or 'uninformative' questions (Boucher and Lewis 1989). Such problems would be compatible with underlying theory of mind problems. The memory difficulties might therefore not be 'true' memory deficits but depend on the way in which the 'memory imprint' is approached.

Third, children with autism perform better than mental-age-matched retarded and normal children in respect to 'concrete' discrimination. However, tasks requiring 'formal' discrimination are more difficult for the child with autism (Maltz 1981). Their concrete way of interpreting and solving problems is often evident throughout life, even in those few with relatively high intellectual functioning.

Fourth, on the WISC, there is a particular test profile with peaks and troughs (Bartak *et al.* 1975, Ohta 1987, Rumsey and Hamburger 1988) in certain areas. A recent study has shown a particular profile also on the Griffiths test (personal data, unpublished). Visuospatial skills show superior results, whereas language-associated and 'intuition/empathy'-associated tests yield extremely low results.

It is the unusual cognitive profile of children with autism that has given rise to the widespread speculation that they are indeed of superior intelligence, and just hiding their phenomenal capacity behind a shell of autism. Unfortunately, a large body of research is agreed that this view of autism is mistaken and that most children with autism, even those showing almost unbelievable splinter skills, are

31

clearly mentally retarded. All have cognitive problems (Rutter 1983).

Summary of diagnostic criteria

There are many children with one or two of the three major criteria proposed for diagnosing autism. What term do we apply to them? Are they autistic, autistic-like, children with autistic features or what? The matter can hardly be regarded as settled.

At the present stage we would argue for an umbrella definition, namely that of 'the autistic syndromes' or, possibly, 'autism and autistic-like conditions', to cover the whole group of severe disorders on the autism spectrum. This term would, clinically, be roughly equivalent to that of 'pervasive developmental disorders', but it would not be conceptually as confusing. Based on the foregoing discussion, all autistic syndromes in our view share these characteristics:

- severe abnormality of reciprocal social relatedness;
- severe abnormality of development of communication, usually prominently noted in abnormalities of the production and, perhaps particularly, comprehension of spoken language;
- rigid and restricted behavioural repertoire and imaginative skills as manifested in elaborate routines, insistence on sameness, restricted play patterns or interests and motor stereotypies.

All symptoms have to be out of phase with the overall intellectual level of the child. For a diagnosis of the 'complete autistic syndrome', 'childhood autism' or just 'autism', all three symptoms have to be present in severe and typical form.

In cases with all three symptoms represented in atypical form or with two of the symptoms in typical form we suggest that 'partial autistic syndrome' or 'autistic-like condition' be diagnosed. This category would equate with 'pervasive developmental disorder not otherwise specified' in the DSM-III-R (APA 1987).

In cases not meeting criteria for these two groups but showing some autistic features we suggest that 'autistic features' be diagnosed.

'Asperger syndrome' might be the diagnostic label selected for certain children falling in one of the above groups. The reader is referred to Chapter 3 for a fuller discussion of this diagnosis.

In autism and autistic-like conditions there is usually (but not always) early onset of the disorder (most often before age 5 years).

Complicating disorders

Mental retardation

A majority of children with classical autism (approximately 67 to 88 per cent) are definitely mentally retarded, *i.e.* they test reliably under IQ 70 (Lotter 1966, Rutter 1978, Wing 1980, Bohman *et al.* 1983, Gillberg 1984*a*, Steffenburg and Gillberg 1986, Gillberg *et al.* 1991). This retardation was previously thought to be a secondary consequence of the affective disturbance, and Kanner (1943, 1949) believed that these were children with potentially superior intelligence. Now, several different lines of research have been followed and the results are in total agreement that many children with autism are indeed mentally retarded (Rutter 1983, Gillberg 1990). This intellectual retardation is not caused by motivational factors in the child and remains relatively stable over the years with or without improvement with regard to the autistic behaviour problems.

It goes without saying that the clinical picture of autism varies somewhat with the intellectual level. Severely mentally retarded children with autism (IQ <50, who constitute about 40 per cent of all children with classical autism) behave differently from mildly retarded or normally intelligent children with autism. Outcome varies with IQ and level of speech development. The speech–language competence, of course, on the whole is closely correlated with the IQ level. Severely retarded children are less likely to have any speech at all, whereas more intelligent children with autism are the ones most likely to demonstrate a wide variety of elaborate repetitive routines and to exhibit islets of special giftedness in circumscribed areas, a symptom once mentioned as central by Kanner, but which, obviously, cannot be as conspicuous in the severely mentally retarded group.

Epilepsy
Some children with autism have early onset seizures. Indeed, infantile spasms are often followed by the development of an autistic syndrome even in infancy (Taft and Cohen 1971, Riikonen and Amnell 1981, Riikonen and Simell 1990). Equally common, however, is the development of any type of epilepsy at or near the time of puberty. One third of all children with autism (Rutter 1970; Gillberg 1984*b*, 1991; Olsson *et al.* 1988) develop seizures. It is a more common phenomenon among those who are also mentally retarded, but it can occur at all levels of intelligence (Gillberg *et al.* 1987). Most children who develop epilepsy in adolescence have not previously shown any outward signs of major neurological abnormality. (For more details on epilepsy in autism, see Chapter 6.)

Vision and hearing impairments
It is often suggested that blindness (especially by way of sensory deprivation) may cause autism and that blindness and autism often coexist (Keeler 1958, Rapin 1979), but there is actually no good evidence to support this view. If autism and blindness are indeed associated, then the association might well stem from some kind of underlying central neurological deficit. A recent study showing a possible increase of autism symptoms in Leber amaurosis (Rogers and Newhart-Larson 1989) has, so far, not been replicated.

Deafness has also been purported to be associated with autism. There is some evidence from population studies for an increased incidence of hearing problems associated with autism (Steffenburg 1991).

It is rather surprising that the possible interrelationships between autism and visual/hearing impairments have attracted so little attention. Many interesting hypotheses might be tested in connection with studies undertaken in order to elucidate this association. For instance, the relative importance of periodic sensory privation versus central brain damage could be evaluated in such studies.

Based on clinical experience, it would seem that hearing impairment and deafness would be more likely than blindness to show a primary connection with autism. Throughout childhood, most children with autism show deviant reactions to sound, whereas deviant reactions to light appear to be less conspicuous. Furthermore, among individuals with autism, there are more clinically proven cases of deafness than of blindness. Nevertheless, in a recent study by Steffenburg (1991), at least half of a population-based group of children with classical autism had major problems in the field of visual acuity (hypermetropia in most cases, myopia in a few and gradually developing blindness in one case).

Other disorders
The autistic syndromes are but behaviourally defined sets of collections of symptoms and it is therefore quite possible to diagnose any kind of disorder in connection with autism. However, cerebral palsy (Schain and Yannett 1960) is only rarely seen in concurrence with autism and related disorders (Gillberg 1984*a*). The fragile X syndrome (Steffenburg and Gillberg 1986), tuberous sclerosis (Lotter 1974), neurofibromatosis (Gillberg and Forsell 1984, Gaffney *et al.* 1989), hypomelanosis of Ito (Åkefeldt and Gillberg 1991), Rett syndrome (Witt-Engerström and Gillberg 1987), achondroplasia (personal case), Moebius syndrome (Ornitz *et al.* 1977, Gillberg and Winnergård 1984), Laurence–Moon–Biedl syndrome (Steffenburg 1991), Williams syndrome (Steffenburg 1991) and Coffin–Lowry syndrome (Bryson *et al.* 1988) have all been reported to cooccur with autism. Later in the book, we will return to a consideration of the possible implications of these connections. (For further details on associated impairments, see Chapter 20.)

Differential diagnosis
Here we need only be concerned with those neurological, developmental and psychiatric syndromes that may cause diagnostic confusion. In the literature, often a whole list of conditions, such as rubella embryopathy, tuberous sclerosis, infantile spasms, Rett syndrome, fragile X syndrome and so on, is presented in the section on differential diagnosis. Since we consider autism to be a set of purely behavioural syndromes, regardless of underlying pathology, we will not enter into such a discussion at this stage.

Deafness
Deaf children may occasionally show some autistic features, though rarely all. In the latter case they should in our view be diagnosed as suffering from deafness and autism.

Blindness
Several authors (*e.g.* Wing 1980) have attested that certain patients who had been

diagnosed as blind for several years were in fact seeing and suffering from autism. Interestingly, there may, in certain cases, be a connection between so-called delayed visual maturation and autistic symptoms (Goodman and Ashby 1990). As with deaf children, children with documented blindness and autism should be diagnosed as blind and as suffering from autism.

Mental retardation
Some children with mental retardation have a number of autistic features without meeting all the necessary criteria for a diagnosis of autism (Haracopos and Kelstrup 1978, Wing and Gould 1979, Gillberg 1983, Gillberg *et al.* 1986). Conversely, children with autism, more often than not, are themselves mentally retarded. Sometimes the dividing line is indeed obscure and the allocation to diagnostic category haphazard. The studies by Wing (1981*b*) are essential reading for anyone interested in this dichotomy.

Emotional deprivation
Retarded children reared in institutions (especially if looked after by a large number of different caretakers) display, like children with autism, abnormalities of social relationships, language and behaviour. However, close inspection and assessment usually makes differential diagnosis easy, since such children are indiscriminate rather than aloof, language-delayed rather than deviant, and show different kinds of behavioural problems. Also, positive environmental stimulation usually leads to quick and continuing development in these cases, quite unlike the relatively minor changes seen in autism in connection with such stimulation.

Infant depression
Children who have developed normally in the first few years of life and who are then separated from their primary carer for an extended period sometimes develop major signs of depression (Spitz 1946). They first protest, then show sadness and withdrawal, but finally slowly adjust to the new situation. Among such children there is possibly an increased risk of depression in adulthood (von Knorring 1983).

Asperger syndrome
Asperger syndrome is no longer considered as a major candidate in differential diagnosis in autism. Rather it should be seen as existing on the autism spectrum, perhaps constituting one variant of high-functioning autism. The following chapter is devoted to Asperger syndrome.

Rett syndrome
Rett syndrome is also sometimes seen as an 'either/or' diagnosis in relation to autism. We argue differently that Rett syndrome and autism quite often co-exist and that in such cases both diagnoses should be made. Rett syndrome is considered further in Chapter 20.

Pervasive developmental disorders (PDD) not otherwise specified (other childhood psychoses)

In the DSM-III (APA 1980), the term 'childhood psychosis' was replaced by 'childhood onset pervasive developmental disorder'. This term was reiterated in the DSM-III-R (APA 1987), which made it clear that, although not widely used in clinical practice, the PDD label was here to stay, at least for some time. Childhood onset PDD was then replaced by PDD not otherwise specified (NOS). Though signifying a more positive approach to autistic-like conditions than the psychosis label (with all its overtones of schizophrenia, insanity, withdrawal from the 'cruel outside world' and so forth), it seemed unwise to introduce the compulsory prefix 'pervasive' (see foregoing text).

Disintegrative disorders

There are instances of disintegrative disorders commencing around the age of 3 to 4 years and usually characterized by restlessness and hyperactivity during the first three to nine months of illness before the child becomes very much like a child with autism. Such cases were often referred to as Heller dementia (Heller 1930) in older literature, as disintegrative psychosis in the 1970s (Evans-Jones and Rosenbloom 1978) and as childhood disintegrative disorders in later writings (*e.g.* WHO 1990). Outcome appears to be at least as poor as in autism, and in a number of instances it is slowly realized that underlying the condition is a progressive neurological disorder.

Childhood schizophrenia

There are also occasional instances of childhood schizophrenia (showing in hallucinating, thought-disordered children, who differ markedly from most children with autism). These cases probably, unlike autism, represent the early onset form of schizophrenia, and rarely commence (at least with typical symptoms) before the age of 7 or 8 years. Some US authors (*e.g.* Asarnow *et al.* 1988) have argued that there are cases with early signs of autism who later develop schizophrenia. This is likely to be very rare.

Other psychiatric conditions

There are quite a number of children with various combinations of deficits in attention, motor control and perception (DAMP), who show several (usually mild) features of autism (Gillberg 1983).

Children with obsessive–compulsive disorders often have severe problems in the field of social relationships. Quite often they show many autistic-like features.

Children and adolescents with Tourette syndrome often have some traits reminiscent of Asperger syndrome (see Chapter 20).

Only rarely does one come across the kind of children described by Mahler and Gosliner (1955) who show a 'clinging' attachment to the mother and in other respects too exhibit an overall arrest of development at the so-called symbiotic stage. These cases are extremely rare, constituting less than 1 per cent of all autism and autistic-like cases seen by us in clinical and population-based studies. It is highly doubtful as to whether they should be grouped as a separate diagnostic category. Most cases of this kind can readily be classified in other categories with the added feature of the conspicuously clinging behaviour.

Comprehensive differential diagnosis
The comprehensive differential diagnosis in respect to autism, autistic-like conditions, Asperger syndrome, emotional deprivation and infant depression is shown in Table 2.2.

It is hoped that the difficulty of diagnosing autistic syndromes has not been understated in the foregoing pages. There are still many unresolved problems. In an era when operational criteria and inter-rater reliability of judgement have come into focus and taken the step from research methodology to clinical necessity, it may seem obsolete to speak of such a thing as experience. Even child psychiatrists only infrequently encounter Kanner autism cases. The cases fulfilling Wing's criteria for the triad of social, language and behavioural impairment occur more frequently, but only those working among the mentally retarded are likely to be aware of the actual number. Clinical experience is a prerequisite seldom mentioned in writings on the diagnosis of autism, and yet this fundamental element is of utmost importance. There is a 'gestalt measure' inherent in the whole concept of autism. The experienced clinician will have no difficulty in selecting the group of children in whom autistic syndromes will be found. S/he may have some trouble deciding whether to diagnose 'infantile autism', 'Asperger syndrome' or 'autistic-like condition', but the Wing category will be easier to discern. The clinically inexperienced researcher on the other hand may have no major difficulty in deciding that a mildly mentally retarded 4-year-old with autistic behaviour does meet DSM-III criteria for infantile autism, but will altogether miss the possibility that a normally intelligent 8-year-old with much communicative speech belongs in that same diagnostic category also. Diagnostic studies concerned with autism and autistic-like conditions require the 'gestalt acumen' of the experienced clinician just as much as everyday clinical work with the people who suffer from autism does.

There will eventually be a need for new concepts and words in the field of autism diagnosis. The discovery of theory of mind deficits in autism might lead to formulations of new broad-band labels such as 'disorders of empathy' (Gillberg 1992a). Nevertheless, autism and the various derivatives of that word will remain with us for many years to come. We believe that the term pervasive developmental disorder will die out because of its conceptual unsoundness. Diagnostic difficulties/confusions have been elegantly discussed by Waterhouse and colleagues (Waterhouse *et al.* 1984, Waterhouse and Fein 1989).

The term 'the autistic syndromes of childhood' may, by some, be taken as further evidence of the diagnostic problems relating to the area. However, at present it is our contention that this label accords best with the current state of

TABLE 2.2

Differential diagnosis in cases with early onset disturbance of social relatedness

Syndrome	Social relationships	Language	Behaviour	Other	Age of onset and course
Autistic syndromes	Period of autistic aloneness; lack of reciprocity; comprehension of human mime and gesture impaired; people treated as objects	Concrete interpretation of language; muteness; echolalia; reversal of personal pronouns	Obsessive insistence on elaborate routines; special stereotypies of hands and arms; toe-walking; lack of interest; failure to meet demands; resistance to change; passivity and overactivity alternating	Abnormal auditory perception	From birth (minority during first 3 years); chronic; usually life-long handicap
Asperger syndrome	Gradual realization that child is uninterested in peers; formal contact; odd, naive appproach devoid of empathy; inability to understand perspective of others	Concrete interpretation of language in spite of superficially well-developed skills; may use 'old-fashioned' metaphorical language	Much like autism though circumscribed interests (astrology, etc.) often more conspicuous	?Mild autism; motor clumsiness; gaucheness; ?'personality' traits	Often not obvious until the age of 3–6 ys; chronic; fair (though restricted) outcome; increased risk for psychiatric problems (depression, paranoia) and bizarre criminality
Disintegrative disorders		Regression to level of echolalia or muteness	Partly same as autism; often extreme degrees of overactivity without purpose	Confusion; variable abnormality of auditory perception	30–48 mths (small minority in the 4–10 yr age range); chronic; usually life-long handicap
Rett syndrome	Isolation and social apraxia in stages II and III; better contact later	No language	Midline hand stereotypies and loss of purposeful hand movements		
Deprivation syndrome	Lack of reticence and distance; always in pursuit of contact; understands human mime and gesture; people not objects	Delayed (not deviant) language development	Extreme overactivity; eats garbage, drinks toilet-water	Quick amelioration if early stimulation	6–30 mths; sensitive to environmental change; fair prognosis if early stimulation
Infant depression	Initial autism followed by accepting relationship with new caregiver; ambivalence upon return to primary caregiver	Initial regression	Apathy followed by adjustment to new demands	Amelioration on return to normal milieu; auditory perception	8–30 mths; highly age-dependent; fair prognosis if promptly treated; ?risk of depression in adult life

knowledge insofar as comprehensive categories are needed. This wording makes clear that, on balance, there is as yet no hard evidence that there exists a qualitatively unique behavioural or aetiological syndrome of autism. Kanner autism does not have more validity than any of the other named syndromes on the autism spectrum (Waterhouse and Fein 1989, Wing 1989, Gillberg 1992*a*).

In the future it may be possible to make a definite distinction between 'inborn' and 'later acquired' forms of autism on some more rational criterion than the rather arbitrary 30 to 36 months onset limit proposed by influential authorities.

As time goes by, we will also be able to distinguish between aetiological and behavioural subsyndromes, and in all probability the autistic syndromes will eventually be replaced by a number of different syndromes (Gillberg 1992*b*).

REFERENCES

Åkefeldt, A., Gillberg, C. (1991) 'Hypomelanosis of Ito in three cases with autism and autistic-like conditions.' *Developmental Medicine and Child Neurology*, **33**, 737–743.
American Psychiatric Association (1980) *Diagnostic and Statistical Manual of Mental Disorders. DSM-III. 3rd Edn.* Washington, DC: APA.
—— (1987) *Diagnostic and Statistical Manual of Mental Disorders. DSM-III-R. 3rd Edn, Revised.* Washington, DC: APA.
Asarnow, J.R., Ben-Meir, S. (1988) 'Children with schizophrenia spectrum and depressive disorders: a comparative study of premorbid adjustment, onset pattern and severity of impairment.' *Journal of Child Psychology and Psychiatry*, **29**, 477–488.
Bartak, L., Rutter, M., Cox, A. (1975) 'A comparative study of infantile autism and specific developmental receptive language disorder. I: The children.' *British Journal of Psychiatry*, **126**, 127–145.
Bleuler, P.E. (1911) *Dementia praecox oder die Gruppe der Schizophrenien.* Leipzig: F. Deuticke. *(Translated 1952 by* Zinkin, J. New York: International University Press.*)*
Bohman, M., Bohman, I.L., Björck, P.O., Sjöholm, E. (1983) 'Childhood psychosis in a northern Swedish county: some preliminary findings from an epidemiological survey'. *In:* Schmidt, M.H., Remschmidt, H. (Eds.) *Epidemiological Approaches in Child Psychiatry, II.* Stuttgart: Thieme, pp. 164–173.
Boucher, J. (1981) 'Memory for recent events in autistic children.' *Journal of Autism and Developmental Disorders*, **11**, 293–302.
—— Lewis, V. (1989) 'Memory impairments and communication in relatively able autistic children.' *Journal of Child Psychology and Psychiatry*, **30**, 99–122.
Bryson, S.E., Clark, B.S., Smith, I.M. (1988) 'First report of a Canadian epidemiologic study of autistic syndromes.' *Journal of Child Psychology and Psychiatry*, **29**, 433–445.
Coleman, M. (1976) *The Autistic Syndromes.* Amsterdam: North Holland.
—— Gillberg, C. (1985) *The Biology of the Autistic Syndromes.* New York: Praeger.
Dahlgren, S.O., Gillberg, C. (1989) 'Symptoms in the first two years of life. A preliminary population study of infantile autism.' *European Archives of Psychiatry and Neurological Sciences*, **238**, 169–174.
DeLong, G.R., Bean, S.C., Brown, F.R. (1981) 'Acquired reversible autistic syndrome in acute encephalopathic illness in children.' *Archives of Neurology*, **38**, 191–194.
Evans-Jones, L.G., Rosenbloom, L. (1978) 'Disintegrative psychosis in childhood.' *Developmental Medicine and Child Neurology*, **20**, 462–470.
Fish, B., Ritvo, E. (1979) 'Psychoses of childhood'. *In:* Noshpitz, V. (Ed.) *Basic Handbook of Child Psychiatry.* New York: Basic Books, pp. 249–303.
Frith, U. (1989) 'Autism and "theory of mind".' *In:* Gillberg, C. (Ed.) *Diagnosis and Treatment of Autism.* New York: Plenum, pp. 33–52.
Gaffney, G.R., Kuperman, S., Tsai, L.Y., Minchin, S. (1989) 'Forebrain structure in infantile autism.'

Journal of the American Academy of Child and Adolescent Psychiatry, **28**, 534–537.

Gillberg, C. (1983) 'Psychotic behaviour in children and young adults in a mental handicap hostel.' *Acta Psychiatrica Scandinavica*, **68**, 351–358.

—— (1984*a*) 'Infantile autism and other childhood psychoses in a Swedish urban region. Epidemiological aspects.' *Journal of Child Psychology and Psychiatry*, **25**, 35–43.

—— (1984*b*) 'Autistic children growing up: problems during puberty and adolescence.' *Developmental Medicine and Child Neurology*, **26**, 125–129.

—— (1986) 'Onset at age 14 of a typical autistic syndrome. A case report of a girl with herpes simplex encephalitis.' *Journal of Autism and Developmental Disorders*, **16**, 369–375.

—— (1989) 'Asperger syndrome in 23 Swedish children.' *Developmental Medicine and Child Neurology*, **31**, 520–531.

—— (1990) 'Autism and pervasive developmental disorders.' *Journal of Child Psychology and Psychiatry*, **31**, 99–119. *(Annotation.)*

—— (1991) 'The treatment of epilepsy in autism.' *Journal of Autism and Developmental Disorders*, **21**, 61–77.

—— (1992*a*) 'The Emanuel Miller Lecture 1991: Autism and autistic-like conditions. Subgroups of disorders of empathy.' *Journal of Child Psychology and Psychiatry*, **33**, 813–842.

—— (1992*b*) 'Subgroups in autism. Are there behavioural phenotypes typical of underlying medical conditions?' *Journal of Intellectual Disability Research*, **36**, 201–214.

—— Ehlers, S., Schaumann, H., Jakobsson, G., Dahlgren, S.O., Lindblom, R., Bågenholm, A., Tjuust, T., Blidner, E. (1990) 'Autism under age 3 years: a clinical study of 28 cases referred for autistic symptoms in infancy.' *Journal of Child Psychology and Psychiatry*, **31**, 921–934.

—— Forsell, C. (1984) 'Childhood psychosis and neurofibromatosis—more than a coincidence?' *Journal of Autism and Developmental Disorders*, **14**, 1–8.

—— Winnergård, I. (1984) 'Childhood psychoosis in a case of Moebius syndrome.' *Neuropediatrics*, **15**, 147–149.

—— Persson, E., Grufman, M., Themnér, U. (1986) 'Psychiatric disorders in mildly and severely mentally retarded urban children and adolescents: epidemiological aspects.' *British Journal of Psychiatry*, **149**, 68–74.

—— Steffenburg, S., Schaumann, H. (1991) 'Autism—epidemiology. Is autism more common now than 10 years ago?' *British Journal of Psychiatry*, **158**, 403–409.

—— —— Jakobsson, G. (1987) 'Neurobiological findings in 20 relatively gifted children with Kanner-type autism or Asperger syndrome.' *Developmental Medicine and Child Neurology*, **29**, 641–649.

Gillberg, I.C. (1991) 'Autistic syndrome with onset at age 31 years: herpes encephalitis as a possible model for childhood autism.' *Developmental Medicine and Child Neurology*, **33**, 920–924.

—— Gillberg, C. (1989) 'Asperger syndrome. Some epidemiological considerations: a research note.' *Journal of Child Psychology and Psychiatry*, **30**, 631–638.

Goodman, R., Ashby, L. (1990) 'Delayed visual maturation and autism.' *Developmental Medicine and Child Neurology*, **32**, 814–819.

Hagerman, R.J. (1989) 'Chromosomes, genes and autism.' *In:* Gillberg, C. (Ed.) *Diagnosis and Treatment of Autism.* New York: Plenum, pp. 105–132.

Haracopos, D., Kelstrup, A. (1978) 'Psychotic behaviour in children under the institutions for the mentally retarded in Denmark.' *Journal of Autism and Childhood Schizophrenia*, **8**, 1–12.

Heller, T. (1930) 'Über Dementia infantilis.' *Zeitschrift für Kinderforschung*, **37**, 661–667.

Hermelin, B., O'Connor, N. (1970) *Psychological Experiments with Autistic Children.* Oxford: Pergamon.

Howlin, P. (1982) 'Echolalic and spontaneous phrase speech in autistic children.' *Journal of Child Psychology and Psychiatry*, **23**, 281–293.

Kanner, L. (1943) 'Autistic disturbances of affective contact.' *Nervous Child*, **2**, 217–250.

—— (1949) 'Problems of nosology and psychodynamics of early infantile autism.' *American Journal of Orthopsychiatry*, **19**, 416–426.

—— Eisenberg, L. (1956) 'Early infantile autism: 1943–1955.' *American Journal of Orthopsychiatry*, **26**, 55–65.

Keeler, W.R. (1958) 'Autistic patterns and defective communication in blind children with retrolental fibroblasia.' *In:* Hoch, P.H., Zubin, J. (Eds) *Psychopathology of Communication.* New York: Grune & Stratton, pp. 64–83.

Lotter, V. (1966) 'Epidemiology of autistic conditions in young children. I: Prevalence.' *Social Psychiatry*, **1**, 124–137.

—— (1974) 'Factors related to outcome in autistic children.' *Journal of Autism and Childhood Schizophrenia*, **4**, 263–277.

Mahler, M.S., Gosliner, B.J. (1955) 'On symbiotic child psychosis: genetic, dynamic and restitutive aspects.' *Psychoanalytic Study of the Child*, **19**, 195–212.

Maltz, A. (1981) 'Comparison of cognitive deficits among autistic and retarded children on the Arthur Adaption of the Leiter International Performance Scale.' *Journal of Autism and Developmental Disorders*, **11**, 413–426.

Masterton, B.A., Biederman, G.B. (1983) 'Proprioceptive versus visual control in autistic children.' *Journal of Autism and Developmental Disorders*, **13**, 141–152.

Mirenda, P.L., Donnellan, A.M., Yoder, D.E. (1983) 'Gaze behaviour: a new look at an old problem.' *Journal of Autism and Developmental Disorders*, **13**, 397–409.

Ohta, M. (1987) 'Cognitive disorders of infantile autism: a study employing the WISC, spatial relationship conceptualization, and gesture imitations.' *Journal of Autism and Developmental Disorders*, **17**, 45–62.

Olsson, I., Steffenburg, S., Gillberg, C. (1988) 'Epilepsy in autism and autistic-like conditions: a population-based study.' *Archives of Neurology*, **45**, 666–668.

Ornitz, E.M. (1983) 'The functional neuroanatomy of infantile autism.' *International Journal of Neuroscience*, **19**, 85–124.

—— (1989) 'Sensory modulation and directed attention.' *Paper presented at Congress of the Federation of Societies of Biological Psychiatry, Jerusalem.*

—— Guthrie, D., Farley, A.J. (1977) 'The early development of autistic children.' *Journal of Autism and Childhood Schizophrenia*, **7**, 207–229.

Rapin, I. (1979) 'Effects of early blindness and deafness on cognition.' *In:* Katzman, R. (Ed.) *Congenital and Acquired Cognitive Disorders.* New York: Raven, pp. 189–245.

Riikonen, R., Amnell, G. (1981) 'Psychiatric disorders in children with earlier infantile spasms.' *Developmental Medicine and Child Neurology*, **23**, 747–760.

—— —— (1990) 'Tuberous sclerosis and infantile spasms.' *Developmental Medicine and Child Neurology*, **32**, 203–209.

Rogers, S.J., Newhart-Larson, S. (1989) 'Characteristics of infantile autism in five children with Leber's congenital amaurosis.' *Developmental Medicine and Child Neurology*, **31**, 598–608.

Rumsey, J.M., Hamburger, S.D. (1988) 'Neuropsychological findings in high-functioning men with infantile autism, residual state.' *Journal of Clinical and Experimental Neuropsychology*, **10**, 201–221.

Rutter, M. (1970) 'Autistic children. Infancy to adulthood.' *Seminars in Psychiatry*, **2**, 435–450.

—— (1978) 'Diagnosis and definition.' *In:* Rutter, M., Schopler, E. (Eds) *Autism: a Reappraisal of Concepts and Treatment.* New York: Plenum, pp. 1–25.

—— (1983) 'Cognitive deficits in the pathogenesis of autism.' *Journal of Child Psychology and Psychiatry*, **24**, 513–531.

—— Schopler, E. (1987) 'Autism and pervasive developmental disorders: concepts and diagnostic issues.' *Journal of Autism and Developmental Disorders*, **17**, 159–186.

Schain, R., Yannet, H. (1960) 'Infantile autism: an analysis of 50 cases and a consideration of certain relevant neuropsychological concepts.' *Journal of Pediatrics*, **57**, 560–567.

Shah, A., Frith, U. (1983) 'An islet of ability in autistic children: a research note.' *Journal of Child Psychology and Psychiatry*, **24**, 613–620.

Siegel, B., Vukicevic, J., Elliott, G.R., Kraemer, H.C. (1989) 'The use of signal detection theory to assess DSM-III-R criteria for autistic disorder.' *Journal of the American Academy of Child and Adolescent Psychiatry*, **28**, 542–548.

Spitz, R.A. (1946) 'Anaclitic depression—an inquiry into the genesis of psychiatric conditions in early childhood.' *Psychoanalytic Study of the Child*, **2**, 313–342.

Steffenburg, S. (1991) 'Neuropsychiatric assessment of children with autism: a population-based study.' *Developmental Medicine and Child Neurology*, **33**, 495–511.

—— Gillberg, C. (1986) 'Autism and autistic-like conditions in Swedish rural and urban areas: a population study.' *British Journal of Psychiatry*, **149**, 81–87.

Taft, L.T., Cohen, H.J. (1971) 'Hypsarrhythmia and childhood autism: a clinical report.' *Journal of*

Autism and Childhood Schizophrenia, **1**, 327–336.

von Knorring, A-L. (1983) *'Adoption Studies on Psychiatric Illness. Epidemiological, Environmental and Genetic Aspects.'* Umeå University Medical Dissertations.

Waterhouse, L., Fein, D. (1989) 'Social or cognitive or both? Crucial dysfunctions in autism.' *In:* Gillberg, C. (Ed.) *Diagnosis and Treatment of Autism.* New York: Plenum, pp. 53–61.

—— —— Nath, J., Snyder, D. (1984) *Pervasive Schizophrenia Occurring in Childhood: a Review of Critical Commentary.* Washington, DC: American Psychiatric Association.

Wing, J.K. (1966) 'Diagnosis, epidemiology, aetiology.' *In:* Wing, J.K. (Ed.) *Early Childhood Autism.* Oxford: Pergamon, pp. 3–49.

Wing, L. (1980) *Early Childhood Autism. 2nd Edn.* Oxford: Pergamon.

—— (1981*a*) 'Asperger's syndrome: a clinical account.' *Psychological Medicine*, **11**, 115–129.

—— (1981*b*) 'Language, social and cognitive impairments in autism and severe mental retardation. *Journal of Autism and Developmental Disorders*, **11**, 33–34.

—— (1989) 'The diagnosis of autism.' *In:* Gillberg, C. (Ed.) *Diagnosis and Treatment of Autism.* New York: Plenum, pp. 5–22.

—— Gould, J. (1979) 'Severe impairments of social interaction and associated abnormalities in children: epidemiology and classification.' *Journal of Autism and Developmental Disorders*, **9**, 11–29.

Witt-Engerström, I., Gillberg, C. (1987) 'Rett syndrome in Sweden.' *Journal of Autism and Developmental Disorders*, **17**, 149–150.

World Health Organisation (1990) *International Classification of Diseases (ICD-10). Draft Version.* Geneva: WHO.

Zetterström, R. (1983) 'Infantile autism—neuropsychological correlates.' *Paper presented at Sävstaholm Conference on Autism. Uppsala, Sweden.*

3
ASPERGER SYNDROME

It is only quite recently that a syndrome originally described by Asperger (1944) has attracted relatively widespread attention in child and adult psychiatry (Gillberg 1985, 1989; Tantam 1988; Szatmari *et al.* 1989*a*) and it was not until 1981 that it received its status as a named syndrome (Wing 1981). There is currently a debate as to whether 'Kanner autism' and 'childhood autistic psychopathy/personality disorder' (the original syndrome name suggested by Asperger) represent overlapping or distinct conditions or whether they exist on a spectrum on which the lowermost portion is represented by Kanner autism and the uppermost section by Asperger syndrome (Frith 1991). Some have argued that the differential diagnosis of Asperger syndrome depends only on IQ, which tends to be low or very low in Kanner autism but normal or high (occasionally very high) in Asperger syndrome. Some appear to believe that the two syndromes exist on a social deficit continuum with Kanner autism again on the lowermost portion and Asperger syndrome in the higher range. Even though both of these continuum approaches have considerable clinical credibility, Kanner autism is sometimes, albeit very rarely, diagnosed in cases with high IQ and Asperger syndrome in cases with low IQ. Also, the social deficits encountered in so-called Asperger syndrome are quite often exceptionally severe, especially if the IQ level is taken into account.

We are aware that distinguishing Asperger syndrome from autism may be an artificial venture and that the two conditions may, in the long run, be treated as one. Nevertheless, so far, the evidence is not unequivocally in favour of such an association. Clinically there is still something to be said for the use of the Asperger label for certain relatively high-functioning individuals with autistic-type empathy deficits and superficially excellent language skills. Research diagnostic criteria for Asperger syndrome—which may well be used in clinical practice also—are presented in Table 3.1. These criteria should not be thought of as an excuse either for separating out Asperger syndrome as a discrete entity different in key aspects from all other syndromes in child psychiatry (including 'autism'), or for extending the autism concept infinitely but inexplicitly to encompass all empathy deficits encountered in psychiatry. Rather, they should be regarded as a tool for distinguishing a group of children and adults with a particular conglomeration of social, communication and behavioural repertoire deficits, who either do not readily meet the clinical criteria for infantile autism or autistic disorder or who, even if they do meet such criteria, for some reason give the impression of being 'too normal' for an autism diagnosis to be appropriate. Superficially, such persons may not seem to be severely disabled, but a more thorough analysis will reveal that they

TABLE 3.I

Diagnostic criteria for Asperger syndrome

1. Severe impairment in reciprocal social interaction
   (at least two of the following)

   (a) inability to interact with peers
   (b) lack of desire to interact with peers
   (c) lack of appreciation of social cues
   (d) socially and emotionally inappropriate behaviour

2. All-absorbing narrow interest
   (at least one of the following)

   (a) exclusion of other activities
   (b) repetitive adherence
   (c) more rote than meaning

3. Imposition of routines and interests
   (at least one of the following)

   (a) on self, in aspects of life
   (b) on others

4. Speech and language problems
   (at least three of the following)

   (a) delayed development
   (b) superficially perfect expressive language
   (c) formal, pedantic language
   (d) odd prosody, peculiar voice characteristics
   (e) impairment of comprehension including misinterpretations
       of literal/implied meanings

5. Non-verbal communication problems
   (at least one of the following)

   (a) limited use of gestures
   (b) clumsy/gauche body language
   (c) limited facial expression
   (d) inappropriate expression
   (e) peculiar, stiff gaze

6. Motor clumsiness: poor performance on neurodevelopmental
   examination

Adapted from Gillberg (1991). All six criteria must be met for confirmation of diagnosis.

---

have extensive empathy problems that warrant further empirical study.

It needs emphasizing that the communication problems included as a diagnostic criterion might seem to differentiate Asperger syndrome as conceptualized in this chapter from that depicted in the draft version of the ICD-10 (WHO 1990). In the latter manual, normal language development will be included as a criterion. Often, however, we are faced with 'clear-cut' Asperger syndrome cases (as described by Asperger himself) reported to have normal or even early language development. In our experience, on closer analysis, all such individuals have been shown to have deviant language development, at least in the context of a group of family members with superior intelligence and/or early language development. There is often a history of 'relatively' late development of language followed by the emergence of perfect language skills, appropriate for an adult rather than for a young child. To be sure, such language development, taken out of its familial context, may be perceived as 'normal' (and may indeed be normal as compared with the average population). However, it is definitely abnormal if analysed in the particular family/social context.

Prevalence
Several Swedish studies (see Gillberg and Gillberg 1989) indicate a population prevalence for Asperger syndrome in school-age children of around 1 to 3 per 1000. Preliminary studies from Göteborg, Sweden (Ehlers, personal communication) and London, England (Wing, personal communication) suggest higher figures. Boys appear to outnumber girls by 5:1 to 15:1. However, in some recent writings (*e.g.* Gillberg 1992*a*, Kopp and Gillberg 1992) it has been suggested that the female phenotype may be slightly different and is perhaps more prevalent than hitherto believed. For instance, one study indicated an increased frequency of Asperger syndrome and similar high-functioning autistic-like conditions in the premorbid history of some girls who developed anorexia nervosa in adolescence (Gillberg and Råstam 1992).

Familial/hereditary factors in Asperger syndrome
No major family, twin or adoption study of Asperger syndrome has been published yet. However, quite a number of clinical studies (e.g. Wing 1981, Gillberg 1989, Szatmari *et al.* 1989*b*) implicate a strong genetic component, with at least 50 per cent of affected cases having a close relative with Asperger syndrome or something very similar. Asperger himself reported that of the approximately 200 cases that he had personally followed for many years, almost all had at least one parent with similar traits. (Asperger also drew attention to possible brain damage in his cases—see below.) Burgoine and Wing (1983) reported on monozygotic male triplets with Asperger syndrome.

A number of family case studies (*e.g.* Bowman 1988, Gillberg 1991) have shown that in certain families there is overlap of autism and Asperger syndrome. For instance, in the family described by Bowman (1988), there was a spectrum of problems in the male first-degree relatives, ranging from severe Kanner autism through Asperger syndrome and mild autistic traits. In the Gillberg (1991) family, the mother (highly intelligent) had Asperger traits, the eldest son had Kanner autism and mild mental retardation, the middle son had mild autistic traits (and his son in turn had Kanner autism) and the youngest son had classical Asperger

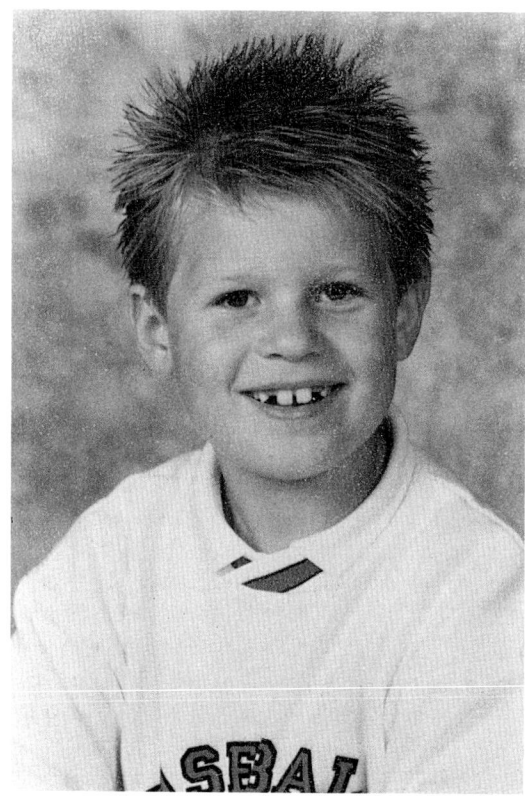

Fig. 3.1. 8-year-old boy with Asperger syndrome with possible semi-dominant semi-recessive mode of inheritance.

syndrome with superior intelligence. The eldest son had been affected by intrauterine rubella infection. The findings suggest that Asperger syndrome might be inherited in a fashion with variable penetrance. The added effects of certain forms of brain damage might produce full-blown autism in such families. Whether the mode of inheritance should be viewed as dominant or not is open to speculation. It appears that at least some cases (like those in the families described by Bowman and Gillberg) may be inherited in a dominant fashion. In other cases, in which both parents show some mild autistic-type traits and the child is quite severely affected, an atypical recessive mode of inheritance might be postulated. The type of 'semi-dominant semi-recessive' pattern purported by Comings (1990) to be common in Tourette syndrome might, theoretically at least, apply in Asperger syndrome also (Fig. 3.1).

A recent controlled population-based study of siblings and parents of children with autism indicated a slight but significant increase in the rate of Asperger syndrome in the first-degree relatives as compared with relatives of normal children and children with learning disorders other than autism (Gillberg *et al.* 1992).

There is a clinical impression that Asperger syndrome cases in some families segregate with obsessive–compulsive personality disorders, Tourette syndrome and simple tics. Except for one study by Comings (1990) supporting this impression, the empirical evidence in this field is lacking. A genetic link with attentional problems, elective mutism and anorexia nervosa has been suggested by a few studies (Gillberg 1989, Gillberg and Gillberg 1989, Råstam 1992), but there is no conclusive evidence.

Even though empirical evidence is largely lacking, the clinical evidence is such that it seems reasonable to conclude that, at least in certain cases, there is an hereditary trait common to autism and Asperger syndrome. Whether this applies to only a few, many, or even most cases with Asperger syndrome remains to be established in population studies making use of modern methodology of twin, family and adoption studies. Asperger syndrome is more common and less severe than autism. In certain instances the cognitive style and obsessional interests may contribute to a 'survival trait' which could even include 'superficially normal family life' in adulthood. An hereditary link between Asperger and Kanner syndromes might account for the persistence of genetic forms of autism in the population. Kanner autism is such a severe disorder that the genetic form would be quickly extinguished if it were inherited only in 'pure' form, unless the genetic variants were all inherited as autosomal recessives. The bulk of the evidence is not in favour of autosomal recessive inheritance in autism/Asperger syndrome (Bolton and Rutter 1990), even though some authors have argued for its importance, at least in a subgroup of patients (see Chapter 18).

Other biological factors in Asperger syndrome
Only occasionally is Asperger syndrome diagnosed in people with mild mental retardation (Gillberg *et al.* 1986). Asperger himself would probably have been reluctant to do this, but it is clear that there are cases with mild mental retardation who better fit the clinical picture described by him than that outlined by Kanner (Wing 1981, Gillberg 1985, Littlejohns *et al.* 1990).

Epilepsy may be marginally more common in Asperger syndrome than in the general population, but it is definitely much less common than in Kanner autism, probably affecting no more than a few per cent of the whole group (Gillberg 1989).

Occasionally, Asperger syndrome—just like autism but less often—may be associated with specific medical conditions, such as fragile X syndrome (Hagerman 1989), tuberous sclerosis (Gillberg 1989), neurofibromatosis (Gaffney *et al.* 1988) and hypothyroidism (Gillberg, I.C. *et al.* 1992).

It also appears that severe perinatal problems may be overrepresented (and perhaps causative or contributory in the pathogenetic chain of events) in a subgroup (Asperger 1944, Wing 1981, Gillberg 1989).

Unilateral brain damage has been proposed to account for the development of some cases of Asperger syndrome on theoretical grounds (Goodman 1989) and on the basis of findings obtained in individual patients (Littlejohns *et al.* 1990). Such

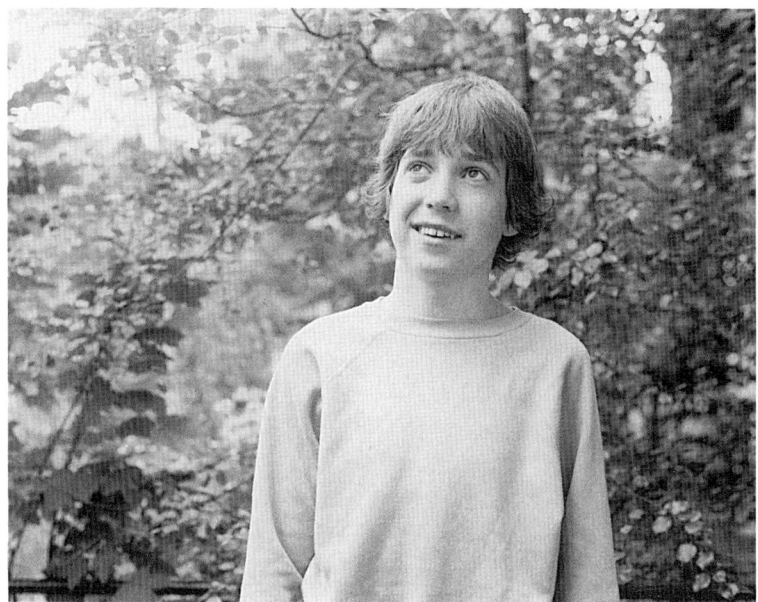

Fig. 3.2. 13-year-old boy with Asperger syndrome and XYY mosaicism.

damage would probably be most likely to affect parts of the temporal and prefrontal areas. Goodman (1989) has suggested that whereas autism would be likely to result from bilateral brain dysfunction, Asperger syndrome could arise on the basis of unilateral dysfunction of the same brain areas. This could be either right- or left-sided if, as hypothesized, social competence and language areas are located, respectively, in these parts of the brain. During early development, these parts, by being interconnected 'mirror images' of each other, could compensate to some extent for damage to the contralateral area (with a subsequent reduction of both functions).

No particular EEG, auditory brainstem response or CSF monoamine or endorphin pattern has yet been reported in Asperger syndrome (Gillberg 1989).

Medical work-up in Asperger syndrome
A full medical and developmental history must be taken in all cases. Medical records from the pre-, peri- and neonatal periods should be analysed. There should be a low threshold for performing chromosomal analysis, particularly with a view to disclosing the fragile Xq27.3 abnormality and other sex chromosome anomalies (Fig. 3.2). Thyroid function should be monitored. Other neurobiological examinations (such as MRI of the cortex—see Chapter 19) should be considered whenever clinical assessment and examination does not reveal a plausible cause.

Treatment/intervention

There are no specific medical treatments currently available for Asperger syndrome. Principles applied to education in autism adhere in Asperger syndrome as well, even though they have to be modified to comply with higher IQ and superficially better social functioning.

Of particular importance is the way in which bizarre interests may have to be dealt with. Many obsessive interests can be turned into something useful. However, extreme interests in areas such as gunpowder, poison, knives or violent sports should not be encouraged, and parents and teachers should be encouraged to seek alternatives in other areas. This is quite often a successful venture, but one which has to be dealt with in thoughtful ways, taking account of all sorts of factors such as family setting and child's IQ, personality and past interest patterns.

Perhaps the most important intervention of all is to make a diagnosis and inform the parents and sometimes the child. Together they will then be able to tell those people, including teachers, who would benefit from knowing that the child's social demeanour is likely to remain relatively stable over many years, regardless of treatment and other interventions. Some might consider this a nihilistic approach, but it is not. To the contrary, it means accepting somebody with a unique personality and a rather unusual set of behavioural traits without feeling the need to change him/her to achieve 'normality' at any cost.

Course and outcome in Asperger syndrome

Outcome in Asperger syndrome is very variable, ranging from excellent to poor (Asperger 1944, Wing 1981, Tantam 1988).

It should be clear that many people with Asperger syndrome never come to the attention of psychiatrists or psychologists. They may be regarded as odd—and even aloof—but they are not perceived as psychiatrically abnormal.

Of those who do attend psychiatric services, it is possible that only a fraction apply for help in childhood. These cases have received a variety of diagnostic labels and it is only during the last decade that they have come to be diagnosed as having Asperger syndrome. 'Old' labels in the field include 'borderline', 'borderline psychosis', 'autistic traits', 'minimal brain dysfunction' and occasionally even 'conduct disorder'. 'Atypical', 'schizoid' and 'schizotypal' are other labels which have been employed by certain groups.

Even among those who do attend child psychiatric services, quite a number have a fair prognosis and lead independent adult lives. They will still be regarded by some as 'highly original', 'eccentric' or 'odd', but such perceived qualities have at least as many positive as negative connotations and therefore can lead to admiration rather than rejection and so may contribute to a good outcome. Their basic style of interaction, their concrete and formalistic treatment of spoken and written language and the narrow interests and routines usually continue relatively unchanged throughout life. A case has been made for Asperger syndrome being associated in rare cases with artistic achievements and even philosophical writings, as exemplified by Béla Bartók and Ludwig Wittgenstein (Gillberg 1992*b*).

Nevertheless, a proportion of young patients diagnosed with Asperger syndrome will grow up to be psychiatric patients or criminal offenders. Many people with Asperger syndrome probably seek psychiatric help for the first time only in adult life. In our experience, 'paranoia', 'depression', 'obsessive–compulsive personality disorder' and 'borderline' are the most common diagnoses given by adult psychiatrists to this group. Some are labelled 'pseudoneurotic schizophrenics'. According to Wing's follow-up, suicide attempts may be relatively common (Wing 1981). Clear-cut classic schizophrenia appears to be very rare, and, so far, there is no evidence for a continuity from childhood Asperger syndrome through adult life schizophrenia. Some of the other diagnoses given may occasionally be correct at the phenomenological level. However, the best help can be provided if the basic 'Asperger traits' are recognized and many of the psychopharmacological treatments of adult psychiatry avoided in this group. The type of criminal offence sometimes encountered in adolescents and adults with Asperger syndrome is usually connected with extreme obsession. It could be anything from poisoning and other variants of 'experimental killing' and arson to bizarre violence (Baron-Cohen 1988, Tantam 1991).

REFERENCES

Asperger, H. (1944) 'Die "autistischen Psychopathen" im Kindesalter.' *Archiv für Psychiatrie und Nervenkrankheiten*, **117**, 76–136.
Baron-Cohen, S. (1988) 'An assessment of violence in a young man with Asperger's syndrome.' *Journal of Child Psychology and Psychiatry*, **29**, 351–360.
Bolton, P., Rutter, M. (1990) 'Genetic influences in autism.' *International Review of Psychiatry*, **2**, 67–80.
Bowman, E.P. (1988) 'Asperger's syndrome and autism: the case for a connection.' *British Journal of Psychiatry*, **152**, 377–382.
Burgoine, E., Wing, L. (1983) 'Identical triplets with Asperger's syndrome.' *British Journal of Psychiatry*, **143**, 261–265.
Comings, D. (1990) *Tourette Syndrome and Human Behavior.* Duarte, CA: Hope Press.
Frith, U. (1991) *Autism and Asperger Syndrome.* Cambridge: Cambridge University Press.
Gaffney, G.R., Kuperman, S., Tsai, L.Y., Minchin, S. (1988) 'Morphological evidence for brainstem involvement in infantile autism.' *Biological Psychiatry*, **24**, 578–586.
Gillberg, C. (1985) 'Asperger's syndrome and recurrent psychosis—a case study.' *Journal of Autism and Developmental Disorders*, **15**, 389–397.
—— (1989) 'Asperger syndrome in 23 Swedish children.' *Developmental Medicine and Child Neurology*, **31**, 520–531.
—— (1991) 'Clinical and neurobiological aspects in six family studies of Asperger syndrome.' *In*: Frith, U. (Ed.) *Autism and Asperger Syndrome.* Cambridge: Cambridge University Press, pp. 122–146.
—— (1992a) 'The Emanuel Miller Lecture 1991: Autism and autistic-like conditions—subgroups of disorders of empathy.' *Journal of Child Psychology and Psychiatry,* **33**, 813–842.
—— (1992b) 'Savant-syndromet.' *In*: Vejlsgaard, R. (Ed.) *Medicinsk årsbok.* Köpenhamn: Munksgaard, pp. 127–131.
—— Gillberg, I.C. (1989) 'Asperger syndrome. Some epidemiological considerations: a research note.' *Journal of Child Psychology and Psychiatry*, **30**, 631–638.
—— Råstam, M. (1992) 'Do some cases of anorexia nervosa reflect underlying autistic-like conditions?' *Behavioural Neurology*, **5**, 27–32.

—— Persson, E., Grufman, M., Themnér, U. (1986) 'Psychiatric disorders in mildly and severely mentally retarded urban children and adolescents: epidemiological aspects.' *British Journal of Psychiatry*, **149**, 68–74.

—— Gillberg, I.C., Steffenburg, S. (1992) 'Siblings and parents of children with autism. A controlled population-based study.' *Developmental Medicine and Child Neurology*, **34**, 389–398.

Gillberg, I.C., Gillberg, C., Kopp, S. (1992) 'Hypothyroidism and autism spectrum disorders.' *Journal of Child Psychology and Psychiatry*, **33**, 531–542.

Goodman, R. (1989) 'Infantile autism: a syndrome of multiple primary deficits?' *Journal of Autism and Developmental Disorders*, **19**, 409–424.

Hagerman, R.J. (1989) 'Chromosomes, genes and autism.' *In:* Gillberg, C. (Ed.) *Diagnosis and Treatment of Autism.* New York: Plenum, pp. 105–132.

Kopp, S., Gillberg, C. (1992) 'Girls with social deficits and learning problems: autism, atypical Asperger syndrome or a variant of these conditions.' *European Child and Adolescent Psychiatry*, **1**, 90–100.

Littlejohns, C.S., Clarke, D.J., Corbett, J.A. (1990) 'Tourette-like disorder in Asperger's syndrome.' *British Journal of Psychiatry*, **156**, 430–433.

Råstam, M. (1992) 'Anorexia nervosa in 51 children and adolescents. Pre-morbid problems and co-morbidity.' *Journal of the American Academy of Child and Adolescent Psychiatry. (In press.)*

Szatmari, P., Bartolucci, G., Bremner, R. (1989*a*) 'Asperger's syndrome and autism: comparison of early history and outcome.' *Developmental Medicine and Child Neurology*, **31**, 709–720.

—— Bremner, R., Nagy, J. (1989*b*) 'Asperger's syndrome: a review of clinical features.' *Canadian Journal of Psychiatry*, **34**, 554–560.

Tantam, D. (1988) 'Asperger's syndrome.' *Journal of Child Psychology and Psychiatry*, **29**, 245–255. *(Annotation.)*

—— (1991) 'Asperger syndrome in adulthood.' *In:* Frith, U. (Ed.) *Autism and Asperger syndrome.* Cambridge: Cambridge University Press, pp. 147–183.

Wing, L. (1981) 'Asperger's syndrome: a clinical account.' *Psychological Medicine*, **11**, 115–129.

World Health Organisation (1990) *International Classification of Diseases (ICD-10). Draft Version.* Geneva: WHO.

4
DIAGNOSIS IN INFANCY

The age of obvious clinical onset in autism can, in rare instances, be as early as the first hour of life. An infant with autism may be born with such severe haptic defensiveness (sensitivity of the tactile system) that the child screams when held; the mother ends up feeding the infant by holding the bottle over the crib (or even tying it with ribbons to the walls of the crib) without actually touching the infant (Coleman 1989). Such infants have great difficulty tolerating breast feeding because of the tactile interaction involved. Instead of being soothed by the mother's touch, it appears to cause the child discomfort or even pain. However, such failure to settle in the mother's arms or lack of 'cuddliness', if not in such an extreme degree, can sometimes be seen in perfectly normal children (Schaffer and Emerson 1964), so this symptom, by itself, cannot be used for screening purposes in detecting infants with autism.

Thus the question arises: are there specific or very high-risk symptoms that can alert the clinical observer to the possibility of an autistic syndrome in a very young infant? In view of the developing understanding of medical aetiologies and their sometimes available specific therapies, this question is no longer limited to an academic exercise. It may be quite helpful to the child if educational intervention, now possibly combined with medical treatment in some cases, can be started very early.

Since autism is a syndrome with multiple aetiologies, it is not anticipated that particular specific signs and symptoms will be present in a high percentage of cases. However, when a combination of signs and symptoms are present in a neonate or a very young child, they may alert the physician and the family. In the experience of the present authors and of other observers in the field of autism, many parents realize that something is seriously wrong with their child from the start or almost from the start (Gillberg 1984). Although it is quite a difficult task in many cases, it is now time for physicians to use what medical knowledge exists to decide if a child is at risk for autism while avoiding undue worry in parents of unusual but normal babies.

Early signs that may signal the risk of developing autism
Most children with autism have no obvious physical stigmata. However, a sophisticated examination of an infant could reveal signs that have differentiated children with and without autism in three studies (Walker 1976, Campbell *et al.* 1978, Links *et al.* 1980). Ear anomalies were a common finding in these studies, including malformations, asymmetrical, soft or pliable ears, adherent lobes and,

especially, low-set ears. (Incidentally, these ear anomalies might well account for some of the association of autism with conductive hearing loss—Smith *et al.* 1988).

Other signs which have been shown to be statistically associated with autism and which might alert the examiner of the infant include hypertelorism, partial syndactyly of the second and third toes, and mouth anomalies (high palate, tongue furrows and smooth/rough spots). Although none of these signs are specific to autism and can be seen in other syndromes, they can be helpful when combined with the clinical symptoms in the very young patient.

Muscular hypotonia in the newborn period may signal a variety of developmental disorders including autism. For instance, in the fragile X syndrome, hypotonia is a fairly common feature, and in 20 per cent of newborns with this syndrome attention was alerted by clinically manifest hypotonia.

Early symptoms that may alert the clinician to the possibility of autism

There are extremely few studies of early symptoms (Arrieta *et al.* 1990, Wolman *et al.* 1990) and even fewer observational records available on people with autism during the first years of life. Such evidence as there is suggests that non-specific symptoms, such as lack of initiative, hyperactivity, sleep problems and feeding difficulties, are often the first to be recognized.

A series of studies is available from Göteborg, Sweden, in which early symptoms have been delineated by both retrospective, current and prospective study (Dahlgren and Gillberg 1989, Gillberg *et al.* 1990). In the Dahlgren and Gillberg study a 130-item questionnaire was filled out by mothers of sex-, age- and IQ-matched mentally retarded and population-representative normal children as well as by the parents of children with autism. The study was retrospective, and the subjects were 7 to 22 years old at the time the parents completed the questionnaire. In the Gillberg *et al.* study, the same questionnaire was used in a study of children with autism who were seen before age 3 years, the mothers completing the questionnaire before the child's third birthday. The children were followed up prospectively, and a diagnosis of autism established after 3 years of age. The results were contrasted with findings obtained in an age-, sex- and IQ-matched comparison group without autistic symptoms. Table 4.1 lists the 28 items which characterized the autism group in either the prospective study only (10 items) or the retrospective study only (8 items) or in both studies (10 items). Two further items pertaining to overall developmental backwardness ('late development' and 'late speech development') also distinguished the autism from the non-autism retarded group in the prospective study. It is of some interest that a number of items, thought to be typical of autism ('loves to spin objects', 'walks on tiptoe', 'turns light on and off', 'does not like to sit on somebody else's knee', 'dislikes change of routine', 'fascinated by sight of running water'), did not discriminate between groups either in the pro- or retrospective study.

The latter study demonstrated that in quite a number of cases of children referred in infancy with a suspicion of autism, it is possible to arrive at a correct

TABLE 4.1

Items discriminating autism from mental retardation and normality under age 3 years

Area/item	Prospective study (Gillberg et al. 1990)	Retrospective study (Dahlgren and Gillberg 1989)
Social		
Appears to be isolated from surroundings	√*	√
Doesn't smile when expected to	√	√
Difficulties getting eye contact	√	√
Doesn't matter much whether Mum or Dad is close by or not	√	
Doesn't like to be disturbed in own world		√
Contented if left alone		√
Communication		
Doesn't try to attract adult's attention to own activity	√	√**
Difficulties imitating movements	√	√
Late speech development	√	
Doesn't point to objects	√	
Doesn't understand what people say	√	
Can't indicate own wishes	√	
Play behaviour		
Doesn't play like other children	√*	√
Occupies self only when alone	√	√
Plays only with hard objects	√	√
Odd attachments to odd objects		√
Perception		
There is (or has been) a suspicion of deafness	√*	√
Empty gaze	√	√**
Overexcited when tickled	√	√
There is something strange about his/her gaze	√	
Interested only in certain parts of objects	√	
Exceptionally interested in things that move	√	
Doesn't listen when spoken to	√	
Strange reactions to sound		√**
Doesn't seem to react to cold		√
Engages in bizarre looking at objects, pattern and movements		√
Rhythmicity		
There are days/periods when s/he seems much worse than usual		√
Severe problems over sleep		√

*3 items with strongest discriminatory power in prospective study.
**3 items with strongest discriminatory power in retrospective study.

diagnosis very early, particularly if the child is also mentally retarded. Also, at least a quarter of children believed to suffer from autism during the first few years of life will later be shown to have other developmental problems, or, in rare instances, to be perfectly normal at follow-up.

Non-specific early problems

Even though overall late development is typical both of children with autism and of children with mental retardation, there were clear trends in the Swedish studies for 'abnormalities of any kind' to have been observed earlier in autism than in mental retardation. This held even if autism cases were compared with non-autism cases with severe mental retardation, provided that comparison across cases was performed at corresponding IQ levels. These findings corroborated those of Short and Schopler (1988).

Sleep problems and a strong tendency for periodicity were noted in the retrospective but not in the prospective study, implying that caution may be warranted as regards generalizability.

There is, quite naturally, considerable overlap in respect of early symptoms in autism and mental retardation. According to a study of schizophrenia with childhood onset (Watkins *et al.* 1988), there may also, in certain cases, be considerable similarity between the early histories of children with school-age onset schizophrenia and infancy-onset autism.

In the Gillberg *et al.* (1990) study, mothers were asked to describe in their own words what they had first noted as possibly abnormal in the child. 'Abnormalities of eye contact' was the single most common type of abnormality reported and had been noted around age 1 to 8 months. A few had worried about 'strange reactions to sound' around age 1 year. Otherwise, no specific symptoms emerged as characteristic of autism. Rather, diffuse concern about something 'not touchable', or 'not graspable', tended to prevail.

However, it is again necessary to point out that in high-functioning children with autism there may be no characteristic (specific or non-specific) signs in infancy.

Early symptoms that may be specific to autism in infancy

Abnormal responses to sensory stimuli tend to represent the most characteristic group of symptoms in autism cases referred in infancy (Ornitz *et al.* 1978, Ornitz 1988, Gillberg 1989). In recent studies by Dahlgren and Gillberg (1989) and Gillberg *et al.* (1990), 10 of 28 possibly specific symptoms of autism belonged in this group (see Table 4.1); this was not an effect of there being more questionnaire items in this category than in the four others (social, communication, play behaviour and rhythmicity).

Except for abnormal perceptual responses, symptoms associated with 'autistic aloneness' and abnormalities of play tend to be those most clearly evident in infants with autistic symptoms.

In a study by Sauvage *et al.* (1987), a relative lack of mimicry and an expressionless face were found to be the most common first signs of autism, at least as judged from home movies. Whether to group such symptoms with social or communication deficits is not yet obvious.

Abnormal babble, widely believed to be an early symptom of autism, has not shown up in recent studies.

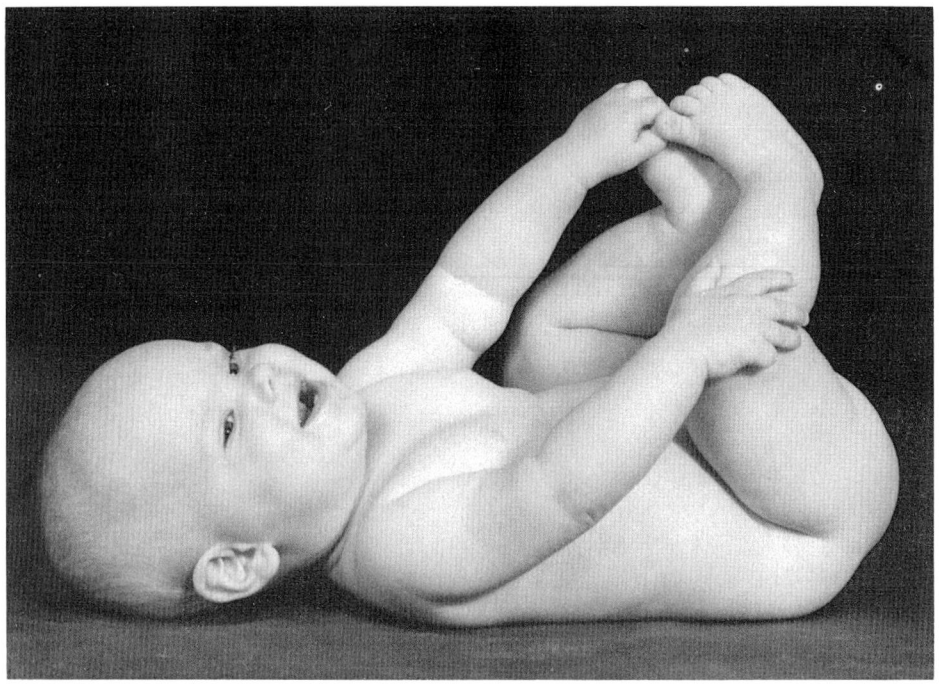

Fig. 4.1. 14-month-old boy with idiopathic autism.

In an ongoing collaborative study between the Department of Psychology at the Institute of Psychiatry in London and the Child Neuropsychiatry Centre in Göteborg, siblings of children with autism are examined at age 18 months with a view to finding symptoms of autism (and in particular symptoms of empathy/theory of mind deficits). Only three out of some 50 examined siblings have yet been diagnosed as suffering from autism; all three could be predicted on the basis of reported deficits in imaginative play behaviours and shared attention at age 18 months (Baron-Cohen *et al.* 1992).

The clinical picture of autism developing in infancy
It appears that about three quarters of children with autism show symptoms and signs of the disorder already in the first 18 to 30 months of life (Gillberg 1989). However, when discussing infancy in autism, it is important to keep in mind the multiple aetiologies and different ages of onset. There are patients in whom one can look in vain for symptoms during early infancy (Fig. 4.1). In such cases, an often rather clear month of onset can be determined in the second or third year of the child's life (Wing 1980). While not disputing the existence of such forms of autism, it is clear that, even in the group with an apparent setback, careful,

detailed, retrospective history-taking with the parents will often reveal that there have been early developmental delays and abnormalities (Wing 1971). Also, there are the high-functioning cases in which it may only become gradually obvious that the child is deviant. The abnormality in the brain which causes autism may well, in certain cases, have been there from before birth, but before a certain age, the nervous system is able to deal with the demands posed by development. Gradually, the brain can no longer fully cope with these demands and the autistic symptoms appear clearly for the first time. In such cases 'autism', even if congenital, will appear to have its onset after infancy.

Many infants with autism show 'no response' or 'no smile'. They may lack the normal anticipatory reactions typical of healthy children about to be picked up by their parents. The abnormal response to sound is often obvious in the second half of the first year, and many children with autism have been thought deaf by persons outside the immediate family (who *know* they cannot be). There may be major sleep problems or the child may be perceived as 'too good to be true', never demanding attention. 'Feeding problems', in both breast- and bottle-fed babies, are very common, the child either displaying sucking difficulties, or holding the head in stiff and strange postures, or, more rarely, actively turning away.

Many children with autism are extremely behaviourally deviant even during this first year of life. They may engage in stereotyped hand movements and be completely passive, not interested in exploring their environment, indeed, showing no initiative whatsoever, and perhaps already fiercely protesting when demands are made or routines changed. A few reject body contact. Many prefer to be left alone.

Toward the end of the first year, the child's lack of initiative and interest in exploring the environment comes into focus. The child will not look for things which disappear out of vision as normal children of that age will do. They do not show shared attention behaviours as early as other children, and one-finger pointing is rarely achieved until several years later. They also fail to develop signs of the emergence of a theory of mind (Frith 1989). In other words, they seem to be unable to understand that other people may have a mind of their own (see also Chapters 2 and 15).

Summary and suggestion for screening in well-baby services
On the basis of the limited empirical study and clinical experience, a screening model for autism in infancy has been suggested (Gillberg 1989). This model (Table 4.2) should not be regarded as an 'exact' device, but rather as a check-list to be used if the child has anything to suggest autism or an autistic-like condition or if the parent is concerned about the child's behaviour or development.

In the future, it will be essential to try to distinguish early symptoms in autism according to the diagnosed underlying medical condition. Finding unifying features in autism will remain important for screening purposes, but differentiation of early symptoms in accordance with underlying aetiology will become crucial if we are to understand brain–behaviour–developmental relationships better.

TABLE 4.2

Screening for autism at the well-baby clinic at ages 10 and 18 months

(1) The following questions to the mother provide a tentative framework for a check-list to be used whenever there is (even mild) suspicion of autistic-like behaviour or autism:

Do you consider your child's eye-to-eye-contact to be normal?
Do you think that s/he listens to you or has normal hearing, or does s/he react only to particular sounds?
If there are or have been any feeding problems or abnormal behaviours in connection with feeding, what were they?
Is s/he comforted by proximity or body contact?
Does s/he oppose body contact?
Does s/he show any interest in his/her surroundings?
Does s/he often smile or laugh quite unexpectedly?
Does s/he prefer to be left alone?
Is your child, on the whole, like other children?

(2) Examine the following features systematically:

Hand stereotypies (including strange looking at or posturing of hands)
Avoidance of gaze contact
Stiff, staring gaze
Rejection of body contact
No or very variable reaction to strong, unexpected noise
Obvious lack of interest (*e.g.* does not show interest in peek-a-boo games)

REFERENCES

Arrieta, M.I., Martinez, B., Criado, B., Simón, A., Salazar, I., Lostao, C.M. (1990) 'Dermatoglyphic analysis of autistic Basque children.' *American Journal of Medical Genetics*, **35**, 1–9.

Baron-Cohen, S., Allen, J., Gillberg, C. (1992) 'Can autism be detected at 18 months? The needle, the haystack and the CHAT.' *British Journal of Psychiatry. (In press.)*

Campbell, M., Geller, B., Small, A.M., Petti, T.A., Ferris, S.H. (1978) 'Minor physical anomalies in young psychotic children.' *American Journal of Psychiatry*, **135**, 573–575.

Coleman, M. (1989) 'Autism: non-drug biological treatments.' *In:* Gillberg, C. (Ed.) *Diagnosis and Treatment of Autism.* New York: Plenum, pp. 219–235.

Dahlgren, S.O., Gillberg, C. (1989) 'Symptoms in the first two years of life. A preliminary population study of infantile autism.' *European Archives of Psychiatry and Neurological Sciences*, **238**, 169–174.

Frith, U. (1989) 'Autism and "theory of mind".' *In:* Gillberg, C. (Ed.) *Diagnosis and Treatment of Autism.* New York: Plenum, pp. 33–52.

Gillberg, C. (1984) 'Infantile autism and other childhood psychoses in a Swedish urban region. Epidemiological aspects.' *Journal of Child Psychology and Psychiatry*, **25**, 35–43.

—— (1989) 'Early symptoms of autism.' *In:* Gillberg, C. (Ed.) *Diagnosis and Treatment of Autism.* New York: Plenum, pp. 23–32.

—— Ehlers, S., Schaumann, H., Jakobsson, G., Dahlgren, S.O., Lindblom, R., Bågenholm, A., Tjuust, T., Blidner, E. (1990) 'Autism under age 3 years: a clinical study of 28 cases referred for autistic symptoms in infancy.' *Journal of Child Psychology and Psychiatry*, **31**, 921–934.

Links, P.S., Stockwell, M., Abichandi, F., Simeon, J. (1980) 'Minor physical anomalies in childhood autism. Part I: Their relationship to pre- and perinatal complications.' *Journal of Autism and Developmental Disorders*, **10**, 273–285.

Ornitz, E. (1988) 'Autism: a disorder of directed attention.' *Brain Dysfunction*, **1**, 309–322.

—— Guthrie, D., Farley, A.J. (1978) 'The early symptoms of childhood autism.' *In:* Serban, G. (Ed.) *Cognitive Defects in the Development of Mental Illness.* New York: Brunner/Mazel.

Sauvage, D., Hameury, L., Adrien, J.L., Larmande, C., Perrot-Beaugerie, A, Barthélémy, C., Peyraud, A. (1987) 'Signes d'autisme avant deux ans. Evaluation et signification.' *Annales de Psychiatrie*, **3**, 418–424.

Schaffer, H.R., Emerson, P.E. (1964) 'The development of social attachments in infancy.' *Monographs of the Society for Research in Child Development*, **94**, 1–77.

Short, A.B., Schopler, E. (1988) 'Factors relating to age of onset in autism.' *Journal of Autism and Developmental Disorders*, **18**, 207–216.

Smith, D.E., Miller, S.D., Stewart, M., Walter, T.L., McConnell, J.V. (1988) 'Conductive hearing loss in autistic, learning-disabled, and normal children.' *Journal of Autism and Developmental Disorders*, **18**, 53–65.

Walker, H. (1976) 'The incidence of minor physical anomalies in autistic children.' *In:* Coleman, M. (Ed.) *The Autistic Syndromes*. Amsterdam: North Holland, pp. 95–116.

Watkins, J.M., Asarnow, R.F., Tanguay, P.E. (1988) 'Symptom development in childhood onset schizophrenia.' *Journal of Child Psychology and Psychiatry*, **29**, 865–878.

Wing, L. (1971) 'Perceptual and language development in autistic children: a comparative study.' *In:* Rutter, M. (Ed.) *Infantile Autism: Concepts, Characteristics and Treatment*. London: Churchill-Livingstone, pp. 173–197.

—— (1980) *Early Childhood Autism. 2nd Edn.* Oxford: Pergamon.

Wolman, S.R., Campbell, M., Marchi, M.L., Deutsch, S.I., Gershon, T.M. (1990) 'Dermatoglyphic study in autistic children and controls.' *Journal of the American Academy of Child and Adolescent Psychiatry*, **29**, 878–884.

5
CLINICAL COURSE AND PROGNOSIS

Autism, like any other developmental disorder, shows changes with respect to prevailing symptomatology with age (Rutter 1978; Wing 1980; Ornitz 1983; Waterhouse *et al.* 1984; Frith 1989, 1991; Wing 1989*b*; Gillberg 1990). This needs repeated emphasis, especially since many children with autism develop in rather different directions. Children who could scarcely be distinguished behaviour-ally at age 18 months may, by the age of 10 years, have developed completely different personalities and symptoms. This is one of the reasons why early recognition and observation is essential for establishing a precise diagnosis. Several years later it may even be impossible to say that the child ever had autism. We have followed at least a dozen children who before 5 years of age showed all the characteristics of Kanner autism, but who ten years later were only a little odd, had some peculiarities of spoken language but had several age peers. By the time these children had reached the age of 7 to 10 years, most people would find it hard to believe that they had ever suffered from autism. The same observation has been made by Chess (1977) in her follow-up of children with autism who had suffered rubella embryopathy. It is possible that it is children such as these who are reported to have been cured by various kinds of intervention.

Infancy and the first few years of life
Home videos and medical history data from parents and other caretakers suggest that non-specific symptoms such as lack of initiative, hyperactivity, sleep problems and feeding difficulties are often the first to be recognized. That such problems are frequent 'first symptoms' in autism was also suggested by two recent systematic studies (Dahlgren and Gillberg 1989, Gillberg *et al.* 1990). These studies further indicated that certain other symptoms might possibly be more specifically associated with autism. These included abnormal responses to sensory stimulation, autistic aloneness and various abnormalities of behaviour and play. These issues are discussed in more detail in Chapter 4.

The preschool years
From about age 2 to 6 years, the typically autistic behaviour patterns are usually most clearly evident. One explanation for this is the fact that many of the children with autism described by Kanner belonged in that age group, and thus the stereo-type of 'Kanner syndrome' is to some extent associated with children of that age.

For most families, the preschool years (and, in some cases, the adolescent years) are the hardest to cope with. The fearful temper tantrums associated with the more extreme forms of insistence on sameness are usually at a peak during this period. Also, most children with autism, after they have started walking unsupported (which they often do on time or only a few months late), become very difficult to manage in that they may be hyperactive, destructive or constantly engaging in repetitive activities, such as endlessly listening to tape recordings or occupying themselves with the tape recorder as a technical device. Some are fascinated by a particular object, such as a set of keys, and will be furious if deprived of it. Motor stereotypies are an extremely common, but not invariable, feature.

Around age 2 years, most normal children have developed some kind of communicative, spoken language, and begin to show a greater interest in other children. The child with autism usually fails to do any of these things and so is, for the first time, recognized as definitely abnormal. Many normal children—and children with autism—experience the birth of a sibling at about this age. It has become popular to attribute the withdrawal of some children with autism to the psychological trauma supposedly connected with this birth. A careful history taking will reveal, however, that the child has already displayed abnormal characteristics, and it is only the demands on normal development, which they cannot live up to, and the comparison with a normal sibling, which makes their abnormalities so much more conspicuous.

In some cases of autism it seems that normal development precedes a period of regression to an autistic state at about the age of 18 to 30 months. It is still unclear what proportion of all autism cases they represent. Some authors would prefer to group them with the cases of childhood disintegrative disorder (Baird *et al.* 1991). Still others maintain that it is possible to separate cases with late onset autism from those with disintegrative disorders (Volkmar and Cohen 1989). As has already been argued in Chapter 4, there is reason to hypothesize that at least some of these cases may be congenital in spite of the fact that obvious symptoms emerge only after a period of seemingly normal development. In other cases, however, it is clear that the autistic syndrome developed after some particular postnatal brain affliction, such as herpes encephalitis (DeLong *et al.* 1981; Gillberg 1986; Gillberg, I.C. 1991).

During the later preschool years, the child with autism quite often shows active avoidance of other children. In all cases there are severe problems in interacting normally, *i.e.* in a reciprocal fashion, with other children. The child may be perceived as suffering from 'extreme autistic aloneness'.

Autistic 'withdrawal' may not be the most striking feature in autism. Some children appear more 'perplexed' and appear not to be able to make sense of the world around them. They may seem to accept proximity to other people, and quite a number actually show, in various odd ways, that they want to interact with other people: they just do not know how to.

Some of the more high-functioning children with autism develop spoken language during the preschool years, although the majority have very little comprehensible speech before age 4 to 5 years. Those who do develop early language skills have a way of talking *at* rather than *with* other people. They appear not to be able to understand that they are talking 'to the inside' of people and not merely repeating phrases which do not require an answer or require only one specific standard reply.

Early school years
During the early school years (about the age of 6 to 11 years) most children with autism, if in an understanding and appropriate environment, gradually become less difficult to manage. The social aloofness usually subsides to some extent, and they become more cooperative. A proportion (perhaps a third) remain quite severely withdrawn throughout childhood. Nevertheless, the vast majority no longer totally avoid other children, even though they cannot relate to them in a manner appropriate to their age.

The degree of development of spoken language at age 5 to 6 years is one of the most significant factors affecting outcome (Rutter 1983). Two children with autism who might appear equally behaviourally deviant around age 3 years may be very different from each other at 7 years: one could appear almost as deviant as at age 3 and without useful language skills, while the other could appear 'odd' but in possession of useful speech and much less deviant than during the preschool years.

On the whole, hyperactivity and temper tantrums are not as frequent during the school years as earlier, and therefore parents, siblings and teachers usually have a relatively calmer period. However, in our experience, this will depend to some extent on whether or not the child has been correctly diagnosed as suffering from autism at the earlier age. Fewer families now live 'in the dark' for years, not knowing what is wrong with their child and constantly oscillating between fear, 'perplexity' and hope. Families receiving an early diagnosis and adequate educational programmes involving the parents report better coping strategies and fewer problems than those who are given the diagnosis later (Bågenholm and Gillberg 1991).

Sleep problems no longer tend to take on such dramatic guises, and although children with autism sometimes still have a greatly reduced need for sleep, they may be able to occupy themselves at night and leave other family members to rest.

There are, of course, exceptions to this rule, and some children with autism, especially those with severe mental retardation (and perhaps also some of the very high-functioning), have major behaviour problems throughout the school years.

Puberty and adolescence
Problems associated with puberty and adolescence in autism have long been disregarded or dealt with only summarily. However, recent studies have shown clearly that the adolescent period may be critical in many cases. Epilepsy, deterioration, aggravation of symptoms and additional psychiatric problems are the most common complications accompanying autism in adolescence. Motor stereo-

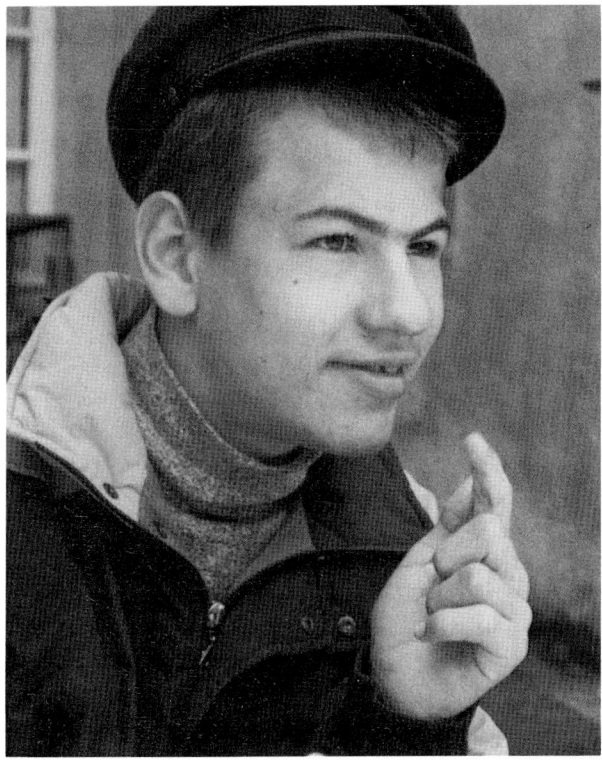

Fig. 5.1. Stereotypies, such as a finger mannerism, can persist into adolescent life.

typies may persist (Fig. 5.1).

A rather small minority of children do improve perceptibly during the teenage period (Kanner 1971). These are usually relatively high-functioning children who have also shown positive development during the early school years (Szatmari *et al.* 1989). Many others go through their teens with no more major behaviour problems than are usually associated with puberty in normal children.

However, among those with mental retardation and borderline intellectual functioning, rather marked physical changes sometimes occur, so that bright-looking children with autism may come out of puberty looking more 'dull'. Very occasionally this can be due to an underlying medical disorder such as tuberous sclerosis or neurofibromatosis which may produce skin problems and other physically visible changes only after infancy and childhood.

Epilepsy
Many youngsters with autism who have not been affected by seizures in childhood will develop epilepsy before adulthood. It seems that 30 to 40 per cent of all people with autism develop epilepsy before the age of 30 years (Rutter 1970, Gillberg and

63

Steffenburg 1987, Olsson *et al.* 1988). At least half of this group have seizure onset around the time of puberty. The risk of epilepsy is higher among people with autism and mental retardation, but the rate is also high in those of normal intelligence (Gillberg *et al.* 1987, Olsson *et al.* 1988).

There has been much controversy as to whether to include children with obvious brain dysfunction in the category of infantile autism. Although the view has become less common during the last decade, some would still argue for the exclusion of those with major neurological impairment. The onset of epilepsy in adolescents with autism who previously demonstrated no signs of neurological dysfunction (and even in children without previous EEG abnormalities) demonstrates the impossibility of such a position. At present, there is still no way of predicting in early childhood (the time when autism is most often diagnosed) just who will experience seizures later in life. However, girls seem to run a slightly higher risk than boys (Gillberg and Steffenburg 1987).

Deterioration
Brown (1969), Rutter (1970) and Gillberg and Schaumann (1981) have all described cases of autism with deterioration in adolescence. According to these studies, an estimated 10 to 30 per cent of children with autism can be expected to show cognitive and behavioural deterioration in puberty, accompanied by regression and a reappearance of many of the symptoms typical of the preschool period (Gillberg 1984*b*).

In the recent follow-up study by Gillberg and Steffenburg (1987), 22 per cent of the whole group showed deterioration (12 per cent of the male and 50 per cent of the female group). In the series of 'infantile psychosis' followed by Brown (1969), 34 per cent of those for whom adequate information was available did less well during puberty than during the early school years and 6 per cent became so disturbed that they required admission to hospital. In the Rutter (1970) study, 12 per cent of the subjects with 'childhood psychosis' deteriorated progressively during adolescence. Several of these simultaneously developed neurological signs and symptoms such as seizures and paralysis of the legs. The development of seizures was also commonly encountered in the Gillberg and Steffenburg (1987) study. However, seizures usually occurred only after a year or two of obvious behavioural deterioration. In the latter study there was also a marked tendency for periodicity in the gradual downhill development. Unfortunately, so far, prospective neurobiological studies of deteriorating autism cases have not been reported. Gillberg and Schaumann (1981) and Gillberg and Steffenburg (1987) have suggested that high maternal age, female sex and a family history of affective disorders might increase the risk of deterioration in puberty in autism.

Aggravation of symptoms not followed by deterioration
At the onset of puberty—or a year before or after—there is often a dramatic aggravation of symptoms such as self-destructiveness, aggressiveness, restlessness

and hyperactivity. In the Göteborg studies, such aggravation has been observed in about half of all subjects with autism or autistic-like conditions. 40 to 50 per cent of those who show aggravation appear to go on to develop frank deterioration (see above), but the remainder, after a few years, begin to improve again. Again there is a marked tendency for periodicity in some cases, with a return to 'normal' for at least weeks or months and then new periods of exacerbation of negative behavioural symptoms. This seems to be particularly common if there is a family history of affective disorder. There is now accumulating evidence that autism may be associated with a family history of affective disorder (Tsai *et al.* 1981, Gillberg 1984*b*, DeLong and Dwyer 1988).

The pubertal symptom aggravation, whether accompanied by deterioration or not, very often prompts some kind of medication (usually prescribed by adult psychiatrists who may know little about autism). In one study, before puberty less than a quarter of children with autism had a medication affecting the nervous system, whereas at age 16 to 23 years, three out of four were given such treatment (Gillberg and Steffenburg 1987).

While most medications prescribed in the pubertal period appear to do little to alter the negative course, our clinical impression has been that lithium can sometimes be effective in controlling pubertal behavioural/'mood' swings in autism (Gillberg 1989, see also Campbell 1989).

It is important to point out that some of the 'pubertal symptom aggravation' may also be the effect of (a) the sheer physical growth and strength of the person with autism, and hence (b) the gradual realization on the part of teachers and parents that some of the behaviours and problems shown by the child with autism will probably continue into adult life and will stand out as even more deviant by virtue of their more abnormal status in an adolescent/adult as compared with a child (*e.g.* problems associated with bladder or bowel function).

Problems associated with sexual maturation
For most individuals with autism puberty is not associated with serious problems connected with sexual maturation. Many parents of girls with autism worry about what might happen in connection with the onset of menstruation. Often these changes are accepted by the child in a very matter of fact way (Wing 1980).

The growth of sexual drive, as a rule, is not accompanied by a corresponding growth in the field of social 'know-how', and this often leads to embarrassing behaviour. This appears to be particularly true of moderately and severely retarded boys with autism, who may expose themselves, masturbate in public and touch other people's genital regions (Gillberg 1984*b*). Such behaviour can, of course, be very embarrassing to those confronted, including parents and siblings. Often, the sexual behaviour is 'interpreted', in more or less sophisticated terms, by 'experts' of various professions. However, one of the most simple explanations is that the young boy with autism is simply doing one of the pleasurable things in life that he knows how to. In autism the behavioural repertoire is very limited (this, indeed, is a diagnostic criterion in the DSM-III-R), and in some cases masturbation may be one of the few activities the person with autism knows how to perform. The social and planning deficits associated with autism preclude the spontaneous 'arrangement' of such activities in ways which will be socially acceptable to other people. It is usually easy to diminish the extent to which the person with autism masturbates by introducing other interesting activities as a substitute. Nevertheless, masturbation activities may occasionally be very difficult to cope with, such as when bottles or other such objects are inserted into the anus, or when the activity becomes 'fixed' in relation to one particular person.

Some people with autism may be involved in unsolicited homo- or heterosexual contacts (Haracopos 1988) for the simple reason that they may be lacking in reticence and suspiciousness to such an extent that they may be taken advantage of sexually.

Problems associated with sexual maturation need to be handled with consistency, common sense and not too much emotion. Medication is usually not indicated.

Inactivity/inertia
The marked overactivity seen in many young children with autism is very often followed by a state of 'underactivity' in adolescence. There may sometimes be an extreme degree of 'psychomotor retardation' and a total or almost total lack of initiative and yet no clear indications of depressive feelings (Rutter 1970).

Depressed mood and depression
Feelings of unhappiness and/or depression are often reported (Wing and Wing 1980, Newson et al. 1982) and may be particularly likely to occur in high-functioning autism or Asperger syndrome (Wing 1981, Tantam 1988). These better-functioning individuals may become painfully aware that they are different from other adolescents. A few develop a strong desire for friendship, but may be totally unable to establish social relationships because they lack the necessary skills.

In families with affective disorder, there is sometimes a typical episode of major depression associated with autism. This might represent a more primary depressive disorder.

Social skills groups, role-playing and videotape feedback followed by systematic training may sometimes be useful when trying to teach youngsters with autism the requirements of social interaction and conversation. Such measures may help alleviate depressive feelings. Occasionally, individual supportive psychotherapy may also be indicated. Medication is rarely used, but tricyclic antidepressants can sometimes help in reducing depressive symptoms in autism.

Adulthood
So far, only a few reports on adults with autism have been published (Kanner 1973; Gillberg 1983, 1992; Wing 1983, 1989b; Gillberg and Steffenburg 1987; Rumsey

and Hamburger 1988; Szatmari *et al.* 1989), but there is growing concern with the continuous psychosocial and psychiatric needs of adults who were diagnosed as suffering from autism in childhood (Schopler and Mesibov 1983).

The 'cures'
It has long been recognized that a small proportion of persons with autism develop into normal, or sometimes highly original though not psychiatrically ill, grown-ups. In most follow-up studies (reviewed in Gillberg 1992) they constitute no more than a few per cent of all persons with autism. They have usually shown positive development very early in childhood, but, occasionally, the amelioration may not come until the pubertal years. Cases such as these are often regarded as related to 'cures' of various kinds rather than as examples of different developmental pathways. However, there is not enough evidence to suggest that interventions in themselves can so dramatically alter the course of autism that it would be reasonable to speak of a cure.

If one concentrates on only the high-functioning individuals with autism—and perhaps particularly on those diagnosed as suffering from Asperger syndrome —then the proportion of cases with a very good outcome increases. Quite a number of such patients actually have a fair prognosis and may be able to hold on to qualified jobs, live independent lives and even marry and raise children (Szatmari *et al.* 1989). Nevertheless, a number of individuals in this group have major psychiatric problems, which are briefly discussed below.

Wing's three broad groups of adults with autism
Wing (1983) outlined three major groups of adults previously diagnosed with childhood autism: (1) the 'aloof' group, (2) the 'passive' group and (3) the 'active but odd' group. Empirical support for this subgrouping has also been provided by studies in Göteborg (Gillberg and Steffenburg 1987).

The 'aloof' group comprises those individuals who retain much or some of the characteristics of autistic aloneness. They will still prefer to be alone and even to withdraw actively from the nearness of other human beings. It may not be as obviously apparent in adult age, but the aloofness shows in the company of others in that individuals with autism do not readily react to other people's questions or approaches. They may quietly withdraw to the seclusion of their own room, where they may play records or just sit and rock incessantly to and fro. If disturbed, they may forcefully push the intruder out of the room, after first having appeared oblivious to the other person's presence for several minutes. Adults in this group cause problems mostly when demands are made. They may be quite easy to 'handle' if they are left completely to themselves. On the other hand, leaving them alone quickly leads to the deterioration of both acquired and self-help skills.

The 'passive' group may also, at a glance, appear aloof. However, approaches by both strangers and well-known people are accepted in a quite friendly manner. They may have 'automatic' imitation skills enabling them to participate in some social activities without appearing extremely odd, so long as reciprocal social interaction is not demanded. As a group, the passive people with autism are those who have the most skills and are most likely to be able to lead relatively independent lives. Changes of routine, at least if introduced in abrupt ways, may be very upsetting to this group, as well as to the aloof and active groups. Because of the overall friendly attitude of the passive people with autism, disturbed behaviour in connection with change may be especially alarming. Unless those living with or caring for these individuals are well informed, tragic mistakes may be made, such as expulsion from a secure group or admission for psychiatric treatment in an emergency ward.

The 'active but odd' group is by far the most difficult. On the surface, adults in this group appear to be totally unlike those in the other two groups, but there is the same lack of reciprocity in all three. The active group tends to approach other people with physical touching if mute, or constant repetitive questioning if speaking. The endless monologues or questioning may seem rather harmless, but anyone who has been confronted with it for any length of time, and learned that answering leads to even further repetitions of the same questions, knows how wearing and frustrating this behaviour is.

Within these three groups there is, of course, very considerable variation. Some persons may show characteristics of more than one 'type', and personality differences naturally play an essential role in all cases.

Periodicity in autism

There are several clinical accounts (Coleman 1976, Wing 1983, Gillberg 1984*a*) and a few systematic studies (*e.g.* Gillberg and Steffenburg 1987) acknowledging a periodic intensification of symptoms in the autistic syndromes. This periodicity may be particularly prominent in puberty (Komoto *et al.* 1984). However, after thorough interviewing of the parents it is often evident that it has been present from the onset in infancy or early childhood. Several authors (see above) have suggested that affective illness might be more common in the families of children with autism than in families of normal children. There is direct or indirect evidence that this might be the case from several different sources (Lotter 1967, Rutter *et al.* 1971, Folstein and Rutter 1977, DeLong and Dwyer 1988, Steffenburg 1991). Early authors generally tended to attribute conditions such as recurrent depression in the parents to reactions against the situation with the affected child. Later writers have considered genetic factors instead. It is likely that an hereditary trait of periodicity exists in some cases of autism in which parents and other relatives have shown major affective disorders.

Overall outcome

There have been a small number of follow-up studies reporting on the overall outcome for children diagnosed as suffering from autism, childhood psychosis or autistic-like conditions. Studies published up to the mid-1970s were closely examined by Lotter (1978). Only a handful of those studies—from the USA (Eisenberg 1956, DeMyer *et al.* 1973), and UK (Creak 1963, Rutter 1970, Lotter 1974)—have presented enough detail to allow conclusions. These studies all yielded remarkably similar results, in spite of the fact that only one (Lotter 1974) was population-based. In the 1980s only one more population-based follow-up study was published (Gillberg and Steffenburg 1987), and this showed results which were consistent with those from the previous studies. In all the studies published, a poor or very poor outcome with regard to social adjustment (characterized by limited independence in social relations) was seen in 61 to 73 per cent of cases followed up to pre-adolescence or early adult life. A good outcome (with near normal or normal social life and acceptable functioning at work or school in spite of certain difficulties in social relationships and oddities in behaviour) was seen in 5 to 17 per cent of cases. In the studies mentioned, 39 to 54 per cent of subjects had been placed in institututions at follow-up.

According to a recent review of the outcome literature in autism, mortality in the age group 2 to 30 years is slightly, but significantly, increased (Gillberg 1992). Even though it is hard to compare mortality rates across Western countries, it appears that mortality in this age group might be increased from about 0.6 per cent in the general population to almost 2 per cent in autism. The higher mortality rate in autism could be accounted for by the association of autism with certain severe medical conditions, such as tuberous sclerosis.

A few (clinic-based) studies on high-functioning people with autism (Rumsey and Hamburger 1988, Szatmari *et al.* 1989) suggest that their outcome may be considerably better, yet severely restricted as compared with people without autism.

All the follow-up studies mentioned above, as well as another from the USA (Goldfarb 1970), agree that the absence of communicative speech at age 5 to 6 years is indicative of a worse long-term overall outcome. However, the single best predictor of outcome is IQ ratings at the time of diagnosis in childhood (Rutter 1970, Gillberg and Steffenburg 1987). Educational functioning in childhood also has relatively good predictive power (DeMyer *et al.* 1973). Other prognostic variables include a lack of reaction to sound in infancy or early childhood (poor outcome), and milder forms of behaviour problems, more schooling and acquisition of specific skills (better outcome).

It might appear from the foregoing discussion that making a reliable prognosis on the basis of diagnostic data obtained at about the age of 5 to 6 years would be fairly easy. However, there are several problems.

Difficulties associated with IQ testing are very common. In the preschool years it may be difficult to test a child with autism at all. Pretest knowledge of the child and special testing skills or experience with autism on the part of the psychologist reduce the problems of testing to a minimum. Freeman (1976) has argued that it is usually possible to accomplish reliable testing of a preschool child with autism. Also, DeMeyer *et al.* (1973) showed that a simple index of educational attainments was a stable predictor of educational outcome. Such measures (*e.g.* the currently widely used Psychoeducational Profile or PEP—Mesibov *et al.* 1980) plus a Vineland interview (Doll 1965) could be added to the test battery in order to strengthen the predictive validity of the IQ factor. Further, it seems that IQ is predictive of overall long-term outcome only for those with ratings <50. Almost all of those who have an IQ <50 before age 5 to 6 years are likely to have a poor, or very poor, prognosis. For those with higher IQ it is much more difficult to make a reliable prediction of outcome. On the whole, though, IQ remains as stable throughout childhood for children with autism as for normal or mentally retarded children (Rutter 1983).

Speech as a prognostic indicator is useful for group effects but not always for individual children. Even in those who show no intelligible speech at 5 years (about half the group with classical autism) there may later be major speech development and a fair overall outcome. Occasionally one comes across a child who unexpectedly starts to talk or communicate at age 10 or even later. One person with a typical history of autism and medical record data to substantiate the diagnosis said nothing for 27 years and then started to write long communicative sentences using a pocket-size typewriter (Sanua 1981).

A considerable minority of children who show deterioration in puberty constitute another problem. As yet we have no way of knowing in advance who they are. It is possible that high maternal age, female sex and a family history of affective disorder might all point in the direction of pubertal aggravation of symptoms and possibly deterioration, but, so far, nothing definite is known in this respect.

On the bright side is the as yet unexplained tendency for a small minority of children with autism to develop in a very hopeful manner, with or without treatment.

Summary
For the most part, we must retain a cautious attitude when discussing outcome in autism with the parents. The majority of children with autism will show deviances and psychiatric impairments throughout life, but others will improve enough to make it possible to lead an (almost) independent adult life. The problem in the individual child is that there is no sure way of knowing to which of these two groups the child will later belong.

In the future it will become increasingly more common to make a prognosis according to the known associated medical diagnosis. It is already clear that outcome in autism with tuberous sclerosis is different from that of autism associated with the fragile X syndrome (Gillberg 1992). A comprehensive state-of-the-art medical work-up will contribute to the refinement of appropriate diagnosis and prognosis in autism.

REFERENCES

Baird, G., Baron-Cohen, S., Bohman, M., Coleman, M., Frith, U., Gillberg, C., Gillberg, C., Howlin, P., Mesibov, G., Peeters, T., *et al.* (1991) 'Autism is not necessarily a pervasive developmental disorder.' *Developmental Medicine and Child Neurology*, **33**, 363–364. *(Letter.)*

Brown, J. (1969) 'Adolescent development of children with infantile psychosis.' *Seminars in Psychiatry*, **1**, 79–89.

Bågenholm, A., Gillberg, C. (1991) 'Psychosocial effects on siblings of children with autism or mental retardation: a population-based study.' *Journal of Mental Deficiency Research*, **35**, 291–307.

Campbell, M. (1989) 'Pharmacotherapy in autism: an overview.' *In:* Gillberg, C. (Ed.) *The Diagnosis and Treatment of Autism.* New York: Plenum, pp. 203–217.

Chess, S. (1977) 'Follow-up report on autism in congenital rubella.' *Journal of Autism and Childhood Schizophrenia*, **7**, 68–81.

Coleman, M. (Ed.) (1976) *The Autistic Syndromes.* Amsterdam: North Holland; New York: Elsevier.

Creak, E.M. (1963) 'Childhood psychosis: a review of 100 cases.' *British Journal of Psychiatry*, **109**, 84–89.

Dahlgren, S.O., Gillberg, C. (1989) 'Symptoms in the first two years of life. A preliminary population study of infantile autism.' *European Archives of Psychiatry and Neurological Sciences*, **238**, 169–174.

DeLong, G.R., Dwyer, J.T. (1988) 'Correlation of family history with specific autistic subgroups; Asperger's syndrome and bipolar affective disease.' *Journal of Autism and Developmental Disorders*, **18**, 593–600.

—— Bean, S.C., Brown, F.R. (1981) 'Acquired reversible autistic syndrome in acute encephalopathic illness in children.' *Archives of Neurology*, **38**, 191–194.

DeMyer, M.K., Barton, S., DeMyer, W.E., Norton, J.A., Allen, J., Steele, R. (1973) 'Prognosis in autism: a follow-up study.' *Journal of Autism and Childhood Schizophrenia*, **3**, 199–246.

Doll, E. (1965) *Vineland Social Maturity Scale. Revised Edition.* Minnesota: American Guidance Service.

Eisenberg, L. (1956) 'The autistic child in adolescence.' *American Journal of Psychiatry*, **112**, 607–612.

Folstein, S., Rutter, M. (1977) 'Infantile autism: a genetic study of 21 twin pairs.' *Journal of Child Psychology and Psychiatry*, **18**, 297–321.

Freeman, B.J. (1976) 'Evaluating autistic children.' *Journal of Pediatric Psychology*, **1**, 18–21.

Frith, U. (1989) *Autism: Explaining the Enigma.* Oxford: Basil Blackwell.

—— (1991) *Autism and Asperger Syndrome.* Cambridge: Cambridge University Press.

Gillberg, C. (1983) 'Psychotic behaviour in children and young adults in a mental handicap hostel.' *Acta Psychiatrica Scandinavica*, **68**, 351–358.

—— (1984*a*) 'Infantile autism and other childhood psychoses in a Swedish urban region. Epidemiological aspects.' *Journal of Child Psychology and Psychiatry*, **25**, 35–43.

—— (1984*b*) 'Autistic children growing up: problems during puberty and adolescence.' *Developmental Medicine and Child Neurology*, **26**, 125–129.

—— (1986) 'Onset at age 14 of a typical autistic syndrome. A case report of a girl with herpes simplex encephalitis.' *Journal of Autism and Developmental Disorders*, **16**, 369–375.

—— (1989) 'The first evulation: treatment begins here.' *In:* Gillberg, C. (Ed.) *Diagnosis and Treatment ofafl3 Autism.* New York: Plenum, pp. 139–149.

—— (1990) 'Autism and pervasive developmental disorders.' *Journal of Child Psychology and Psychiatry*, **31**, 99–119. *(Annotation.)*

—— (1992) 'The Emanuel Miller Lecture 1991: Autism and autistic-like conditions—subgroups of disorders of empathy.' *Journal of Child Psychology and Psychiatry*, **33**, 813–842.

—— Schaumann, H. (1981) 'Infantile autism and puberty.' *Journal of Autism and Developmental Disorders*, **11**, 365–371.

—— Steffenberg, S. (1987) 'Outcome and prognostic factors in infantile autism and similar conditions: a population-based study of 46 cases followed through puberty.' *Journal of Autism and Developmental Disorders*, **17**, 273–287.

—— —— Jakobsson, G. (1987) 'Neurobiological findings in 20 relatively gifted children with Kanner-type autism or Asperger syndrome.' *Developmental Medicine and Child Neurology*, **29**, 641–649.

—— Ehlers, S., Schaumann, H., Jakobsson, G., Dahlgren, S.O., Lindblom, R., Bågenholm, A.,

Tjuust, T., Blidner, E. (1990) 'Autism under age 3 years: a clinical study of 28 cases referred for autistic symptoms in infancy.' *Journal of Child Psychology and Psychiatry*, **31**, 921–934.

Gillberg, I.C. (1991) 'Autistic syndrome with onset at age 31 years: herpes encephalitis as a possible model for childhood autism.' *Developmental Medicine and Child Neurology*, **33**, 920–924.

Goldfarb, W.A. (1970) 'A follow-up investigation of schizophrenic children treated in residence.' *Psychosocial Process*, **1**, 9–64.

Haracopos, D. (1988) *What About Me? Autistic Children and Adults.* Copenhagen: Andonia.

Kanner, L. (1971) 'Follow-up study of eleven children originally reported in 1943.' *Journal of Autism and Childhood Schizophrenia*, **1**, 119–145.

—— (1973) *Childhood Psychosis. Initial Studies and New Insights.* Washington, DC: V.H. Winston.

Komoto, J., Usui, S., Hirata, J. (1984) 'Infantile autism and affective disorders.' *Journal of Autism and Developmental Disorders*, **14**, 81–84.

Lotter, V. (1967) 'Epidemiology of autistic conditions in young children. II. Some characteristics of the parents and children.' *Social Psychiatry*, **1**, 163–173.

—— (1974) 'Factors related to outcome in autistic children.' *Journal of Autism and Childhood Schizophrenia*, **4**, 263–277.

—— (1978) 'Follow-up studies.' *In:* Rutter, M., Schopler, E. (Eds) *Autism: A Reappraisal of Concepts and Treatment.* New York: Plenum, pp. 475–495.

Mesibov, G.B., Schopler, E., Schaffer, B., Landrus, R. (1980) *Individualized Assessment and Treatment for Autistic and Developmentally Disabled Children. Adolescent and Adult Psychoeducational Profile (AAPEP).* Austin, TX: Pro-Ed.

Newson, E., Dawson, M., Everard, P. (1982) *The Natural History of Able Autistic People: the Management and Functioning in a Social Context. (Summary of Report to DHSS.)*

Olsson, I., Steffenburg, S., Gillberg, C. (1988) 'Epilepsy in autism and autistic-like conditions: a population-based study.' *Archives of Neurology*, **45**, 666–668.

Ornitz, E.M. (1983) 'The functional neuroanatomy of infantile autism.' *International Journal of Neuroscience*, **19**, 358–366.

Rumsey, J.M., Hamburger, S.D. (1988) 'Neuropsychological findings in high-functioning men with infantile autism, residual state.' *Journal of Clinical and Experimental Neuropsychology*, **10**, 201–221.

Rutter, M. (1970) 'Autistic children. Infancy to adulthood.' *Seminars in Psychiatry*, **2**, 435–450.

—— (1978) 'Diagnosis and definition.' *In:* Rutter, M., Schopler, E. (Eds) *Autism: A Reappraisal of Concepts and Treatment.* New York: Plenum, pp. 1–25..

—— (1983) 'Cognitive deficits in the pathogenesis of autism.' *Journal of Child Psychology and Psychiatry*, **24**, 513–531.

—— Bartak, L., Newman, S. (1971) 'Autism—a central disorder of cognition and language?' *In:* Rutter, M. (Ed.) *Infantile Autism: Concepts, Characteristics and Treatment.* London: Churchill Livingstone, pp. 148–171.

Sanua, V.D. (1981) 'Cultural changes and psychopathology in children: with special reference to infantile autism.' *Acta Paedopsychiatrica*, **47**, 133–142.

Schopler, E., Mesibov, G.B. (1983) *Autism in Adolescents and Adults.* New York: Plenum.

Steffenburg, S. (1991) 'Neuropsychiatric assessment of children with autism: a population-based study.' *Developmental Medicine and Child Neurology*, **33**, 495-511.

Szatmari, P., Bartolucci, G., Bremner, R., Bond, S., Rich, S. (1989) 'A follow-up study of high-functioning autistic children.' *Journal of Autism and Developmental Disorders*, **19**, 213–225.

Tantam, D. (1988) 'Asperger's syndrome.' *Journal of Child Psychology and Psychiatry*, **29**, 245–255. *(Annotation.)*

Tsai, L., Stewart, M.A., August, G. (1981) 'Implication of sex differences in the familial transmission of infantile autism.' *Journal of Autism and Developmental Disorders*, **11**, 165–173.

Volkmar, F.R., Cohen, D.J. (1989) 'Disintegrative disorder or "late onset" autism.' *Journal of Child Psychology and Psychiatry*, **30**, 717–724.

Waterhouse, L., Fein, D., Nath, J., Snyder, D. (1984) *Pervasive Schizophrenia Occurring in Childhood: A Review of Critical Commentary.* Washington, DC: American Psychiatric Association.

Wing, J.K., Wing, L. (1980) 'Provision of services.' *In:* Wing, L. (Ed.) *Early Childhood Autism. 2nd Edn.* Oxford: Pergamon.

Wing, L. (1980) *Early Childhood Autism. 2nd Edn.* Oxford: Pergamon.

72

—— (1981) 'Asperger's syndrome: a clinical account.' *Psychological Medicine*, **11**, 115–129.

—— (1983) 'Social and interpersonal needs.' *In:* Schopler, E., Mesibov, G.B. (Eds) *Autism in Adolescents and Adults.* New York: Plenum, pp. 337–354.

—— (1989*a*) 'The diagnosis of autism.' *In:* Gillberg, C. (Ed.) *Diagnosis and Treatment of Autism.* New York: Plenum, pp. 5–22.

—— (1989*b*) 'Autistic adults.' *In:* Gillberg, C. (Ed.) *Diagnosis and Treatment of Autism.* New York: Plenum, pp. 419–432.

6
EPILEPSY

Autism and autistic-like conditions are associated with epilepsy (Schain and Yannet 1960, Lotter 1967, Rutter 1970, Kanner 1971, Ornitz 1973, Deykin and MacMahon 1979, Fish and Ritvo 1979, Wing 1980, Shirataki *et al.* 1982, Bohman *et al.* 1983, Gillberg 1984*a,b*, Gillberg and Steffenburg 1987, Olsson *et al.* 1988, Ritvo *et al.* 1990, Volkmar and Nelson 1990).

Epilepsy in classical forms of autism is reported in between 1:7 and 1:3 children, the frequency rising in accordance with the length of the follow-up period. Epilepsy in autistic-like conditions may be even more common, possibly affecting 35 to 45 per cent of cases (Gillberg and Steffenburg 1987, Olsson *et al.* 1988). In his first report, Kanner (1943) stated that one of the 11 children diagnosed by him as suffering from autistic disturbances of affective contact was affected by epilepsy, whereas at follow-up in adult life (Kanner 1971) two were said to suffer from epilepsy. Similarly, Rutter (1970), Lotter (1974), Deykin and MacMahon (1979), Corbett (1982) and Gillberg and Steffenburg (1987) have all found an increase in the rate of epilepsy with increasing age.

The rise in frequency appears to be particularly pronounced around the time of puberty (Rutter 1970, Gillberg and Steffenburg 1987). However, epilepsy is also relatively common in prepubertal children with infantile autism. Two recent studies, one population survey (Olsson *et al.* 1988) and the other clinic-based (Volkmar and Nelson 1990), suggested that about half of those children with autism who also develop epilepsy do so in the first few years of life. Another recent study (Ritvo *et al.* 1990) found that the onset of epilepsy in autism was very often in the first three years of life. These studies cast some doubt on the notion of a specific link between autism and adolescent onset epilepsy. Also, it remains to be settled whether the rate of epilepsy continues to rise, albeit at a very slow rate, throughout the entire life span. An interesting finding of these recent studies has been the association of autism with epilepsy even in the absence of mental retardation.

The rate of 14 to 42 per cent (mostly 25 to 35 per cent) for epilepsy among adults who were diagnosed in childhood as suffering from autism (all intellectual abilities counted) should be compared with 0.5 per cent among the general population (Corbett 1983), 3 to 12 per cent among mildly mentally retarded subjects (Rutter *et al.* 1970, Hagberg and Kyllerman 1983) and 18 to 32 per cent among the severely mentally retarded (Corbett 1983). It should also be noted that the prevalence rate for epilepsy in severe mental retardation includes a fraction with autism and autistic-like conditions. Thus, the incidence is decidedly higher than among the normal population and may even be higher than among indiscriminate groups of people with mental retardation. The frequency of epilepsy in autism (regardless of IQ level) is almost definitely considerably higher than in 'non-autistic' severe mental retardation (Gillberg *et al.* 1986).

Epilepsy is more common among the more severely mentally retarded subjects with autism (Rutter 1970, Corbett 1983, Olsson *et al.* 1988), but it is not uncommon in mildly mentally retarded youngsters with autism and occurs relatively often in high-functioning cases also (Gillberg *et al.* 1987, Ritvo *et al.* 1990).

We may sum up some of the existing evidence by saying that (1) the association between autism and epilepsy is indisputable and suggests brain dysfunction in many cases of autism; (2) there is possibly a relatively steep rise in the frequency of epilepsy around the time of puberty (possibly, but not conclusively, steeper than in non-autism mental retardation), suggesting hormonal influences on the development of epilepsy or the provocation of seizures in a brain which can no longer keep pace with accelerating demands for development around the time of puberty; and (3) it appears that the connection between autism and epilepsy might be rather specific, and not only mediated via the common denominator of mental retardation.

The third of these statements is slightly speculative at present, but is supported by both the higher rate of epilepsy among children with autism than among those with non-autism mental retardation (at least if groups of children with autism are matched for IQ on a pair-wise basis with a non-autism comparison group) and its possibly more specific appearance in association with puberty.

It should be mentioned here that many children with autism showing no gross signs of neurological damage (apart from mental retardation and autism) in infancy and early childhood unexpectedly develop epilepsy around the time of puberty.

The interpretation of EEGs, particularly regarding slowing and background abnormalities, remains controversial. As reviewed by Tsai *et al.* (1985), the majority of children with autism in the literature have shown EEG abnormalities whether they had seizures or not. In this overview, focal location was most often in the temporal lobe. Dorenbaum *et al.* (1987) found no correlation between EEG findings and speech performance.

Type of epilepsy
Given the ample evidence that autism and autistic-like conditions are associated with epilepsy, it is surprising that so little descriptive literature discusses the type or severity of this associated condition. At the time of a survey of the area by Corbett (1982), no study was available detailing the subcategories of epilepsy in autism: the first such (population-based) study was published in the late 1980s (Olsson *et al.* 1988).

Infantile spasms
There is evidence that children with infantile spasms have an increased risk compared with otherwise normal children of developing autism or autistic-like

behaviour (Knobloch *et al.* 1956, Schain and Yannet 1960, Kolvin *et al.* 1971, Taft and Cohen 1971, Riikonen and Amnell 1981, Corbett 1982). This increase is not produced merely by way of mental retardation, as is evidenced by the higher rate of autism in infantile spasms (16 per cent according to the Riikonen and Amnell study) than in mental retardation (4 to 6 per cent of cases with severe mental retardation appear to have classical autism according to Gillberg 1984*a*, Gillberg *et al.* 1986), and underlined further by the fact that a small proportion of children with infantile spasms do not become mentally retarded. However, infantile spasms are also associated with tuberous sclerosis (Riikonen and Simell 1990), which, in turn, is also associated with autism (Hunt and Dennis 1987). The nature of this trifold connection is poorly understood, but it is reasonable to assume that tuberous sclerosis (whether clinically diagnosed or not) may underlie both infantile spasms and autism in these cases. It has still not been settled what proportion of children with the combination of autism and infantile spasms have tuberous sclerosis.

Complex partial seizures (psychomotor/temporal lobe epilepsy)
Corbett (1982) was possibly the first author to suggest that complex partial seizures (psychomotor epilepsy with temporal lobe affliction) might be under-reported in autism because of diagnostic difficulties arising when such seizures affect non-communicative children. This was confirmed in a population study of epilepsy in prepubertal children with autism and autistic-like conditions (Olsson *et al.* 1988) in which complex partial seizures were reported in 71 per cent of those who had had onset of seizures in early childhood. Epilepsy occurred in 20 per cent of those with autism and in 41 per cent of those with an autistic-like condition. Generalized tonic–clonic seizures had also been very common, but epilepsy of this type usually occurred in conjunction with complex partial seizures or as 'sequelae' after infantile spasms. In a study of young people (aged 16 to 23 years) with autism and similar conditions, 35 per cent had epilepsy, and three quarters of these had pubertal onset (Gillberg and Steffenburg 1987). Of those with prepubertal onset, the majority had 'psychomotor epilepsy'. A case-report of a young girl with autistic behaviour and a complex seizure disorder with very uncharacteristic staring spells and temporal lobe discharge on the EEG (Gillberg and Schaumann 1983) demonstrates the difficulty of arriving at a correct diagnosis in the field. The girl's autistic behaviour and the staring spells promptly disappeared after treatment with valproic acid, and the EEG normalized almost completely.

In the Swedish studies, EEG abnormalities in cases with the combination of autism–epilepsy were most often generated from the temporal lobes and phylogenetically older parts of the brain. In cases with unilateral predominance of the abnormality, this was right-sided as often as left-sided.

The relationship between autistic-like problems and psychomotor epilepsy is further illustrated by the follow-up studies of Ounsted and associates in Oxford, England, who found 'temporal lobe epilepsy' to predispose to later 'psychosis' in boys with a left-sided EEG abnormality (Lindsay *et al.* 1979).

Myoclonic epilepsies of early childhood (minor motor seizures)

Excluding the infantile spasms category, myoclonic epilepsies of childhood (Lennox 1945, Gastaut *et al.* 1966) have not regularly been reported as common in infantile autism. However, some authors have described classic cases of autism in connection with minor motor epilepsy (Boyer *et al.* 1981, Gillberg *et al.* 1984), and it appears that in clinical practice with severely mentally retarded persons with autism, minor motor epilepsy is relatively common. Gillberg and associates (1984*b*) described a boy with autism and severe and frequent minor motor seizures who became seizure-free on medication with valproic acid, and thereafter quickly grew out of his most severe autistic and language disturbances.

In the two population-based studies from Göteborg detailing type of epilepsy (Gillberg and Steffenburg 1987, Olsson *et al.* 1988), minor motor seizures were fairly common, both in the group with classic autism and in that with autistic-like conditions. However, they usually occurred in cases showing a multitude of other kinds of seizures as well. The total pooled group of 90 cases with autism and autistic-like conditions from the two studies contained only one case (the boy reported in Gillberg *et al.* 1984) with minor motor seizures as the only type of epilepsy. A total of 30 of the 90 cases in this pooled group had developed epilepsy at the time of the study (subjects ranged from 2 to 23 years of age). Of these, eight (9 per cent) had myoclonic epilepsies of childhood other than infantile spasms. Four (4 per cent) had had infantile spasms.

Childhood absence epilepsy (petit mal)

Childhood absence epilepsy (petit mal), another form of subcortically generated epilepsy, has been reported to 'masquerade' as autism in an 8-year-old boy who had almost continuous bilateral synchronous 3Hz spike and wave activity on the EEG (Gillberg and Schaumann 1983). This boy improved dramatically—both psychiatrically and neurologically—with ethosuximide monotherapy. Except in the Ritvo *et al.* (1990) study, petit mal has not been mentioned frequently in the literature on autism. Nevertheless, of the substantial number of individuals with autism who show combinations of several different kinds of seizures several show 'atypical absences', even though these are not, on average, classified with any of the easily categorized seizure types. There are also children and adolescents who show staring spells which may be difficult to differentiate from 'autistic-type staring' without epileptogenic correlate.

Generalized tonic–clonic seizures (grand mal)

Generalized tonic–clonic seizures are the most frequent form of epilepsy in the general population. According to the study by Olsson *et al.* (1988), they are relatively common in children and adolescents with autism. However, in the general population, generalized tonic–clonic seizures often appear as the only type of epilepsy in the individual patient. In autism they are usually associated with other kinds of epilepsy. For instance, 'uncomplicated' grand mal epilepsy (*i.e.*

generalized tonic–clonic seizures not associated with other kinds of epilepsy) occurred in only three of the 30 cases with epilepsy in the pooled group from Olsson *et al.* (1988) and Gillberg and Steffenburg (1987), but 18 of the 30 showed generalized tonic–clonic seizures in association with other types of epilepsy. In these latter cases, individual seizures were often 'triggered' by complex partial seizures, which were then followed by secondary generalized tonic–clonic seizures.

Autism, epilepsy and other disorders

A number of disease entities that are found in patients with autistic syndromes predispose to seizures. Thus, if a child with autism develops seizures, these entities should be specifically sought if the child has not already had a firm diagnosis or, at least, an adequate work-up.

If an infant displays the infantile spasms syndrome there are a variety of possibilities to be considered (Jeavons and Bower 1964). Those also currently included in the autistic syndromes are tuberous sclerosis, neurofibromatosis, phenylketonuria and minor hydrocephalus.

In seizures appearing at a somewhat later age, the differential diagnosis changes. If the child is a girl, Rett syndrome should be considered: 70 to 80 per cent of this group develop epilepsy, and the median age of onset is 4 years (Hagberg *et al.* 1983). If the child is a boy, the possibility of the fragile X syndrome, which often coincides with autism and sometimes with epilepsy, should be considered. It has been suggested that brainstem dysfunction, muscular hypotonia, complex partial seizures and autism might be specifically associated with this chromosomal syndrome (Gillberg *et al.* 1986*b*). Purine disorders are associated with seizures in children (Coleman *et al.* 1974), therefore purine metabolism should be evaluated in children with autism who develop epilepsy. Therapies available for purine patients include a new class of anticonvulsants, specific to the purine disorder (Coleman *et al.* 1986, 1989).

Antiepileptic treatment in autism

There are no adequately controlled studies relevant to the topic of anticonvulsive pharmacological treatment either in autism or in epilepsy associated with autism. There is one systematic study of open drug trials in autism associated with epilepsy (Gillberg 1991). That study, and anecdotal clinical reports, suggest that some of the best antiepileptic drugs (phenytoin, phenobarbitone and, in particular, the benzo-diazepines) may be detrimental to the behavioural status of the child with autism and epilepsy. Instead, carbamazepine and valproic acid should often be considered drugs of first choice. These two drugs—with supposedly 'psychotropic' properties (Gualtieri *et al.* 1987)—might be of special benefit since behaviour is only rarely adversely affected.

Drug treatment aimed at alleviating a seizure disorder in autism should be tried only if the child has two or more major seizures a year, and even in such cases an individual decision has to be taken. Reduction of environmental stimuli may sometimes serve as an adjunct.

In the child with autism who has no clear-cut clinical signs of epilepsy, but has unclassifiable spells of absent-mindedness, 'rolling' of the eyes, etc., plus an EEG with epileptogenic discharge, we would suggest a three- to six-month trial with a suitable anticonvulsant drug.

If the child with autism and epilepsy is for some reason also in need of a neuroleptic drug, which seems often to be the case in puberty (Gillberg and Steffenburg 1987), pimozide, haloperidol and thioridazine appear to be the most useful, because of their relative lack of epileptogenic properties (see also Chapter 22).

It is again important to point out the occasional concurrence of purine disorders, autism and epilepsy, so that such abnormalities can be ruled out or identified and treated appropriately.

It is quite possible that research into the area of anticonvulsive treatment in autism might prove valuable. The possibility of a relatively strong correlation between autism and complex partial seizures makes systematic study of such drugs particularly warranted.

Antiepileptic surgery

People with 'hard-to-treat' seizures are now often worked up with a view to possible neurosurgery. Among the population with such therapy-resistant epilepsy, autistic symptoms are likely to be common, but there are no systematic data available so far, although one study of this connection is under way in Göteborg. Whether or not children with severe epilepsy and autism would derive beneficial effects on behaviour from neurosurgical treatment leading to control of seizures is an open question.

Summary

In conclusion, one can only be amazed that so little scientific progress has been made in the field of epilepsy in autism, especially since this association has been amply documented for the last 20 years or so. Autism *is* associated with epilepsy, and the nature of this association needs much more elucidation in the future.

REFERENCES

Bohman, M., Bohman, I.L., Björck, P.O., Sjöholm, E. (1983) 'Childhood psychosis in a northern Swedish county: some preliminary findings from an epidemiological survey.' *In:* Schmidt, M.H., Remschmidt, H. (Eds) *Epidemiological Approaches in Child Psychiatry, II.* Stuttgart: Thieme, pp. 164–173.
Boyer, J-P., Deschatrette, A., Delwarde, M. (1981) 'Autisme convulsif?' *Pédiatrie*, **5**, 353–368.
Coleman, M. (1989) 'Autism: non-drug biological treatments.' *In:* Gillberg, C. (Ed.) *Diagnosis and Treatment of Autism.* New York: Plenum, pp. 219–236.
—— Landgrebe, M., Landgrebe, A. (1974) 'Progressive seizures with hyperuricosuria reversed by allopurinol.' *Archives of Neurology*, **31**, 238–242.
—— —— —— (1986) 'Purine seizure disorders.' *Epilepsia*, **23**, 263–269.

Corbett, J. (1982) 'Epilepsy and the electroencephalogram in early childhood psychoses.' *In:* Wing, J.K., Wing, L. (Eds) *Handbook of Psychiatry, Vol. 3.* London: Cambridge University Press, pp. 198–202.

—— (1983) 'Epilepsy and mental retardation: a follow up study.' *In:* Parsonage, M. (Ed.) *Advances of Epileptology. XIVth Epilepsy International Symposium, August 1982.* New York: Raven Press, pp. 207–214.

Deykin, E.Y., MacMahon, G. (1979) 'Viral exposure and autism.' *American Journal of Epidemiology*, **109**, 628–638.

Dorenbaum, D., Mencel, E., Blume, W.T., Fisman, S. (1987) 'EEG findings and language patterns in autistic children: clinical correlations.' *Canadian Journal of Psychiatry*, **32**, 31–34.

Fish, B., Ritvo, E. (1979) 'Psychoses of childhood.' *In:* Noshpitz, V. (Ed.) *Basic Handbook of Child Psychiatry.* New York: Basic Books, pp. 249–303.

Gastaut, H., Roger, J., Soulayrol, R., Tassinari, C.A., Regis, H., Dravet, C., Bernard, R., Pinsard, N., Saint-Jean, M. (1966) 'Childhood epileptic encephalopathy with diffused slow spike-waves.' *Epilepsia*, **7**, 139–179.

Gillberg, C. (1984a) 'Autistic children growing up: problems during puberty and adolescence.' *Developmental Medicine and Child Neurology*, **26**, 125–129.

—— (1984b) 'Infantile autism and other childhood psychoses in a Swedish urban region. Epidemiological aspects.' *Journal of Child Psychology and Psychiatry*, **25**, 35–43.

—— (1991) 'The treatment of epilepsy in autism.' *Journal of Autism and Developmental Disorders*, **21**, 61–77.

—— Schaumann, H. (1983) 'Epilepsy presenting as infantile autism? Two case studies.' *Neuropediatrics*, **14**, 206–212.

—— Steffenburg, S. (1987) 'Outcome and prognostic factors in infantile autism and similar conditions: a population-based study of 46 cases followed through puberty.' *Journal of Autism and Developmental Disorders*, **17**, 273–287.

—— Winnergård, I., Wahlström, J. (1984) 'The sex chromosomes—one key to autism? An XXY case of infantile autism.' *Applied Research in Mental Retardation*, **5**, 353–360.

—— Persson, E., Grufman, M., Themnér, U. (1986a) 'Psychiatric disorders in mildly and severely mentally retarded urban children and adolescents: epidemiological aspects.' *British Journal of Psychiatry*, **149**, 68–74.

—— —— Wahlström, J. (1986b) 'The autism-fragile-X syndrome (AFRAX): a population-based study of ten boys.' *Journal of Mental Deficiency Research*, **30**, 27–39.

—— Steffenburg, S., Jakobsson, G. (1987) 'Neurobiological findings in 20 relatively gifted children with Kanner-type autism or Asperger syndrome.' *Developmental Medicine and Child Neurology*, **29**, 641–649.

Gualtieri, T., Evans, R.W., Patterson, D.R. (1987) 'The medical treatment of autistic people. Problems and side effects.' *In:* Schopler, E., Mesibov, G. (Eds) *Neurobiological Issues in Autism.* New York: Plenum, 374–388.

Hagberg, B., Kyllerman, M. (1983) 'Epidemiology of mental retardation—a Swedish survey.' *Brain and Development*, **5**, 441–449.

—— Aicardi, J., Dias, K., Ramos, O. (1983) 'A progressive syndrome of autism, dementia, ataxia and loss of purposeful hand use in girls: Rett syndrome: a report of 35 cases.' *Annals of Neurology*, **14**, 471–479.

Hunt, A., Dennis, J. (1987) 'Psychiatric disorder among children with tuberous sclerosis.' *Developmental Medicine and Child Neurology*, **29**, 190–198.

Jeavons, P.M., Bower, B.D. (1964) *Infantile Spasms. Clinics in Developmental Medicine No. 15.* London: The Spastics Society Medical Education and Information Unit with Heinemann Medical.

Kanner, L. (1943) 'Autistic disturbances of affective contact.' *Nervous Child*, **2**, 217–250.

—— (1971) 'Follow-up study of eleven children originally reported in 1943.' *Journal of Autism and Childhood Schizophrenia*, **1**, 119–145.

Knobloch, H., Rider, R., Harper, P., Pasamanick, B. (1956) 'Neuropsychiatric sequelae of prematurity.' *Journal of the American Medical Association*, **161**, 581–585.

Kolvin, I., Ounsted, C., Roth, M. (1971) 'Studies in the childhood psychoses. V: Cerebral dysfunction and childhood psychoses.' *British Journal of Psychiatry*, **118**, 407–414.

Lennox, W.G. (1945) 'The petit mal epilepsies: their treatment with tridione.' *Journal of the American*

Medical Association, **129**, 1069–1073.

Lindsay, J., Ounsted, C., Richards, P. (1979) 'Long-term outcome in children with temporal lobe seizures. III: Psychiatric aspects.' *Developmental Medicine and Child Neurology*, **21**, 630–636.

Lotter, V. (1967) 'Epidemiology of autistic conditions in young children. II: Some characteristics of the parents and children.' *Social Psychiatry*, **1**, 163–173.

—— (1974) 'Factors related to outcome in autistic children.' *Journal of Autism and Childhood Schizophrenia*, **4**, 263–277.

Olsson, I., Steffenburg, S., Gillberg, C. (1988) 'Epilepsy in autism and autistic-like conditions: a population-based study.' *Archives of Neurology*, **45**, 666–668.

Ornitz, E.M. (1973) 'Childhood autism: a review of the clinical and experimental literature.' *California Medicine*, **118**, 21–47.

Riikonen, R., Amnell, G. (1981) 'Psychiatric disorders in children with earlier infantile spasms.' *Developmental Medicine and Child Neurology*, **23**, 747–760.

—— Simell, O. (1990) 'Tuberous sclerosis and infantile spasms.' *Developmental Medicine and Child Neurology*, **32**, 203–209.

Ritvo, E.R., Freeman, B.J., Pingree, C., Mason-Brothers, A., Jorde, L.B., Jenson, W.R., McMahon, W.M., Petersen, P.B., Mo, A., Ritvo, A. (1990) 'The UCLA-University of Utah epidemiologic survey of autism: prevalence.' *American Journal of Psychiatry*, **146**, 194–199.

Rutter, M. (1970) 'Autistic children. Infancy to adulthood.' *Seminars in Psychiatry*, **2**, 435–450.

—— Graham, P., Yule, W. (1970) *A Neuropsychiatric Study in Childhood. Clinics in Developmental Medicine Nos 35/36.* London: Spastics International Medical Publications with Heinemann Medical; Philadelphia: J.B. Lippincott.

Schain, R., Yannet, H. (1960) 'Infantile autism: an analysis of 50 cases and a consideration of certain relevant neuropsychological concepts.' *Journal of Pediatrics*, **57**, 560–567.

Shirataki, S., Kuromaru, S., Hanada, M., Sugiura, Y., Yamada, T., Ushida, S., Shimada, S. (1982) 'Longterm follow-up of 13 autistic children.' *Paper presented at the International Conference on Child Psychiatry, Dublin, Ireland.*

Taft, L.T., Cohen, H.J. (1971) 'Hypsarrhythmia and childhood autism: a clinical report.' *Journal of Autism and Childhood Schizophrenia*, **1**, 327–336.

Tsai, L.Y., Tsai, M.C., August, G.J. (1985) 'Brief report: implication of EEG diagnoses in the subclassification of infantile autism.' *Journal of Autism and Developmental Disorders*, **15**, 339–344.

Volkmar, F.R., Nelson, D.S. (1990) 'Seizure disorders in autism.' *Journal of the American Academy of Child and Adolescent Psychiatry*, **29**, 127–129.

Wing, L. (1980) *Early Childhood Autism.* Oxford: Pergamon.

PART II

REVIEW OF THE GENERAL LITERATURE

7
PREVALENCE OF AUTISM AND
AUTISTIC-LIKE CONDITIONS

Prevalence rates from the major epidemiological studies of autism and autistic-like conditions are listed in Table 7.1. The first population-based study was conducted by Victor Lotter (1966, 1967), who found 'nuclear' autism (corresponding to the clinical syndrome described by Kanner) in 2.0 per 10,000 children in the county of Middlesex, England (a total of 15 cases). 'Non-nuclear' autism (closely resembling classic Kanner cases but with a few atypical traits) was found in another 2.5 per 10,000 children. A third group, comprising 3.3 per 10,000, contained individuals with some but not all of the characteristics of autism. Thus, Lotter found 7.8 per 10,000 children in the 8- to 10-year age range (as at 1 January 1964) who suffered from autism or autistic-like conditions. 56 per cent of the children with nuclear and non-nuclear autism had tested performance IQ <50, and only 19 per cent had performance IQ ⩾70 (Wing 1980). Verbal IQs were not tested, implying that full-scale IQs would most likely have been even lower, as verbal capacity is particularly limited in most children with autism.

Lotter's study included a thorough search of all schools and other institutions known to care for 8- to 10-year-old children, and even now, 25 years later, his investigation is considered by many as 'standard'.

Prior to Lotter's study, Rutter (1966) had discovered 4.4 'psychotic' children per 10,000 in the 8- to 10-year-old population in Aberdeen, Scotland.

Lotter's finding of four to five clear cases of autism/childhood psychosis per 10,000 children was later confirmed by three different epidemiological studies: in Århus, Denmark (Brask 1970); London, England (Wing and Gould 1979); Göteborg, Sweden (Gillberg 1984); and the state of Utah, USA (Ritvo *et al.* 1989).

The National Institutes of Health Perinatal Collaborative Prospective Study (Torrey *et al.* 1975) also found the same frequency. Clinically based surveys (Treffert 1970, Steinhausen *et al.* 1986) yielded somewhat smaller numbers, but the figures are not widely discrepant.

However, there is now growing evidence that autism might be more common than previously believed (Gillberg *et al.* 1991a).

First, in a study of a handicapped population aged under 15 years, Wing and Gould (1979) found the 'triad of social, language and behavioural impairments' (see Chapter 2) in 21 per 10,000 children (including both nuclear and non-nuclear autism plus other 'triad' cases).

Second, Wing and Gould's findings were later confirmed in a study of all 13- to 17-year-old children with mental retardation in Göteborg (Gillberg *et al.* 1986). In

TABLE 7.1

Epidemiological studies of autism and autistic-like conditions. Prevalence (n per 10,000 age-specific) and boy:girl ratios (in brackets)

Study	Country	Nuclear autism[1]	Non-nuclear autism/autistic-like conditions/other childhood psychosis	Autism and autistic-like conditions combined	Asperger syndrome	Total triad
Lotter (1966)	England	2.0 (2.8:1)	2.5 (2.4:1)	4.5 (2.6:1)	—	7.8 (2.0:1)
Brask (1970)	Denmark	—	—	4.3 (1.4:1)	—	—
Wing et al. (1976); Wing and Gould (1979)	England	2.0 (6:1)	2.9 (10:0)	4.9 (16:1)	1.7[2] (3.8:1)[3]	21.2 (2.7:1)
Bohman et al. (1983)	Sweden	3.0	3.0	6.1 (1.6:1)	—	—
Gillberg (1983b)	Sweden	—	—	—	—	69 (7:1)
Gillberg (1984)	Sweden	2.0 (3.3:1)	1.9 (1.1:1)	4.0 (1.8:1)	0.4 (3:1)	—
Steffenburg and Gillberg (1986)	Sweden	4.7 (5.4:1)	2.8 (1.0:1)	7.5 (2.4:1)	1.9 (12:1)	—
Gillberg et al. (1986)	Sweden	—	—	—	—	19[4] (2.5:1)
Bryson et al. (1988)	Canada	—	—	10.1 (2.5:1)	—	—
Gillberg and Gillberg (1989)	Sweden	—	—	—	26[2] (3:0)	—
Tanoue et al. (1988)	Japan	—	—	13.8 (4.1:1)	—	—
Sugiyama and Abe (1989)	Japan	—	—	13.0	—	21.1
Cialdella and Mamelle (1989)	France	—	—	4.5 (2.3:1)	—	9.2 (2.1:1)
Gillberg et al. (1991a)	Sweden	8.4 (3.7:1)	3.2 (0.8:1)	11.6 (2.8:1)	—	—

[1]Social aloofness and elaborate routines, both to a marked extent.
[2]Minimum figure.
[3]Sex ratio computed on basis of clinic sample.
[4]Mental retardation screening population.

that study, 20 per 10,000 children had the combination of mental retardation and the triad (including nuclear and non-nuclear autism).

Third, in an epidemiological study of deficits in attention, motor control and perception (DAMP) in unselected 7-year-olds, Gillberg (1983a) found that 69 per 10,000 children were affected by 'psychotic behaviour'. This term is no longer used by the Swedish group, and 'autistic traits' is now preferred. All the children classified in this way have 'triad symptoms'. Also, on the basis of a number of epidemiological studies in Göteborg, Gillberg and Gillberg (1989) concluded that Asperger syndrome (closely related to 'high-functioning' autism) occurred at a minimum frequency of 26 per 10,000 children in the school-age period. A total population study of Asperger syndrome in Göteborg (Ehlers, personal communication) suggests that this syndrome affects at least 0.9 per cent of all school-age boys. The cases with Asperger syndrome also have triad symptoms.

Fourth, Bohman and his associates (Bohman *et al.* 1983) in the northern-most part of Sweden found 6.1 per 10,000 children with 'childhood psychosis'. Bohman's group now refer to the cases in this study as suffering from 'autistic disorder' (von Knorring 1991).

Fifth, there are several reports from Japan that 'infantile autism' occurs in 13 to 16 per 10,000 children (Ishii and Takahashi 1982, Tanoue *et al.* 1988, Sugiyama and Abe 1989).

Finally, quite a number of recent studies from Canada, France and Sweden (see Table 7.1) have yielded prevalence figures considerably higher than in the early studies.

What sense can one make of these partly conflicting findings? First of all, the possibility remains that different diagnostic criteria have been applied in the different studies. This issue has already been discussed in Chapter 2 and will not be elaborated upon here, except to say that the studies reporting lower figures are more likely to have focused on only the most 'Kanner-typical' and severely impaired cases of autism. The low-frequency studies reported above conform to acceptable epidemiological standards, and there is little reason to assume that any large percentage of 'classical' cases considered to suffer from autism and mild/moderate mental retardation (including a large proportion with IQs under, but close to, 50) would have been missed in the screening or diagnostic procedure. These are the typical 'Kanner autism' cases corresponding to Kanner's original description (Kanner 1943). It should be clear that the stereotype of Kanner autism may apply specifically only to the type of children Kanner described. Thus, very severely retarded and very bright children with 'autism' might well have slightly different phenotypes. Girls may have different autism phenotypes than boys. Constitutional personality differences not associated with autism may also influence the clinical picture (Gillberg 1992). In the Göteborg studies, in spite of an overall increase in the rate of autism (according to currently accepted definitions of autism), the prevalence of Kanner autism with IQ in the 50–70 range has not increased across three population studies performed in 1980 (Gillberg 1984), 1984 (Steffenburg and Gillberg 1986) and 1988 (Gillberg *et al.* 1991a). However, the frequency of severely mentally retarded and normally intelligent children with autism has increased. This is likely to be due to better detection of cases, rather than to an actual increase, considering the stable rate of cases with mild mental retardation (who, after many years of discussion about the 'Kanner stereotype', were easier to identify already in the first screening studies). In the severely retarded group there is also the possibility that because more children who have sustained severe brain damage now survive, the rate of severe autism with severe retardation might be on the increase. The possibility that a high prevalence of autism in children born to immigrant parents might have contributed to higher overall prevalence rates is discussed below.

Five Swedish epidemiological studies of 'autism/childhood psychosis' performed in the same era by authors who have discussed diagnostic criteria and case-finding methods in some detail are of particular interest in this context (Bohman *et al.* 1983, Gillberg 1984, Steffenburg and Gillberg 1986, Lögdahl 1989, Gillberg *et al.* 1991*a*). The study by Gillberg (1984) yielded an age-specific prevalence figure of 4.0 per 10,000 for autism and autistic-like conditions (with half being classic Kanner autism cases). Gillberg also reported four to five times as many children with mental retardation with similar, though not quite characteristic, autistic-type symptomatology (Gillberg *et al.* 1986). In the two later studies from Göteborg, the prevalence rose to 7.5 per 10,000 in 1984 and 11.6 per 10,000 in 1988 (see below). Bohman *et al.* (1983), on the other hand, reported an age-specific prevalence of 6.1 per 10,000 for autism and autistic-like conditions (collectively referred to as 'childhood psychosis' in the original studies, later termed 'autistic disorder') from a rural area in the northernmost part of Sweden at the time when Gillberg reported 4.0 per 10,000 in southwestern Sweden. According to a Scandinavian–Finnish study of twins with autism (Steffenburg *et al.* 1989) it appears that autism in twins is considerably more prevalent in northern Scandinavia and Finland (which are predominantly rural areas) than in the southern parts of these countries (which are more urban in character), suggesting that autism might be more common in rural than in urban areas. However, contradictory evidence in this respect is available in the Gillberg *et al.* (1991*a*) study, in which the prevalence of autism and autistic-like conditions was 11.6 per 10,000 in the urban region, but only 7.2 per 10,000 in the rural area. Some of the difference between urban and rural areas in the latter study could have been accounted for by more comprehensive screening coverage in the urban area, but it does seem unlikely that the true prevalence in the rural county of Bohuslän would be higher than in the city of Göteborg. One possible interpretation is that in spite of general agreement that autism is a relatively rare disorder, prevalence may in fact vary quite considerably from one region to another. This would seem to be reasonable considering the multiple aetiologies including a number of specific medical conditions which may well vary in frequency in different areas. Thus, the difference in prevalence between various parts of Sweden may not be so much associated with rural–urban distinctions but with other regional characteristics (*e.g.* certain hereditary conditions or genetic factors operating in some regions and not in others). The Lögdahl (1989) study reported a prevalence of 9.0 per 10,000 children who suffered from 'childhood psychosis', using a definition which corresponds to autism and autistic-like conditions in other studies. Her study was based in central Sweden with a mixture of rural and urban areas.

The study by Wing and Gould (1979), reporting 21 per 10,000 children with the triad of social, language and behavioural impairments (see above), is one of the best epidemiological studies in the field of childhood autism so far. These authors used clearly defined criteria, and the prevalence of nuclear autism cases corresponds with that of most other studies. Other authors have highlighted the similarities between autism and other kinds of disturbances of social relatedness in mental retardation (*e.g.* Corbett 1983), but this London study and the study from Göteborg (Gillberg *et al.* 1986) are the only surveys so far (possibly excepting the Danish study from institutions for the mentally retarded by Kelstrup and Haracopos, 1978) in which this borderline group has been awarded the status of an empirically based prevalence figure. The Wing and Gould study is a landmark in that it showed that, although Kanner autism could be identified among the triad patients, there was no indication that they differed in any clinically meaningful way from other cases on the spectrum. The validity of Kanner syndrome has been seriously challenged by this study.

Sibling rank

There is still no clear consensus with regard to birth order of children with autism. Early studies (Despert 1951, Kanner 1954, Rimland 1964) suggested a high number of first-born children, but later reports (Lotter 1967, Wing 1980*a*) have yielded conflicting results. On balance, it seems reasonable to assume that the Tsai and Stewart (1983) position of more first and late-born (fourth or later) children in autism may turn out to be correct. Jones and Szatmari (1988) have proposed that so-called genetic stoppage might be in operation in autism. Genetic stoppage implies that if a child with a severe disability such as autism is born into a family it often leads to the parents deciding either to refrain from having further children or to limit themselves to having only one more (hopefully healthy) child.

Social class

From as early as Kanner's first account of autism (1943), there has been a notion—which has sometimes taken on mythological qualities—that children with autism come from the upper social classes (see discussion in Chapter 1). Kanner, in all probability, saw a highly selected population of children with autism. Wing (1980*a*), Andersson and Wadensjö (1981), Gillberg and Schaumann (1982), Bohman *et al.* (1983), Steffenburg and Gillberg (1986), Lögdahl (1989), Cialdella and Mamelle (1989) and Gillberg *et al.* (1991*a*), in population studies of autism, found no indication whatsoever of a trend towards upper social class in autism. Brask (1970), on the basis of her epidemiological sample, reported no upper social class bias. Lotter (1967) is the only student of autism epidemiology who found a *slight* social class bias. Taken together, the bulk of the evidence does not favour a high social class bias in autism. It is hoped that the endless, often pointless arguments about social class in autism will come to an end. There is nothing very substantial to suggest that autism has anything to do with social class. That clinic-based samples may be biased in favour of higher social class is uninformative regarding social class in autism generally. The possibility remains that among the relatively brighter children with autism, social class might be somewhat higher. This, in turn, might mean no more than that among the normal child population high intelligence and high social class show some correlation.

Sex ratios

Most studies of autism report a boy:girl ratio of 3:1 or 4:1 (see Rutter 1985). It appears that in cases exactly fitting Kanner's description this ratio may be considerably higher: Wing and Gould (1979) reported a 16:1 ratio and Gillberg *et al.* (1991*a*) a 13:1 ratio in the groups with the most typical Kanner-type profiles. Nevertheless, population-based studies report lower ratios when all levels of IQ are included and nuclear and non-nuclear cases are pooled. Thus, the boy:girl ratio in such studies usually ranges from around 1.5:1 (Brask 1970, Bohman *et al.* 1983) to around 2.8:1 (Lotter 1966, Wing and Gould 1979, Lögdahl 1989, Gillberg *et al.* 1991). There is a tendency for some of the Scandinavian studies to show particularly 'low' boy:girl ratios. Thus, a ratio of 1.5:1 was reported in twins with autism by Steffenburg *et al.* (1989). The reasons for these studies showing discrepant sex ratios are unclear.

In Asperger syndrome, the boy:girl ratio tends to be even higher than in classical autism. However, population-based studies detailing results in this respect have not yet been published.

Wing (1980*b*), and others before and after, have documented that the overrepresentation of boys with autism is less pronounced in the severely mentally retarded group. Thus, in her group of 74 children with the triad, the boy:girl ratios were 1.1:1, 1.3:1 and 14.2:1 in the IQ ranges of 0–19, 20–49 and ≥50, respectively. Similar, though less pronounced trends have been reported by most authors in the field. These trends could suggest that whereas boys are (genetically?) much more prone to developing autism, more severe brain damage would be required for the development of autism in girls.

Mental retardation

All studies to date agree that the vast majority of children with autism and autistic-like conditions are also mentally retarded (see Rutter 1983) and test reliably in the IQ range <70 (Clark and Rutter 1979, Rutter 1983). 70 to 90 per cent of the children included in various studies are described as clearly mentally retarded, whereas only about 10 per cent are of average (or in rare instances, above average) intelligence.

Many Kanner autism cases, in spite of severe overall mental retardation, have an 'islet' of special ability, which does not represent a signal symptom of hidden superior talents, but is rather to be taken as the only intact functioning area in an otherwise extremely deviant child (Shah and Frith 1983).

Our concepts relating to the combination of autism and mental retardation may have to change considerably over the next decade if, as currently seems quite likely, the Asperger phenotype becomes 'incorporated' in the inclusive category of autism. Asperger syndrome is probably substantially more common than Kanner autism, and since mental retardation is rare in Asperger syndrome (Gillberg and Gillberg 1989) the pooled Kanner/Asperger group would still show mental retardation at an increased level compared with the general population, though no longer in the majority of cases.

Epilepsy
One quarter to one third of all people with autism develop seizures at some time before adulthood (see Chapter 6). Infantile spasms and complex partial seizures are possibly more frequent than in other populations.

Other disorders
There are several references in the literature (*e.g.* Keeler 1958, Fraiberg 1977, Rapin 1979, Wing 1980*b*) to the high incidence of blindness and deafness in autism. However, there is little in the way of scientific evidence to support this view, and, although clinically credible, claims for a connection between visual/auditory deprivation and autism await definitive scientific study. A longitudinal study in the New York area by Rapin found 61 cases of autism among 1150 hearing-impaired children (5.3 per cent), but the authors of this report (Jure *et al.* 1991) cautioned that this did not represent data on the prevalence of autism in hearing-impaired children generally as Rapin's sample was drawn from three clinically biased populations. According to a recent study by Steffenburg (1991), it appears that visual and hearing deficits may be very common in autism, even though blindness and deafness appear to be rare.

Dysphasia may also be common in autism, but empirical evidence is lacking so far. That there is considerable overlap between certain kind of speech–language disorders and autism is not a matter of dispute, but it is unclear where the boundaries are (Bishop 1989). For instance, so called semantic–pragmatic disorders often overlap with Asperger syndrome, and the majority of people with Asperger syndrome would probably be classified as suffering from a semantic–pragmatic disorder.

Epidemiological and clinical studies strongly suggest that tuberous sclerosis, neurofibromatosis, the fragile X syndrome, Rett syndrome and Moebius syndrome may all be associated with autism in a stronger than chance fashion. Steffenburg (1991), in a population based study, demonstrated that more than one in three people with nuclear autism had an associated known medical syndrome, in many cases revealed only after extensive neurobiological/medical work-up. Table 7.2 lists those disorders that have been reported in various epidemiological studies as being associated with autism, thereby pointing toward a neurobiological basis for the development of autism.

TABLE 7.2

Associated medical conditions in autism

Medical condition	Important reference
Fragile X syndrome	Hagerman (1989)
Other sex chromosome anomalies	Hagerman (1989)
Marker chromosome syndrome	Gillberg et al. (1991b)
Other chromosome anomalies	Hagerman (1989)
Tuberous sclerosis	Hunt and Dennis (1987)
Neurofibromatosis	Gillberg and Forsell (1984)
Hypomelanosis of Ito	Gillberg and Åkefeldt (1991)
Goldenhar syndrome	Landgren et al. (1992)
Rett syndrome	Coleman and Gillberg (1985)
Moebius syndrome	Ornitz et al. (1977)
Phenylketonuria	Friedman (1969)
Lactic acidosis	Coleman and Blass (1985)
Hypothyroidism	Gillberg, I.C. et al. (1992)
Rubella embryopathy	Chess et al. (1971)
Herpes simplex encephalitis	Gillberg (1986)
Cytomegalovirus infection	Stubbs (1976)
Williams syndrome	Reiss et al. (1985)
Duchenne muscular dystrophy	Komoto et al. (1984)

Summary

Most of the early epidemiological studies concluded that autistic syndromes occur somewhere in the range of four to five children per 10,000. Recent studies suggest that the frequency might be considerably higher, of the order of 10 to 13 per 10,000. (If Asperger syndrome is conceptualized as an autistic syndrome, then prevalence figures are definitely much higher than previously reported.) Nuclear Kanner autism cases possibly account for half to three quarters of all cases with autistic syndromes reported in the literature to date. There is a larger group of mentally retarded and clumsy/attention-deficient children who show autistic features without meeting all the specific criteria for autism. Many children with typical autism are mentally retarded, and only about one in ten have a clearly normal level of intelligence. Epilepsy affects about one in three people with autism by adulthood. A number of associated disorders are common in autism. Girls are less frequently affected by 'classic' Kanner autism than boys, but the behavioural phenotype might differ slightly across sexes, so the prevalence figures for girls reported in the literature may be too low. This may be particularly true in the relatively brighter group of people with autism with IQ levels >50, in which females are reported to be very rare.

REFERENCES

Åkefeldt, A., Gillberg, C. (1991) 'Hypomelanosis of Ito in three cases with autism and autistic-like conditions.' *Developmental Medicine and Child Neurology*, **33**, 735–741.

Andersson, L., Wadensjö, K. (1981) *Early Childhood Psychosis in Malmöhus län.* Lund: Social-avdelningen. *(In Swedish.)*

Bishop, D.V. (1989) 'Autism, Asperger's syndrome and semantic-pragmatic disorder: where are the boundaries?' *British Journal of Disorders of Communication*, **24**, 107–121.

Bohman, M., Bohman, I.L., Björck, P.O., Sjöholm, E. (1983) 'Childhood psychosis in a northern Swedish county: some preliminary findings from an epidemiological survey.' *In:* Schmidt, M.H., Remschmidt, H. (Eds) *Epidemiological Approaches in Child Psychiatry, II.* Stuttgart: Thieme, pp. 164–173.

Brask, B.H. (1970) 'A prevalence investigation of childhood psychosis.' *Paper presented at the 16th Scandinavian Congress of Psychiatry.*

Bryson, S.E., Clark, B.S., Smith, I.M. (1988) 'First report of a Canadian epidemiological study of autistic syndromes.' *Journal of Child Psychology and Psychiatry*, **29**, 433–445.

Chess, S., Korn, S.J., Fernandez, P.B. (1971) *Psychiatric Disorders of Children with Congenital Rubella.* New York: Brunner/Mazel.

Cialdella, P., Mamelle, N. (1989) 'An epidemiological study of infantile autism in a French department (Rhône): a research note.' *Journal of Child Psychology and Psychiatry*, **30**, 165–175.

Clark, P., Rutter, M. (1979) 'Task difficulty and task performance in autistic children.' *Journal of Child Psychology and Psychiatry*, **20**, 271–285.

Coleman, M., Blass, J.P. (1985) 'Autism and lactic acidosis.' *Journal of Autism and Developmental Disorders*, **15**, 1–8.

—— Gillberg, C. (1985) *The Biology of the Autistic Syndromes.* New York: Praeger.

Corbett, J. (1983) 'An epidemiological approach to the evaluation of services for children with mental retardation.' *In:* Remschmidt, M.H. (Ed.) *Epidemiological Approaches in Child Psychiatry.* Stuttgart: Thieme.

Despert, J.L. (1951) 'Some considerations relating to the genesis of autistic behaviour in children.' *American Journal of Orthopsychiatry*, **21**, 335–350.

Fraiberg, S. (1977) *Insights from the Blind. Comparative Studies of Blind and Sighted Infants.* New York: Basic Books.

Friedman, E. (1969) 'The autistic syndrome and phenylketonuria.' *Schizophrenia*, **1**, 249–261.

Gillberg, C. (1983*a*) 'Perceptual, motor and attentional deficits in Swedish primary school children. Some child psychiatric aspects.' *Journal of Child Psychology and Psychiatry*, **24**, 377–403.

—— (1983*b*) 'Psychotic behaviour in children and young adults in a mental handicap hostel.' *Acta Psychiatrica Scandinavica*, **68**, 351–358.

—— (1984) 'Infantile autism and other childhood psychoses in a Swedish urban region. Epidemiological aspects.' *Journal of Child Psychology and Psychiatry*, **25**, 35–43.

—— (1986) 'Onset at age 14 of a typical autistic syndrome. A case report of a girl with herpes simplex encephalitis.' *Journal of Autism and Developmental Disorders*, **16**, 369–375.

—— (1991) 'Outcome in autism and autistic-like conditions.' *Journal of the American Academy of Child and Adolescent Psychiatry*, **30**, 375–382.

—— (1992) 'The Emanuel Miller Lecture 1991: Autism and austistic-like conditions—subgroups of disorders of empathy.' *Journal of Child Psychology and Psychiatry*, **33**, 813–842.

—— Forsell, C. (1984) 'Childhood psychosis and neurofibromatosis—more than a coincidence?' *Journal of Autism and Development Disorders*, **14**, 1–8.

—— Schaumann, H. (1982) 'Social class and infantile autism.' *Journal of Autism and Developmental Disorders*, **12**, 223–228.

—— Persson, E., Grufman, M., Themnér, U. (1986) 'Psychiatric disorders in mildly and severely mentally retarded urban children and adolescents: epidemiological aspects.' *British Journal of Psychiatry*, **149**, 68–74.

—— Steffenburg, S., Schaumann, H. (1991*a*) 'Autism: epidemiology: is autism more common now than 10 years ago?' *British Journal of Psychiatry*, **158**, 403–409.

—— —— Wahlström, J., Gillberg, I.C., Sjöstedt, A., Martinsson, T., Liedgren, S., Eeg-Olofsson, O. (1991*b*) 'Autism associated with marker chromosome.' *Journal of the American Academy of Child and Adolescent Psychiatry*, **30**, 489–494.

Gillberg, I.C., Gillberg, C. (1989) 'Asperger syndrome. Some epidemiological considerations: a research note.' *Journal of Child Psychology and Psychiatry*, **30**, 631–638.

—— —— Kopp, S. (1992) 'Hypothyroidism and autism spectrum disorders.' *Journal of Child Psychology and Psychiatry*, **33**, 531–542.

Hagerman, R.J. (1989) 'Chromosomes, genes and autism.' *In:* Gillberg, C. (Ed.) *Diagnosis and*

Treatment of Autism. New York: Plenum, pp. 105–132.

Hunt, A., Dennis, J. (1987) 'Psychiatric disorder among children with tuberous sclerosis.' *Developmental Medicine and Child Neurology*, **29**, 190–198.

Ishii, T., Takahashi, O. (1982) 'Epidemiology of autistic children in Toyota City, Japan. Prevalence.' *Paper presented at the World Child Psychiatry Conference, Dublin.*

Jones, M.B., Szatmari, P. (1988) 'Stoppage rules and genetic studies of autism.' *Journal of Autism and Developmental Disorders*, **18**, 31–40. [*Erratum:* **18**, 477.]

Jure, R., Rapin, I., Tuchman, R.F. (1991) 'Hearing-impaired autistic children.' *Developmental Medicine and Child Neurology*, **33**, 1062–1072.

Kanner, L (1943) 'Autistic disturbances of affective contact.' *Nervous Child*, **2**, 217–250.

—— (1954) 'To what extent is early childhood autism determined by constitutional inadequacies?' *Proceedings of the Association for Research in Nervous and Mental Diseases*, **33**, 378–385.

Keeler, W. R. (1958) 'Autistic patterns and defective communication in blind children with retrolental fibroplasia.' *In:* Hoch, P.H., Zubin, J. (Eds) *Psychopathology of Communication.* New York: Grune & Stratton, pp. 64–83.

Kelstrup, A., Haracopos, D. (1978) 'Psychotic behavior in children under the institutions for the mentally retarded in Denmark.' *Journal of Autism and Developmental Disorders*, **8**, 1–12.

Komoto, J., Udsui, S., Otsuki, S., Terao, A. (1984) 'Infantile autism and Duchenne muscular dystrophy.' *Journal of Autism and Developmental Disorders*, **14**, 191–195.

Landgren, M., Gillberg, C., Strömland, K. (1992) 'Goldenhar syndrome and autistic behaviour.' *Developmental Medicine and Child Neurology. (In press.)*

Lögdahl, K. (1989) *The Prevalence of Autism in a Swedish County. Report to Sörmland County Authorities. (In Swedish.)*

Lotter, V. (1966) 'Epidemiology of autistic conditions in young children. I. Prevalence.' *Social Psychiatry*, **1**, 124–137.

—— (1967) *The Prevalence of the Autistic Syndrome in Children.* London: University of London Press.

Ornitz, E.M., Guthrie, D., Farley, A.J. (1977) 'The early development of autistic children.' *Journal of Autism and Childhood Schizophrenia*, **7**, 207–229.

Rapin, I. (1979) 'Effects of early blindness and deafness on cognition.' *In:* Katzman, R. (Ed.) *Congenital and Acquired Cognitive Disorders.* New York: Raven, pp. 189–245.

Reiss, A.L., Feinstein, C., Rosenbaum, K.N., Borengasser-Caruso, M.A., Goldsmith, B.M. (1985) 'Autism associated with Williams syndrome.' *Journal of Pediatrics*, **106**, 247–249.

Rimland, B. (1964) *Infantile Autism.* New York: Appleton-Century-Crofts.

Ritvo, E.R., Freeman, B.J., Pingree, C., Mason-Brothers, A., Jorde, L.B., Jensen, W.R., McMahon, W.M., Petersen, P.B., Mo, A., Ritvo, A. (1990) 'The UCLA–University of Utah epidemiologic survey of autism: prevalence.' *American Journal of Psychiatry*, **146**, 194–199.

Rutter, M. (1966) 'Behavioural and cognitive characteristics of a series of psychotic children.' *In:* Wing, J.K. (Ed.) *Early Childhood Autism.* Oxford: Pergamon, pp. 51–81.

—— (1983) 'Cognitive deficits in the pathogenesis of autism.' *Journal of Child Psychology and Psychiatry*, **24**, 513–531.

—— (1985) 'Infantile autism and other pervasive developmental disorders.' *In:* Rutter, M., Hersov, L. (Eds) *Child and Adolescent Psychiatry: Modern Approaches.* Oxford: Blackwell Scientific, pp. 545–566.

Shah, A., Frith, U. (1983) 'An islet of ability in autistic children: a research note.' *Journal of Child Psychology and Psychiatry*, **24**, 613–620.

Steffenburg, S. (1991) 'Neuropsychiatric assessment of children with autism: a population-based study.' *Developmental Medicine and Child Neurology*, **33**, 495–511.

—— Gillberg, C. (1986) 'Autism and autistic-like conditions in Swedish rural and urban areas: a population study.' *British Journal of Psychiatry*, **149**, 81–87.

—— —— Hellgren, L., Andersson, L., Gillberg, I.C., Jakobsson, G., Bohman, M. (1989) 'A twin study of autism in Denmark, Finland, Iceland, Norway and Sweden.' *Journal of Child Psychology and Psychiatry*, **30**, 405–416.

Steinhausen, H.C., Göbel, D., Breinlinger, M., Wohlleben, B. (1986) 'A community survey of infantile autism.' *Journal of the American Academy of Child Psychiatry*, **25**, 186–189.

Stubbs, E.G. (1976) 'Autistic children exhibit undetectable hemagglutination-inhibition antibody titers despite previous rubella vaccination.' *Journal of Autism and Childhood Schizophrenia*, **6**, 269–274.

Sugiyama, T., Abe, T. (1989) 'The prevalence of autism in Nagoya, Japan: a total population study.' *Journal of Autism and Developmental Disorders*, **19**, 87–96.

Tanoue, Y., Oda, S., Asano, F., Kawashima, K. (1988) 'Epidemiology of infantile autism in southern Ibaraki, Japan; differences in prevalence in birth cohorts.' *Journal of Autism and Developmental Disorders*, **18**, 155–166.

Torrey, E.F., Hersh, S.P., McCabe, K.D. (1975) 'Early childhood psychosis and bleeding during pregnancy: a prospective study of gravid women and their offspring.' *Journal of Autism and Childhood Schizophrenia*, **5**, 287–297.

Treffert, D.A. (1970) 'Epidemiology of infantile autism.' *Archives of General Psychiatry*, **22**, 431–438.

Tsai, L.Y., Stewart, M.A. (1983) 'Etiological implication of maternal age and birth order in infantile autism.' *Journal of Autism and Developmental Disorders*, **13**, 57–65.

von Knorring, A-L. (1991) 'Outcome in autism.' *Svensk Medicin*, **23**, 34–36.

Wing, L. (1980a) 'Childhood autism and social class: a question of selection.' *British Journal of Psychiatry*, **137**, 410–417.

—— (1980b) 'Sex ratios in early childhood autism and related conditions.' *Psychiatry Research*, **5**, 129–137.

—— Gould, J. (1979) 'Severe impairments of social interaction and associated abnormalities in children: epidemiology and classification.' *Journal of Autism and Developmental Disorders*, **9**, 11–29.

—— Yeates, S.R., Brierley, L.M., Gould, J. (1976) 'The prevalence of early childhood autism: comparison of administrative and epidemiological studies.' *Psychological Medicine*, **6**, 89–100.

8
GENETIC FACTORS*

In the 20th century, advances in medical techniques have revolutionized the quality of life and the understanding of disease mechanisms. This process has increased in pace as the century has advanced, and in the understanding of inherited disease progress has recently been particularly rapid.

A good example is the study of familial autism. As the detection of enzyme defects by biochemical methods has accelerated, specific enzyme errors have been found in more and more disease entities with a subgroup of patients with autism. In the last decade, the pulse of development has quickened because of the introduction of molecular biological and, more particularly, recombinant DNA techniques. Results of these developments can be seen in Chapters 16, 17 and 20. These new approaches are already providing powerful and precise definitions for inherited psychoneurological disorders such as autism.

As we learn more about normal development, abnormal development becomes easier to define. The new techniques have the potential to define genetic regulatory events that underlie cellular differentiation and tissue development in brain embryogenesis. Equally fascinating is the new information showing how sensory input has a role to play in selecting which groups of neurons survive into adult life to form the underlying cognitive and personality structures.

When something has gone wrong with the genetic information encoding the components of the CNS, several major patterns emerge. One is mental retardation. At present about 20 per cent of individuals with an IQ between 51 and 70 and about half of those with IQ $\leqslant 50$ can be assigned diagnoses (genetic, infectious, etc.) with present technology (Costeff *et al.* 1983, Hagberg and Kyllerman 1983). There is a great deal more work to be done, since a further 20 per cent or more may have a genetic aetiology detectable by various types of study, including that of family history.

Another pattern is the autistic spectrum with its now classic diagnostic criteria (see Chapter 2). It is currently believed that a genetic disease underlies 10 to 20 per cent of all autism cases, although it is likely that this figure will rise as contemporary techniques are applied to more cases. The current figure has been arrived at by an analysis of epidemiological studies, including population-based twin and family studies (Bolton and Rutter 1990, Gillberg 1992). It includes cases associated with a well-defined underlying medical disorder (such as tuberous sclerosis and the fragile X syndrome) as well as other genetic cases in which an underlying clear aetiology remains to be established.

*A glossary of genetic terms used in this book is given as an Appendix (p. 307).

Genetic factors in autism not associated with specific medical conditions
There are now two population-based twin studies, several family studies and several single-family case studies indicating that some cases of autism have an important hereditary root even when there are no associated specific medical conditions yet identified.

Twin studies in autism
Folstein and Rutter (1977) reported the first nationwide systematic twin study in autism and found a 36 per cent autism concordance rate in monozygotic (MZ) twins and a 0 per cent concordance rate in same-sex dizygotic (DZ) twins. When they extended the phenotype to include other cognitive disorders, the concordance rate rose to over 80 per cent in the MZ twins but to only 10 per cent in the DZ sets. In their follow-up study, Bolton and Rutter (1990) reported that almost all of the cognitively impaired MZ twins who were not diagnosed as suffering from autism in the first study subsequently showed significant difficulties with reciprocal social interaction. The findings were interpreted as showing the considerable influence of a genetic component in autism. There was also an increased rate of perinatal hazards in the non-concordant autism twin cases, which could suggest that some autism cases could be produced by perinatally acquired brain damage, or that some children are already at risk when they enter the perinatal period with its stressful events on the fetus.

In a Nordic population-based twin study, Steffenburg *et al.* (1989) reported an 89 per cent concordance rate for autism in MZ twins and a 0 per cent concordance rate for same-sex DZ twins who did not have the fragile X syndrome (one male and one female MZ pair and one set of MZ triplets showed clear or possible fragile X syndrome). If cognitive impairment of any kind was included in concordance estimates, the MZ twins remained at the same level, whereas in the DZ group the rate rose to 30 per cent. Perinatal hazards were associated with non-concordance cases of autism, just as in the Folstein and Rutter (1977) study. The male-to-female ratio was relatively low in the Nordic study. Sex ratios lower than those reported from clinical surveys of autism have been noted in several population studies (Lotter 1966, Brask 1970, Bohman *et al.* 1983). In the Nordic twin sample, boy:girl ratios were close to 3:1 in southern parts of Scandinavia, but actually tended towards the reverse in the northernmost parts. Regardless of whether the results were analysed pooled or separately for north and south Scandinavia (including Finland), the major conclusions remained unaffected. The Nordic twin study yielded results which supported the conclusion of the Folstein and Rutter (1977) study that genetic factors are important in some cases of autism.

Bolton and Rutter (1990) also reported that a new twin study is showing concordance rates for autism in MZ twins which are in between those of that group's first twin study and those of the Nordic study, although at the time of writing this book, their results have not yet been published.

In summary, the available population-based twin studies strongly suggest an important genetic component in some cases of autism. Whether autism *per se* or some broader autism phenotype is inherited cannot yet be determined. However, there are a number of problems with twin studies, which we shall not dwell on here except to say that twin studies alone are not sufficient to determine either the extent to which a disorder is inherited in non-twin cases or the possible mode of inheritance.

There are also a number of other twin studies in the field of autism, but the majority of these refer to single pairs, very small numbers, or samples in which selection bias may have been introduced. The twin studies by Ritvo *et al.* (1985) indicate a strong genetic component in autism. The concordance in MZ twins was almost identical to that of the Nordic study. The Ritvo *et al.* study included a reasonably large sample, but because it was recruited from families belonging to an autism support group, selection factors may have been introduced which could detract from the possibility of generalization. For instance, as would be expected in volunteer samples, there was an excess of MZ twins. Also, the data analysis included opposite-sex twin pairs. Because of the well-established excess of males in population samples of autism, twin studies examining same-sex pairs separately are to be preferred.

Family studies in autism and autistic-like conditions (including Asperger syndrome)
There have been many studies of an epidemiological character that have reported a rate of autism of around 3 per cent in siblings of probands with autism (see Smalley *et al.* 1988). This represents a 60- to 100-fold increase over the general population prevalence if the 'old' population rates (see Chapter 7) are used for comparison or a 15- to 30-fold increase if the results from the more recent population studies are used instead. Further, given the limited evidence that genetic stoppage may be in operation in autism (Jones and Szatmari 1988), the rate of multiple-case families appears to be considerably higher than chance. Ritvo *et al.* (1985) accumulated volunteer families with autism in two or more siblings. Using segregation analysis of their case material they concluded that autosomal recessive inheritance could account for their findings. However, the excess of males is difficult to account for. It is clear that there are several different autism subgroups, including the fragile X–autism and tuberous sclerosis–autism subgroups, both of which show inheritance patterns which are not autosomal recessive. On the basis of the available evidence it seems prudent to conclude that in a subgroup of patients with autism, an autosomal recessive pattern of inheritance may exist (see also below and Chapter 16).

Bolton and Rutter (1990) found higher rates of cognitive and social interaction disorders in the siblings of children with autism. They concluded that it is likely that what is inherited in autism is a broader phenotype characterized by specific cognitive problems involving both language and social abnormalities. However, the study by Steffenburg (1991), which compared the rate of cognitive disorder in the first-degree relatives of children with autism and that in children from the general population who did not exhibit overt signs of deficits in attention, motor control and perception, did not yield any difference between the groups in this respect. However, 9 per cent of the children with autism but none of the comparison children had a father with Asperger syndrome (one of the children with autism also had a brother with Asperger syndrome). Thus, the available evidence as regards exactly what it is that is inherited is contradictory (see also August *et al.* 1981, DeLong and Dwyer 1988, Wolff *et al.* 1988, Freeman *et al.* 1989, MacDonald *et al.* 1989, Silliman *et al.* 1989, Piven 1990, for further illustration of the divided findings in this area).

Family case studies
Several single-family case studies implicate genetic factors in certain families in which children with autism are born. Several of these (*e.g.* Gillberg 1985, 1989, 1991*a*; Bowman 1988) implicate genetic overlap between classic Kanner autism and Asperger syndrome and also occasionally suggest a link with affective disorders.

Autism in families with learning disorders
In families with the fragile X syndrome there are individuals (often females) with dyslexia and other learning disorders, others with emotional avoidance and shyness but not autism (often females, sometimes males) and others still with clear autistic features, autistic-like conditions or autism in the Kannerian sense of the word (Hagerman 1989). This pattern is sometimes seen in non-fragile-X families also. Some of these latter families are likely to have 'low count' fragile X, which may not be disclosed or would only be discovered after molecular genetic analysis.

Autism in families with psychiatric disorders
The possibility that autism might be familially associated with anorexia nervosa has been mentioned by Gillberg (1985), who described several males with second- and third-degree female relatives with teenage onset anorexia nervosa. The social aloofness and obsessive desire for preservation of sameness seen in many young female patients with anorexia nervosa were proposed as possible clinical/genetic links. In Steffenburg's (1991) population study, 3 per cent of the group with classical autism had a paternal aunt with anorexia nervosa, and 24 per cent of the group with autistic-like conditions had maternal aunts or first-cousins with that disorder. A recent population study of teenage anorexia nervosa by Råstam (1992) presented evidence that high-functioning autism/Asperger syndrome and anorexia nervosa might be overlapping conditions in certain cases. Individual case studies have been published of anorexia nervosa occurring in patients with autism (Stiver and Dobbins 1980, Rothery and Garden 1988). Recently, phenylketonuria (PKU) was described in connection with anorexia nervosa (Clarke and Yapa 1991). A connection between high serum phenylalanine concentrations and the development of anorexia nervosa was suggested. It may be relevant that untreated PKU has been reported to be associated with autism in a large number of cases.

A number of case studies and clinical epidemiological studies have indicated an association of autism and affective disorder in near relatives (Gillberg 1985, Gillberg and Steffenburg 1987, DeLong and Dwyer 1988, Piven 1990). The nature of such a possible association is poorly understood. The criteria for a diagnosis of affective disorder have rarely been explicit in the published studies so far. Gillberg (1984) and Gillberg and Steffenburg (1987) have suggested that affective disorder in the near relatives might predispose the individual with autism to pubertal mood swings and even frank deterioration. DeLong and Dwyer (1988) and certain case studies (Gillberg 1985, 1991a) implicate a common genetic underlying trait which can predispose to affective disorder in one individual and autism in another, particularly in the more high-functioning cases (or those currently often diagnosed as suffering from Asperger syndrome). The possibility that some of the overlap between the affective disorders and autism could be accounted for by the presence of the fragile X syndrome was highlighted by Hagerman (1989) and Steffenburg (1991).

Autism and schizophrenia: are there genetic links?
There is no convincing systematic evidence that autism and schizophrenia are clinically or genetically linked. However, it is clear that a small proportion of cases diagnosed as suffering from Asperger syndrome in childhood are given labels like 'schizophrenia', 'schizophrenia-like disorder' or 'non-specific psychosis' in early adult life (Wing 1981, Tantam 1988). Asperger (1944) reported that one of more than 200 cases seen by himself developed clear signs of schizophrenia. This would be an indication of the prevalence being no higher in Asperger syndrome than in the general population. Also, the cases reported by Wing (1981) and Tantam (1988) were 'atypical' in many ways, and it is possible that the fact that adult psychiatrists are unfamiliar with the concept of Asperger syndrome may lead to 'misdiagnoses' of schizophrenia. Follow-up into adulthood of the 'schizoid' children originally reported by Wolff and Chick (1980) (some of whom are likely to be within the autism spectrum/Asperger group) has revealed that only a very few have developed symptoms compatible with a diagnosis of schizophrenia (Wolff 1992).

The follow-up studies of autism that have been published to date do not indicate that autism 'predisposes' to the development of schizophrenia in adulthood (Gillberg 1991b). Nevertheless, cases with atypical but clearly autism-associated symptomatology are occasionally being diagnosed as 'childhood schizophrenia', and the follow-up of such cases indicates continued atypical autism symptoms in a considerable proportion of cases (Watkins *et al.* 1988). This does not necessarily indicate overlap between autism and schizophrenia at the aetiological level. However, it does bring out the fact that we need to be aware that at the symptomatic level current concepts and strict operational definitions of autism and schizophrenia cannot always provide a firm basis for distinction of the two. Furthermore, the claim that autism and schizophrenia are totally distinct conditions might turn out to have been premature (Frith and Frith 1991).

Types of genetic patterns seen in patients with autism

When a syndrome has many different aetiologies (as in autism), it can hardly be expected that all, or even most, of the patients with genetic aetiologies to their disease process would have a single genetic pattern. Analyses by statistical methods of family aggregation patterns of a mixed group of individuals with autism are interesting but of limited information. In the study by Jorde *et al.* (1990) the pattern of affected relatives was not consistent (which is what you would expect in a disorder of multiple aetiologies); the single largest genetic pattern noted was compatible with autosomal recessive inheritance. In autism, as in mental retardation, attempts to use statistics to determine genetic factors are complicated by the 'stoppage' effect which often truncates family size after the affected child is born (Jones and Szatmari 1988). In reality, there simply is no substitute for working up each patient and each family to discover the particular genetic mode in that family.

A number of genetic patterns are well-established in the medical literature, and there appears to be at least one disease where autistic symptoms have been described which fits most of these patterns. In fact, a careful analysis of the aetiological heterogeneity of autism may help explain findings such as the greater proportion of males than females with the syndrome. To take one example, there seems (although some contradictory evidence exists) to be a higher proportion of boys than girls with autism and the fragile X syndrome (Fig. 8.1).

Chromosome patterns

There are a number of aberrations of whole or pieces of chromosomes as a result of which a disease entity occurs that may include autistic symptomatology (see Chapter 16). The most common patterns reported are *partial deletions* of chromosomes: an example is the 'cri-du-chat' syndrome with a deletion of the short arm of the fifth chromosome (5p– syndrome) (Cantu *et al.* 1990). A *marker chromosome* (extra material from the long arm of chromosome 15) has been described in association with a specific autistic syndrome (Gillberg *et al.* 1991). Another example of extra chromosomal material is a *partial trisomy* involving chromosome 8 (Ritvo *et al.* 1990). Using chromosomal karyotyping techniques, a *fragile site* (Xq27.3) has been found in quite a number of individuals with autism (Cohen *et al.* 1991).

Mendelian genetic patterns

A *sex-linked recessive* pattern of inheritance is the likely mode of transmission in individuals with autistic features and the Lujan–Fryns syndrome (Gurrieri and Neri 1991). The fragile X syndrome, originally classified as having a sex-linked recessive pattern of inheritance, does not strictly meet such genetic criteria (Shapiro 1991). (For a discussion of the genetics of the fragile X syndrome, see Chapter 16.) The *autosomal recessive* pattern can be seen in the children with PKU who, before the introduction of regular screening for the condition or of medical testing of

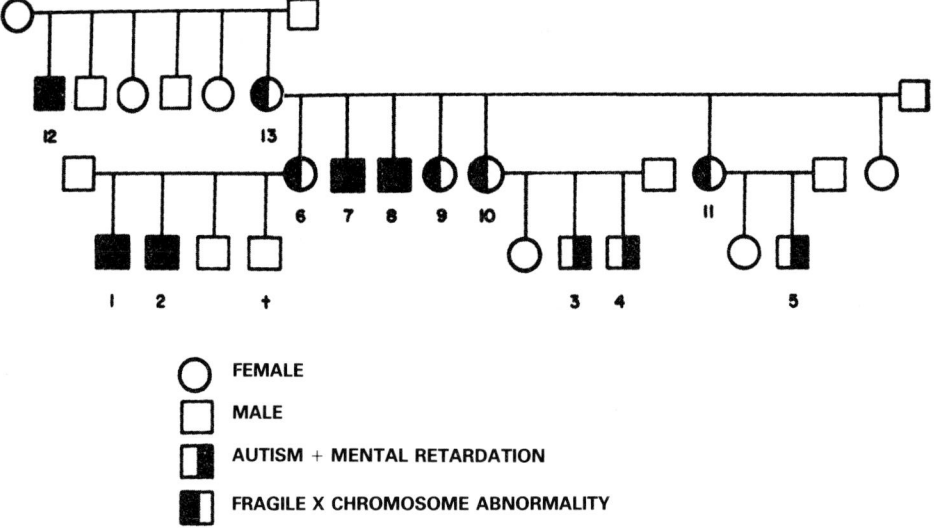

Fig. 8.1. Family with several fragile X positive males with autism. Case 1 is a severely mentally retarded 10-year-old boy with classic Kanner autism. Case 2, his 14-year-old brother, is moderately mentally retarded and has autism and psychomotor epilepsy. These brothers have one healthy brother; one elder brother was stillborn. Their mother (6) is fragile X positive, shy, and has articulation problems. Two of her brothers (7,8) are fragile X positive, moderately mentally retarded adults who have autism with aloofness, insistence on sameness and echolalia. Three of her four sisters are fragile X positive (9,10,11). Two of these have two moderately retarded sons (3,4) and one mildly retarded son (5), respectively, all three of whom have autism. These three boys have not been chromosomally examined. The maternal grandmother (13) is fragile X positive and retains speech/language problems. One of her brothers (12) has autism, is moderately mentally retarded and shows the fragile X chromosome abnormality. The great-grandparents are dead.

children with autism, were mistaken for 'neurologically intact' Kanner autism children (Friedman 1969). An example of the *autosomal dominant* diseases (which include the majority of the genetic diseases of the nervous system) is seen in the subgroup of patients with autism and neurofibromatosis.

In spite of the many patterns of genetic disease already described in patients with autistic symptoms, the majority of patients with a likely genetic disease have yet to have their specific chromosome or gene error identified. A massive, but exciting, task lies ahead.

Genetic counselling in autism
With the growing data base relating genetic factors to autism, parents and siblings of children with autism now often request genetic counselling.

At present, accurate genetic counselling in autism is possible only in the considerable minority of cases in which a clear cause has been established. For instance, if autism is associated with an hereditary genetic disorder such as the

102

fragile X syndrome, tuberous sclerosis, neurofibromatosis or PKU, the risk for recurrence in the family is linked with the risk for that particular disorder. Such cases of autism associated with a medical condition with a reasonably well established risk of recurrence represented 20 per cent of the whole autism group in the Steffenburg (1991) population study from Göteborg. In order to be able to provide appropriate genetic counselling in this subgroup, a comprehensive medical work-up should be conducted first in each case.

There is another autism subgroup in which the autistic symptomatology is linked to disease processes currently thought to be, in many instances, of a non-genetic (or at least 'non-inherited') character (such as Moebius syndrome). In such cases the risk of recurrence in future family members appears to be very small.

Also, when the comprehensive work-up has revealed severe peri- or postnatal damage leading to neurological complications (including autism) and when there is no clear family history of neuropsychiatric disorders thought to be associated with autism (autism, Asperger syndrome or cognitive/social cognitive disorders of other types), it is likely that the risk of recurrence is very low. Nevertheless, caution is warranted in such cases, both because family histories of related disorders may be inaccurate and because we do not know exactly which spectrum of disorders in the neuropsychiatric domain may be implicated in the broader autism phenotype (Gillberg 1992). Furthermore, the possibility that autosomal recessive inheritance patterns (which would be less likely to signal as a positive family history) might coincide with severe peri- or postnatal brain damage (for specific or coincidental reasons) means that considerable caution is warranted and that it is inappropriate to say that the risk is no higher than for people in the general population.

In the remaining 'cryptogenic' cases—currently constituting at least half of all cases with autism (51 per cent according to the Steffenburg study)—the recurrence risk is even more difficult to predict. Within this group is a subgroup which is likely to have a strong genetic component, *viz*. that in which a close relative has autism or Asperger syndrome. According to the available data, around 3 to 6 per cent of individuals with cryptogenic autism have a sibling with autism/Asperger syndrome (6 per cent in the Steffenburg study) and around 10 to 30 per cent have a parent with autism/Asperger syndrome (11 per cent in the Steffenburg study) or some cognitive or social cognitive disorder currently believed to be associated genetically with autism (16 per cent in the Steffenburg study). According to a number of family case studies, the recurrence risk for autism/Asperger syndrome might be very high if one of the parents has high-functioning autism or Asperger syndrome (Gillberg 1991*a*). In particular, it appears that if pre-, peri- or postnatal brain damage is added to the genetic risk factor, autism rather than milder Asperger variants might result.

In the other cryptogenic cases, where no close family member has an autism spectrum disorder, there is really no sound basis for genetic counselling except to quote the available figures for multiple incidence in a sibship (3 to 5 per cent), adding the qualification that the risk is likely to be lower than that. However, even this statement has to be tempered with the information that because of the possibility of genetic stoppage in autism, the available figures for multiple incidence among siblings might be an underestimate.

REFERENCES

Asperger, H. (1944) 'Die autistischen Psychopathen im Kindesalter.' *Archiv für Psychiatrie und Nervenkrankheiten*, **117**, 76–136.

August, G.J., Stewart, M.A., Tsai, L. (1981) 'The incidence of cognitive disabilities in the siblings of autistic children.' *British Journal of Psychiatry*, **138**, 416–422.

Bohman, M., Bohman, I.L., Björck, P.O., Sjöholm, E. (1983) 'Childhood psychosis in a northern Swedish county: some preliminary findings from an epidemiological survey.' *In:* Schmidt, M.H., Remschmidt, H. (Eds) *Epidemiological Approaches in Child Psychiatry, II.* Stuttgart: Thieme, pp. 164–173.

Bolton, P., Rutter, M. (1990) 'Genetic influences in autism.' *International Review of Psychiatry*, **2**, 67–80.

Bowman, E.P. (1988) 'Asperger's syndrome and autism: the case for a connection.' *British Journal of Psychiatry*, **152**, 377–382.

Brask, B.H. (1970) 'A prevalence investigation of childhood psychosis.' *Paper presented at the 16th Scandinavian Congress of Psychiatry.*

Cantu, E.S., Stone, J.W., Wing, A.A., Langee, H.R., Williams, C.A. (1990) 'Cytogenetic survey for autistic fragile-X carriers in a mental retardation center.' *American Journal of Mental Retardation*, **94**, 442–447.

Clarke, D.J., Yapa, P. (1991) 'Phenylketonuria and anorexia nervosa.' *Journal of Mental Deficiency Research*, **35**, 165–170.

Cohen, I.L., Vietze, P.M., Sudhalter, V., Jenkins, E.D., Brown, W.T. (1991) 'Effects of age and communication level on eye contact in fragile X males and non-fragile X autistic males.' *American Journal of Medical Genetics*, **38**, 498–502.

Costeff, H., Cohen, B.E., Weller, L. (1983) 'Relative importance of genetic and nongenetic etiologies in idiopathic mental retardation: estimates based on analysis of medical histories.' *Annals of Human Genetics*, **47**, 83–93.

DeLong, G.R., Dwyer, J.T. (1988) 'Correlation of family history with specific autistic subgroups; Asperger's syndrome and bipolar affective disease.' *Journal of Autism and Developmental Disorders*, **18**, 593–600.

Folstein, S., Rutter, M. (1977) 'Infantile autism: a genetic study of 21 twin pairs.' *Journal of Child Psychology and Psychiatry*, **18**, 297–321.

Freeman, B.J., Ritvo, E.R., Mason-Brothers, A., Pingree, C., Yokota, A., Jenson, W.R., McMahon, W.M., Petersen, P.B., Mo, A., Schroth, P. (1989) 'Psychometric assessment of first-degree relatives of 62 autistic probands in Utah.' *American Journal of Psychiatry*, **146**, 361–364.

Friedman, E. (1969) 'The autistic syndrome and phenylketonuria.' *Schizophrenia*, **1**, 249–261.

Frith, C.D., Frith, U. (1991) 'Elective affinities in autism and schizophrenia.' *In:* Bebbington, P. (Ed.) *Social Psychiatry, Theory, Methodology and Practice.* New Brunswick, NJ: Transaction Books, pp. 65–88.

Gillberg, C. (1984) 'Autistic children growing up: problems during puberty and adolescence.' *Developmental Medicine and Child Neurology*, **26**, 125–129.

—— (1985) 'Asperger's syndrome and recurrent psychosis—a case study.' *Journal of Autism and Developmental Disorders*, **15**, 389–397.

—— (1989) 'Asperger syndrome in 23 Swedish children.' *Developmental Medicine and Child Neurology*, **31**, 520–531.

—— (1991a) 'Clinical and neurobiological aspects in six family studies of Asperger syndrome.' *In:* Frith, U. (Ed.) *Autism and Asperger Syndrome.* Cambridge: Cambridge University Press, pp. 122–146.

—— (1991b) 'Outcome in autism and autistic-like conditions.' *Journal of the American Academy of Child and Adolescent Psychiatry*, **30**, 375–382.

—— (1992) 'Savant-syndromet.' *In:* Vejlsgaard, R. (Ed.) *Medicinsk årsbok*, Köpenhamn: Munksgaard, pp. 127–131.

—— Steffenburg, S. (1987) 'Outcome and prognostic factors in infantile autism and similar conditions: a population-based study of 46 cases followed through puberty.' *Journal of Autism and Developmental Disorders*, **17**, 273–287.

—— —— Wahlström, J., Sjöstedt, A., Gillberg, I.C., Martinsson, T., Liedgren, S., Eeg-Olofsson, O. (1991) 'Autism associated with marker chromosome.' *Journal of the American Academy of Child and Adolescent Psychiatry*, **30**, 489–494.

Gurrieri, F., Neri, G. (1991) 'A girl with the Lujan-Fryns syndrome.' *American Journal of Medical Genetics*, **38**, 290–291.

Hagberg, B., Kyllerman, M. (1983) 'Epidemiology of mental retardation—a Swedish survey.' *Brain and Development*, **5**, 441–449.

Hagerman, R.J. (1989) 'Chromosomes, genes and autism.' *In:* Gillberg, C. (Ed.) *Diagnosis and Treatment of Autism.* New York: Plenum, pp. 105–132.

Jones, M.B., Szatmari, P. (1988) 'Stoppage rules and genetic studies of autism.' *Journal of Autism and Developmental Disorders*, **18**, 31–40. [*Erratum*: **18**, 477.]

Jorde, L.B., Mason-Brothers, A., Waldmann, R., Ritvo, E.R., Freeman, B.J., Pingree, C., McMahon, W.M., Petersen, B., Jenson, W.R., Mo, A. (1990) 'The UCLA–University of Utah epidemiologic survey of autism: genealogical analysis of familial aggregation.' *American Journal of Medical Genetics*, **36**, 85–88.

Lotter, V. (1966) 'Epidemiology of autistic conditions in young children. I. Prevalence.' *Social Psychiatry*, **1**, 124–137.

Macdonald, H., Rutter, M., Howlin, P., Rios, P., Le-Conteur, A., Evered, C., Folstein, S. (1989) 'Recognition and expression of emotional cues by autistic and normal adults.' *Journal of Child Psychology and Psychiatry*, **30**, 865–877.

Piven, J., Gayle, J., Chase, G.A., Fink, B., Landa, R., Wzorek, M.M., Folstein, S.E. (1990) 'A family history study of neuropsychiatric disorders in the adult siblings of autistic individuals.' *Journal of the American Academy of Child and Adolescent Psychiatry*, **29**, 177–183.

Råstam, M. (1992) 'Anorexia nervosa in 51 children and adolescents. Pre-morbid problems and co-morbidity.' *Journal of the American Academy of Child and Adolescent Psychiatry. (In press.)*

Ritvo, E.R., Freeman, B.J., Mason-Brothers, A., Mo, A., Ritvo, A.M. (1985) 'Concordance of the syndrome of autism in 40 pairs of afflicted twins.' *American Journal of Psychiatry*, **142**, 74–77.

—— Freeman, B.J., Pingree, C., Mason-Brothers, A. Jorde, L.B., Jensen, W.R., McMahon, W.M., Petersen, P.B., Mo, A., Ritvo, A. (1990) 'The UCLA–University of Utah epidemiologic survey of autism: prevalence.' *American Journal of Psychiatry*, **146**, 194–199.

Rothery, D.J., Garden, G.M. (1988) 'Anorexia nervosa and infantile autism.' *British Journal of Psychiatry*, **153**, 714. *(Letter.)*

Shapiro, L.R. (1991) 'The fragile X syndrome: a peculiar pattern of inheritance.' *New England Journal of Medicine*, **325**, 1736–1738.

Silliman, E.R., Campbell, M., Mitchell, R.S. (1989) 'Genetic influences in autism and assessment of metalinguistic performance in siblings of autistic children.' *In:* Dawson, G. (Ed.) *Autism.* New York: Guilford Press.

Smalley, S.L., Asarnow, R.F., Spence, M.A. (1988) 'Autism and genetics. A decade of research.' *Archives of General Psychiatry*, **45**, 953–961.

Steffenburg, S. (1991) 'Neuropsychiatric assessment of children with autism: a population-based study.' *Developmental Medicine and Child Neurology*, **33**, 495–511.

—— Gillberg, C., Hellgren, L., Andersson, L., Gillberg, I.C., Jakobsson, G., Bohman, M. (1989) 'A twin study of autism in Denmark, Finland, Iceland, Norway and Sweden.' *Journal of Child Psychology and Psychiatry*, **30**, 405–416.

Stiver, R.L.S., Dobbins, J.P. (1980) 'Treatment of atypical anorexia nervosa in public school: an autistic girl.' *Journal of Autism and Developmental Disorders*, **10**, 67–73.

Tantam, D. (1988) Asperger's syndrome.' *Journal of Child Psychology and Psychiatry*, **29**, 245–255. *(Annotation.)*

Verkerk, A.J.M.H., Pieretti, M., Sutcliffe, J.S., Fu, Y-H., Kuhl, D.P.A., Pizzuti, A., Reiner, O., Richards, S., Victoria, M.F., Zhang, F., *et al.* (1991) 'Identification of a gene (FMR-1) containing a CGG repeat coincident with a breakpoint cluster region exhibiting length variation in fragile X

105

syndrome.' *Cell*, **65**, 905–914.

Watkins, J.M., Asarnow, R.F., Tanguay, P.E. (1988) 'Symptom development in childhood onset schizophrenia.' *Journal of Child Psychology and Psychiatry*, **29**, 865–878.

Wing, L. (1981) 'Asperger's syndrome: a clinical account.' *Psychological Medicine*, **11**, 115–129.

Wolff, S. (1992) 'Psychiatric morbidity and criminality in "schizoid" children grown-up: a record survey.' *European Child and Adolescent Psychiatry. (In press.)*

—— Chick, J. (1980) 'Schizoid personality in childhood: a controlled follow-up study.' *Psychological Medicine*, **10**, 85–100.

—— Narayan, S., Moyes, B. (1988) 'Personality characteristics of parents of autistic children: a controlled study. *Journal of Child Psychology and Psychiatry*, **29**, 143–153.

9
PRECONCEPTION, PRENATAL AND PERINATAL STUDIES

Children with a disease entity whose symptoms often become apparent in early infancy are in a group of patients for whom the preconception and prenatal histories of the parents may have direct relevance to the child's illness. In this chapter, evidence from the literature reviewing preconception and prenatal histories of the parents of children with autism will be summarized.

Preconception factors
In 1976, at the Children's Brain Research Clinic in Washington, DC, 78 children with autism were studied, along with 78 age- and sex-matched controls (Coleman 1976). One of the criteria for eligibility to participate in the project for both patients and controls involved an elaborate six-page questionnaire to be filled out by the parents. The information was, of course, retrospective. Since the patients and controls ranged up to the age of 22 years, some very old information was required, and thus the questionnaire—particularly concerning preconception and prenatal history—was bound to be incomplete. However, since the limitations of this retrospective study might be assumed to apply equally to the parents of both the children with autism and the control children, there was nevertheless a value in raising certain basic questions.

Analysis of the preconception histories indicated two areas where there was a statistically significant difference between the parents of children with autism and controls.

One of these areas was exposure to chemicals. In 20 families of the autism patients an unusual amount of exposure to chemicals had occurred during the preconception period. In four of these families, both the mother and the father had been exposed to chemicals, seven of the eight working professionally as chemists. However, since the parents in this project were self-selected to participate in one of the first large biochemical studies ever performed on children with autism, it is possible that chemists, familiar with biochemical problems, might have selectively joined in this particular study.

In an attempt to answer this question of self-selection by the parents, a second study was done by another investigator (Felicetti 1981). This new study took a group of 20 unselected autism patients who were enrolled in a residential setting that could provide necessary services. These were compared with 20 retarded, non-autistic children in the same setting, and with a control group of 20 normal children in the nearby community. The parents of all three groups then filled out an elaborate preconception history questionnaire. Felicetti reported that parents who had been exposed to chemical toxins accounted for 21 per cent of the autism group compared with 2.7 per cent of the retarded control group and 10 per cent of the normal control group, again a statistically significant finding despite the relatively small number of patients under study. In this second study, five of the parents of the children with autism were found to be professional chemists.

The best type of research for producing accurate information is a prospective study. Such a study was the Collaborative Perinatal Study at the National Institutes of Health (NIH) (Niswander and Gordon 1972) where 55,908 pregnancies were followed prospectively, starting in early pregnancy and continuing after the child was born and up to 7 years of age. From this population, 14 children were identified who conformed to the syndrome of infantile autism. Torrey *et al.* (1975) matched this group with two control groups: one of normal children and one of neurologically and behaviourally normal children with low IQs. The controls were matched for race, sex, habitat (that is, they were from the same section of the country) and socioeconomic factors. The preconception occupations of the parents in each of these groups were analysed by Marcus and Broman (unpublished manuscript): they found a higher incidence of occupations involving exposure to chemicals among the parents of the children with autism.

These studies raised the possibility of preconception exposure factors in parents of children with autism. What would be useful next is a prospective study of a population of chemists and other workers exposed to chemical toxins. Moreover, future studies need to have a much greater number of participants so that the results will not be skewed by small numbers. Until then, the 'chemical connection' in autism remains a challenging hypothesis.

In the 1976 study at the Children's Brain Research Clinic, the other statistically significant difference in preconception histories between the parents of children with autism and controls concerned the presence of hypothyroidism. Five fathers and 11 mothers of the 78 patients with autism reported having thyroid disease prior to conception, and in two cases both parents had a diagnosis of hypothyroidism at some time before the conception of the child, whereas in the control group only one father and three mothers reported a diagnosis of hypothyroidism. Although thyroid disease has not been reported as increased in patients with autism (see Chapter 19), the finding does have another possible implication. Many cases of hypothyroidism in adults are caused by autoimmune disease, and the role of autoimmune factors in autism is currently an active area of research (see Chapter 11). One study in Göteborg (Gillberg *et al.* 1992) has suggested that maternal hypothyroidism in pregnancy or prior to conception might be linked to the development of autism in the child in certain cases.

The study group from the NIH Collaborative Perinatal Study (Torrey *et al.* 1975) evaluated a number of preconception factors determined from the records and the mother's memory of the pregnancy. The variables looked at included the mother's history of irregular menstrual periods and dysmenorrhoea, previous X-rays, past illnesses, transfusions and immunizations, and the maternal age at the time of delivery. They also included the history of stillbirths and spontaneous abortions prior to the birth of the studied child and in the subsequent seven-year period. In none of these variables was any statistically significant difference found between the parents of the children with autism and the two sets of controls.

In 1983, Funderburk *et al.* looked again at some of the questions addressed by the Torrey *et al.* study using a larger patient group, this time in a retrospective survey. They studied 61 patients, 51 of whom either met the criteria of autism or had autistic features or language disorders not specified. The other 10 patients had a diagnosis of either classic or atypical psychosis. For control data, these authors used three previously reported surveys of normal infants born during the same period as the patients in the study and in comparable statewide or metropolitan areas. Comparing their patient group to the three published control groups, they found that 13.1 per cent of the parents of the children with autism/psychosis had experienced a problem with infertility, and 11.5 per cent of mothers had had more than two spontaneous abortions. These rates were considerably higher than in the control populations where infertility affected only 3.7 per cent and more than two spontaneous abortions 5.2 per cent.

Gillberg and Gillberg (1983) reported a study of 25 children with a diagnosis of autism and a comparison group of non-autistic children of the same sex, born in the same obstetrics department. The pre- and perinatal conditions under which these children were born were evaluated, using an optimality concept of Prechtl (1980). One factor studied in the preconception maternal history was the record of more than two spontaneous abortions prior to the pregnancy with the index child. Not found in the control group, this history was present in one mother of a child with autism.

The Gillberg and Gillberg study also showed a statistically significant increase in mean maternal age in the autism group, confirming an earlier study by Gillberg (1980). However, this is an area where the medical literature is divided. Arajärvi *et al.* (1964), Treffert (1970), and Finegan and Quarrington (1979) all found evidence of increased maternal age in their surveys. In contrast, Lotter (1966), Torrey *et al.* (1975), Wiedel and Coleman (1976) and Steinhausen *et al.* (1986) reported no difference in maternal age between the mothers of autism patients and controls.

One theory suggests that the disparities in these reports are based on differences in the diagnoses of the autistic syndromes, a problem confronting all the material reviewed in this book. Another possibility is that, since autism is a disorder of many aetiologies, different subgroups of the syndrome vary in number from one study group to another. Gillberg (1984) has suggested that the aetiologies of the autistic syndromes may show wide regional variation, as is the case with mental retardation syndromes.

Increasing maternal age is associated with a large number of central nervous syndromes of childhood, ranging from Down syndrome (Pueschel and Rynders

1982) to syndromes involving deficits in attention, motor control and perception (Gillberg *et al.* 1982). As knowledge advances, the relevant question will be which of the many diagnostic subgroups of the autistic spectrum are associated with older maternal age?

Prenatal factors

Prenatal events that occur during the gestation of a child who later is diagnosed as having autism have been studied in several surveys.

The one conducted by the NIH Collaborative Perinatal Study (see above) is the only prospective study of these variables in the literature. Of 15 factors examined, only one prenatal event was identified that appeared to be significantly associated with the subsequent development of infantile autism, namely maternal uterine bleeding during pregnancy. Of the 14 mothers in the study, nine had some bleeding compared with five of the low-IQ control group and four of the normal-IQ control group. The authors noted that the distribution by trimesters was probably as important as the incidence of bleeding in these mothers. There was a significant amount of early and especially mid-trimester bleeding among mothers who subsequently delivered children with autism, whereas in the control groups, mid-trimester bleeding was extremely rare (p<0.01).

There have been a number of retrospective studies examining prenatal complications associated with autism (or autism and childhood schizophrenia) (see Chapter 15). Sometimes the studies have not singled out gestational bleeding as an individual variable, and are accordingly very difficult to interpret. In the study by Harper and Williams (1974), gestational bleeding was separated out as a sign of threatened abortion, and was said to occur significantly more often among children with autism than among physically ill children, but not more frequently among children with autism than among emotionally disturbed children. Deykin and MacMahon (1979) retrospectively compared 173 children with autism with an unaffected sibling control group and found maternal bleeding in 16 per cent of gestations in the autism group but in only 7 per cent in the sibling control group. In the study by Gillberg and Gillberg (1983), bleeding during pregnancy was found significantly more commonly in the autism than in the control group. The Campbell *et al.* (1978) study found a spectacular 71 per cent bleeding before the third trimester in their autism group, compared to 49 per cent for sibling controls.

To date, bleeding during pregnancy, particularly during the mid-trimester, is the main finding that seems to stand out from the literature regarding gestational factors related to autism. There are, of course, many children with autism whose mothers did not bleed during pregnancy. [Torrey *et al.* (1975) caution that it is difficult to interpret a result in any individual case since, in their study, the only woman who had a confirmed case of rubella during pregnancy and also bled in the third trimester had a child who was in the group of normal IQ controls!] In the Funderburk *et al.* (1983) study referred to earlier, increased gestational exposure to hormones was noted: in some (but not all) of the autism cases, the reason for the administration of hormones appears to have been maternal bleeding.

Theoretically, it is interesting to speculate on the meaning of mid-trimester bleeding. If bleeding occurs concurrently with or shortly after the lesion occurs to the fetus, it might help suggest why many children with autism are so normal in appearance. If, in fact, the insult that struck the CNS of these infants occurred after the first trimester, then this was after the formation of the face was more or less complete. However, the second trimester is a very important time for brain differentiation and growth. This would explain how there could be brain problems in such normal looking, attractive children as those whose pictures are seen throughout this book.

In the Gillberg and Gillberg (1983) study, signs of clinical dysmaturity* and pre- or post-term birth were other single factors that were significantly more common in the autism group than in the control group. These authors found, however, that if one looks at the overall picture such as is seen in the optimality/reduced optimality concept, one gets a clearer picture of the perinatal complications in children with autism. 48 per cent of the children with infantile autism had reduced optimality scores above the 95th percentile for the control group. Boys and girls had equally high values. One very interesting finding was that all the children with autism showing reduced optimality in the peri- and neonatal period also had reductions in prenatal optimality.

Bryson *et al.* (1988) reported similar findings with regard to obstetric suboptimality in a population-based series of Canadian children with autism. According to a Japanese study by Shiotsuki *et al.* (1986), children with autism had significantly greater reductions of optimality in the pre-, peri- and neonatal periods than children with 'minimal brain damage' and control children with febrile seizures. A US report on a group of clinical patients (Levy *et al.* 1988) claimed that those with mental retardation were more affected by prenatal risks than were those with autism. However, the representativeness of the samples in that study is questionable. To the contrary, the Gillbergs and their co-workers presented data showing normal children to have low and children with autism to have very high reductions of optimality in the pre- and perinatal periods, with children in teenage psychosis, mental retardation and DAMP groups (in that order) being placed in between the extremes (Table 9.1).

Recently, Lord *et al.* (1991) reported on 46 high-functioning children with autism (23 male, 23 female; non-verbal IQ>60) with respect to pre- and perinatal findings (using data from medical records and maternal reports), as compared to non-autistic sibling controls. Like other authors they found a significantly raised incidence of non-optimal factors, but these were mostly related to birth order and a gestation >42 weeks. Their total reduced optimality score for male subjects (4.0) is not widely discrepant from the figure of 4.8 found among high-functioning males

---

*Taken here to mean small for gestational age (though birthweights not necessarily <2 SD below the mean), with peeling skin.

TABLE 9.1

Reduced optimality* in total population groups of normal children and children with various disorders

Group	N	Reduced optimality score†	SD	Reference
Normal	55	2.2	1.8	Gillberg *et al.* (1986)
	130	2.3	1.7	Gillberg *et al.* (1990)
	51	2.6	1.3	Gillberg and Rasmussen (1982)
Teenage psychosis	55	3.0	2.0	Gillberg *et al.* (1986)
Mental retardation	130	3.4	1.8	Gillberg *et al.* (1990)
Deficits in attention, motor control and perception (DAMP)	42	4.1	2.0	Gillberg and Rasmussen (1982)
Autism	25	5.6	2.5	Gillberg and Gillberg (1983)

*According to the method described in Gillberg and Gillberg (1983). Evaluation of medical records done blind in respect to child's diagnosis.
†The same checklist of 29 obstetric/perinatal conditions was used in all 5 groups. Possible reduced optimality scores range from 0–29.

with autism in Sweden (Gillberg *et al.* 1987).

In understanding these results, it is interesting to compare them with recent investigations of reduced optimality in cerebral palsy (Kyllerman *et al.* 1982). These findings reveal that children with infantile autism, although having reduced optimality in the perinatal period, are not so heavily affected on optimality scores as those suffering from dyskinetic cerebral palsy. Although cerebral palsy is generally thought to be associated with birth asphyxia, there is pathological evidence to suggest that a major portion of CNS lesions present at birth are due to processes of *prenatal* origin that have occurred well in advance of labour (Towbin 1969). Like children with autism, the majority of children later diagnosed as having cerebral palsy are of normal birthweight and term gestational age (Ellenberg and Nelson 1979). Thus, in this chapter, where we emphasize the evidence that there is a suboptimal perinatal period in many patients with autism, we do not necessarily imply that birth injury *per se*, rather than earlier gestational events of metabolic predisposition, puts a fetus at risk for perinatal morbidity.

In utero studies
Prenatal diagnosis of some of the genetic subgroups that are associated with autism is now a reality. In the case of chromosomal syndromes, it has been demonstrated that the fragile X chromosome can be identified in cultured amniotic fluid cells (Jenkins *et al.* 1981, Shapiro *et al.* 1982). It can also be detected prenatally through fetoscopy using short-term leukocyte cultures (Webb *et al.* 1981). With the discovery of the fragile X gene locus we may soon have more sophisticated tools for prenatal diagnosis of the fragile X syndrome.

In the metabolic subgroups found in the autistic syndromes, the identification of a specific enzyme abormality is possible if the enzyme is present in fibroblasts. Even in the case of phenylketonuria (where the enzyme in error—phenylalanine hydroxylase—is an hepatic enzyme not present in fibroblasts), the possibility of prenatal identification has been announced using recombinant DNA techniques (Woo *et al.* 1983).

Tuberous sclerosis and neurofibromatosis are two further candidates for which prenatal DNA diagnosis may be possible within the next few years. At the time of writing, however, such prenatal diagnostic measures have not been developed.

REFERENCES

Arajärvi, T., Alanen, Y.O., Viitamäki, R.O. (1964) 'Psychoses in childhood.' *Acta Psychiatrica Scandinavica*, **174** (Suppl.), 1–93.

Bryson, S.E., Smith, I.M., Eastwood, D. (1988) 'Obstetrical suboptimality in autistic children.' *Journal of the American Academy of Child and Adolescent Psychiatry*, **27**, 418–422.

Campbell, M., Hardesty, A.S., Burdock, E.I. (1978) 'Demographic and perinatal profile of 105 autistic children: a preliminary report.' *Psychopharmacology Bulletin*, **14**, 36–39.

Coleman, M. (Ed.) (1976) *The Autistic Syndromes*. Amsterdam: North Holland; New York: Elsevier.

Deykin, E.Y., MacMahon, G. (1979) 'Viral exposure and autism.' *American Journal of Epidemiology*, **109**, 628–638.

Ellenberg, J., Nelson, K. (1979) 'Birth weight and gestational age in children with cerebral palsy or seizure disorders.' *American Journal of Diseases of Children*, **133**, 1044–1049.

Felicetti, T. (1981) 'Parents of autistic children: some notes on a chemical connection.' *Milieu Therapy*, **1**, 13–16.

Finegan, J-A., Quarrington, B. (1979) 'Pre-, peri-, and neonatal factors and infantile autism.' *Journal of Child Psychology and Psychiatry*, **20**, 119–128.

Funderburk, S.J., Carter, J., Tanguay, P., Freeman, B.J., Westlake, J.R. (1983) 'Parental reproductive problems and gestational hormonal exposure in autistic and schizophrenic children.' *Journal of Autism and Developmental Disorders*, **13**, 325–332.

Gillberg, C. (1980) 'Maternal age and infantile autism.' *Journal of Autism and Developmental Disorders*, **10**, 293–297.

—— (1984) 'On the relationship between epidemiological and clinical samples.' *Journal of Autism and Developmental Disorders*, **14**, 214–217. *(Letter.)*

—— Gillberg, I.C. (1983) 'Infantile autism: a total population study of reduced optimality in the pre-, peri-, and neonatal period.' *Journal of Autism and Developmental Disorders*, **13**, 153–166.

—— Rasmussen, P. (1982) 'Perceptual, motor and attentional deficits in six-year-old children. Screening procedure in pre-school.' *Acta Paediatrica Scandinavica*, **71**, 121–129.

—— Trygstad, O., Foss, I. (1982) 'Childhood psychosis and urinary excretion of peptides and protein associated peptide complexes.' *Journal of Autism and Developmental Disorders*, **12**, 229–241.

—— Wahlström, J., Forsman, A., Hellgren, L., Gillberg, I.C. (1986) 'Teenage psychosis—epidemiology, classification and reduced optimality in the pre-, peri- and neonatal periods.' *Journal of Child Psychology and Psychiatry*, **27**, 87–98.

—— Steffenburg, S., Jakobsson, G. (1987) 'Neurobiological findings in 20 relatively gifted children with Kanner-type autism or Asperger syndrome.' *Developmental Medicine and Child Neurology*, **29**, 641–649.

—— Enerskog, I., Johansson, S. (1990) 'Mental retardation in urban children: a population study of reduced optimality in the pre-, peri- and neonatal periods.' *Developmental Medicine and Child Neurology*, **32**, 230–237.

Gillberg, I.C., Gillberg, C., Kopp, S. (1992) 'Hypothyroidism and autism spectrum disorders.' *Journal of Child Psychology and Psychiatry*, **33**, 531–542.

Harper, J., Williams, S. (1974) 'Early environmental stress and infantile autism.' *Medical Journal of Australia*, **1**, 341–346.

Jenkins, E.C., Brown, W.T., Duncan, C.J., Brooks, J., Ben-Yishay, M., Giordano, F.M., Nitowsky, H.M. (1981) 'Feasibility of fragile X chromosome prenatal diagnosis demonstrated.' *Lancet*, **2**, 1292. *(Letter.)*

Kyllerman, M., Bager, B., Bensch, J., Bille, B., Olow, I., Voss, H. (1982) 'Dyskinetic cerebral palsy. I: Clinical categories, associated neurological abnormalities and incidences.' *Acta Paediatrica Scandinavica*, **71**, 543–550.

Levy, S., Zoltak, B., Saelens, T. (1988) 'A comparison of obstetrical records of autistic and nonautistic referrals for psychoeducational evaluations.' *Journal of Autism and Developmental Disorders*, **18**, 573–581.

Lord, C., Mulloy, C., Wendelboe, M., Schopler, E. (1991) 'Pre- and perinatal factors in high-functioning females and males with autism.' *Journal of Autism and Developmental Disorders*, **21**, 197–209.

Lotter, V. (1966) 'Epidemiology of autistic conditions in young children. I. Prevalence.' *Social Psychiatry*, **1**, 124–137.

Niswander, K.R., Gordon, M. (1972) *The Women and their Pregnancies*. Washington, DC: US Government Printing Office. (DHEW pub'n no. 73–379.)

Prechtl, H.F. (1980) 'The optimality concept.' *Early Human Development*, **4**, 201–205.

Pueschel, S.M., Rynders, J.E. (1982) *Down's Syndrome: Advances in Biomedicine and the Behavioral Sciences*. Cambridge, MA: Ware Press.

Shapiro, L.R., Wilmot, P.L., Brenholz, P., Leff, A., Martino, M., Harris, G., Mahoney, M., Hobbins, J.C. (1982) 'Prenatal diagnosis of fragile X chromosome.' *Lancet*, **1**, 99–100.

Shiotsuki, Y., Otaki, E., Yamaguchi, Y., Katafuchi, Y., Matsuishi, T., Yamashita, F. (1986) 'Pregnancy, delivery and neonatal complications in infantile autism, mental retardation and minimal brain dysfunction in children.' *Brain and Development*, **8**, 796.

Steinhausen, H-C., Göbel, D., Breinlinger, M., Wohlleben, B. (1986) 'A community survey of infantile autism.' *Journal of the American Academy of Child and Adolescent Psychiatry*, **25**, 186–189.

Torrey, E.F., Hersh, S.P., McCabe, K.D. (1975) 'Early childhood psychosis and bleeding during pregnancy: a prospective study of gravid women and their offspring.' *Journal of Autism and Childhood Schizophrenia*, **5**, 287–297.

Towbin, A. (1969) 'Cerebral hypoxic damage in fetus and newborn. Basic patterns and their clinical significance.' *Archives of Neurology*, **20**, 35–43.

Treffert, D.A. (1970) 'Epidemiology of infantile autism.' *Archives of General Psychiatry*, **22**, 431–438.

Webb, T., Butler, D., Insley, J., Weaver, J.B., Green, S., Rodeck, C. (1981) 'Prenatal diagnosis of Martin-Bell syndrome associated with fragile site Xq27-28.' *Lancet*, **2**, 1423. *(Letter.)*

Wiedel, L., Coleman, M. (1976) 'The autistic and control population of this study. Demographic, historical and attitudinal data.' *In*: Coleman, M. (Ed.) *The Autistic Syndromes*. Amsterdam: North Holland; New York: Elsevier, pp. 11–20.

Woo, S.L.C., Lidsky, A.S., Güttler, F., Chandra, T., Robson, K.J.H. (1973) 'Cloned human phenylalanine hydroxylase gene allows prenatal diagnosis carrier detection of classical phenylketonuria.' *Nature*, **306**, 151–155.

10
BIOCHEMISTRY

Study of the biochemistry of the autistic syndromes has been an interesting process to watch historically; the parallels to the study of mental retardation are striking. Both autism (a behavioural disorder) and mental retardation (a cognitive disorder) are non-specific syndromes that present in early childhood—the expression of the final common pathway in the CNS of many different disease entities. Both disciplines suffer from the fact that the brain is most difficult to study directly with biochemical tools and that inferences about brain function are made from studies of other body tissues and fluids.

In the mid-19th century, most children with mental retardation were thought to have the same disease. J. Langdon Down, who distinguished trisomy 21 children (he called them 'mongols') from children with infant hypothyroidism and other forms of retardation (then all called 'cretins') began a major surge forward in the field of differentiating separate diseases of mental retardation (Down 1866). From then on, biochemical studies in mental retardation were divided into two different focuses: those seeking general (retardation) abnormalities and those seeking specific (individual disease entity) abnormalities. In the hindsight of history, it is clear to see that those tirelessly teasing out specific abnormalities patient by patient were more successful. By finding out exactly what biochemical abnormality caused a particular form of mental retardation, today some children are saved from a lifetime of mental handicap (*e.g.* infant hypothyroidism, phenylketonuria).

The biochemical studies on autism patients are also divided into two groups: those looking for a single or at least general abnormality, and those looking for specific diagnostic biochemical subgroups (metabolic errors) that might lead to individualized treatments. The results of the latter studies to date are reviewed in Chapter 17.

In this chapter we look at the studies published or under way examining the fluids and tissues of autism patients as a whole. Is there a single biochemical denominator for autism? Rationale for these studies includes trying to delineate the possible common final neurochemical pathway in the brain that functions poorly in all autism patients as well as the hope that such studies mght lead to the development of drugs tailored to treating autistic behavioural disturbances in general (see Chapter 22).

Studies of serotonin (5-hydroxytryptamine, 5-HT) metabolism (Fig. 10.1)
In a recent review of neurochemistry in the field of autism, Cook (1990) pointed out that the most consistent finding has been that over 25 per cent of children and

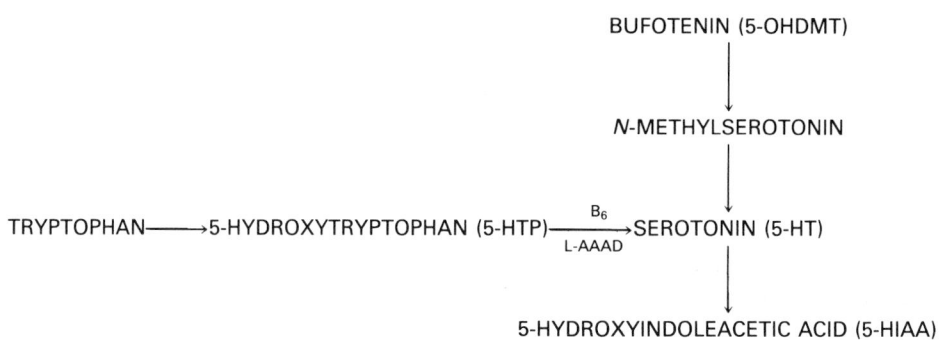

Fig. 10.1. Metabolic pathway of serotonin.

adolescents with autism are hyperserotoninaemic and that the hyperserotonin-aemia has been found to be familial. With a tinge of frustration, he also pointed out that after 29 years of investigation, the mechanism of hyperserotoninaemia has not been determined. It was in 1961 that Schain and Freedman first reported increased whole blood serotonin in six out of 23 children with infantile autism. The finding of increased whole blood or platelet serotonin in more than a quarter of children with autism has turned out to be quite robust and often replicated (Table 10.1).

Hyperserotoninaemia is not just a finding in autism—it has been reported in chronic schizophrenia (Freedman *et al.* 1981), Huntington chorea (Belendiuk *et al.* 1980) and motor neuron disease (Belendiuk *et al.* 1981). Serotonin abnormalities as measured by blood studies are an old story in generalized studies of mental retardation also. Some of the retarded patients with a variety of disease entities have been found to have hyperserotoninaemia (kernicterus, leukodystrophy, lipidosis, mucopolysaccharidosis, dysautonomia, Schilder disease, rubella embryo-pathy, infant hypothyroidism, infantile spasms, tuberous sclerosis) or hyposero-toninaemia (trisomy 21, histidinaemia, deLange syndrome, phenylketonuria) (references summarized in Coleman 1973*a,b*). Note that some of these diseases are also included in the autistic spectrum (Table 10.2).

In fact, when a child with autism is found to have an abnormal level of serotonin, both systemic diseases and diseases of the CNS need to be considered. Serotonin is present in several different body tissues—the enterochromaffin system of the gastrointestinal tract, the spleen, the blood platelets, the thyroid, the lung, and the central and peripheral nervous systems. When serotonin is measured in the blood, it is not a direct measurement of CNS serotonin. Haverback and Davidson (1958) studied an adult patient with resection of the large and small intestine and demonstrated that 97 per cent of his whole blood serotonin and 75 per cent of his urinary 5-hydroxyindolacetic acid (5-HIAA, the end-product of serotonin meta-bolism) originated from the intestines. CNS serotonin is made *de novo* from tryptophan; Bertaccini (1960) has shown that in the rat the total removal of the

TABLE 10.1

Endogenous serotonin levels reported in persons with autism

Study	Patients (Controls)*	Medium tested	Results
Schain and Freedman (1961)	23 (12 + 4)	Whole blood	6/23 patients had elevated serotonin
Ritvo et al. (1970)	24 (36)	Whole blood	Higher in patients (p<0.006)
Yuwiler et al. (1971)	7 (4)	Whole blood	No significant difference; circadian rhythmicity not observed
Campbell et al. (1974)	11 (6)	Platelet-rich plasma	No significant difference
Suemitsu et al. (1974)	6 (6)	Serum	Higher in patients (p<0.05)
Goldstein et al. (1976)	72 (71)	Whole blood	Higher in patients (p<0.01)
Takahashi et al. (1976)	30 (30 + 45)	Platelet pellet	Higher in patients (p<0.02)
Hanley et al. (1977)	27 (23 + 6)	Whole blood	Higher in patients (p<0.01)
Hoshino et al. (1979)	42 (20)	Serum	Higher in patients (p<0.05)
Douay et al. (1980)	10 (11)	Whole blood	Higher in patients (p<0.01)
Hoshino et al. (1984)	37 (39)	Whole blood	Higher in patients (p<0.02)
Anderson et al. (1987)	40 (87)	Whole blood	Higher in patients (p<0.001)
Babcock et al. (1987)	30 (106)	Whole blood	Higher in patients (p<0.05); maturational decline with age missing in children with autism
Ferrari et al. (1987)	22 (22)	Whole blood	Higher in patients (p<0.05)
Minderaa et al. (1987)	36 (27)	Whole blood	Higher in patients (p<0.01)
Geller et al. 1988)	19 (26)	Whole blood	Patient level within limits of controls
Launay et al. (1988)	22 (22)	Whole blood	Higher in patients (p<0.02)
Abramson et al. (1989)	57 (17)	Whole blood	Higher in patients (p<0.001); serotonin levels segregate by families
Minderaa et al. (1989)	17 (20)	Whole blood	Higher in patients (p<0.02)
Piven et al. (1991)	28 (10)	Platelet-rich plasma	Levels highest in familial autism

*Two sets of controls = normal + neurologically impaired.

gastrointestinal tract has very little effect on brain serotonin, in spite of decreasing blood, spleen and lung levels.

Thus, the serotonin in the brain is not being measured directly. High serotonin levels in the blood do not necessarily mean high levels in the brain itself. In fact, there is a report of a child who had a degenerative disease (leukodystrophy) and many high blood serotonin values during life, but in whom a serotonin level well below that of a normal control brain was measured in the CNS on autopsy (Coleman et al. 1977). There is evidence that central serotoninergic responsivity is reduced, based on a study of altered serotonin-mediated responses in a small sample of young adult males with autism; this central effect seen with fenfluramine-induced prolactin release is negatively correlated with whole blood serotonin content (McBride et al. 1989a). One hypothesis, based in part on the pharmacology of epilepsy, suggests that high levels of blood serotonin signal that some type of

TABLE 10.2

**Disease entities to consider in
patients with autism with
abnormal serotonin levels**

Hyperserotoninaemia
    Infant hypothyroidism
    Maternal rubella
    Tuberous sclerosis
    Williams syndrome

Hyposerotoninaemia
    Phenylketonuria
    Cornelia deLange syndrome

compensatory mechanism is in process at the platelet binding site for functionally low levels of serotonin at neuronal binding sites in the brain itself.

There is little evidence so far that the rate of serotonin metabolism is altered in individuals with autism. 5-HIAA, the final metabolite for more than 95 per cent of serotonin, has been studied in both the urine and CSF of patients with autism (Leckman *et al.* 1980, Winsberg *et al.* 1980, Gillberg *et al.* 1983, Gillberg and Svennerholm 1987, Minderaa *et al.* 1987), and serotonin itself has been studied in urine (Jouve *et al.* 1986, Anderson *et al.* 1989). These recent studies are generally not suggestive of increased metabolic turnover of the serotonin pathway, which could account for the findings of hyperserotoninaemia in autism. Studies of enzymes in the serotonin pathway (summarized by Anderson *et al.* 1990) have also not been helpful in explaining the hyperserotoninaemia. One study (Launay *et al.* 1988) does dispute the general consensus, suggesting evidence for a metabolic origin of hyperserotoninaemia (Winsberg *et al.* 1980).

In the blood, more than 99 per cent of the serotonin is in the platelet, a cell that can be used as a partial model for the serotoninergic neuron (Paasonen 1968). Both platelets and neurons transport serotonin in an energy-dependent process, store it in subcellular organelles of similar electron-microscopic appearance and metabolize serotonin in a similar way (Pletscher 1968). A recent study focusing on the plasma ultrafiltrate of autism patients and family members found that the increased serotonin in the whole blood of children with autism appears to be due solely to elevation of platelet serotonin (Cook *et al.* 1988). A great deal of work has been done on how the platelet handles serotonin uptake, storage and release in patients with autism; there are excellent recent summaries of this extensive literature (Anderson *et al.* 1990, Cook 1990).

There are multiple receptor subtypes for serotonin; they have been classified into three 'families' of receptor subtypes in the CNS (Peroutka *et al.* 1990). The only serotonin-receptor binding site that has been characterized on the platelet to date is the 5-HT$_2$ binding site (Leysen *et al.* 1984); studies conducted on subjects with autism have failed to find a significant correlation between whole blood serotonin and 5-HT$_2$ receptor binding site B$_{MAX}$ (McBride *et al.* 1989*b*; Perry *et al.* 1991). (Autoantibodies to a 5-HT$_{1A}$ receptor have been reported in one patient with autism—Todd and Ciaranello 1985.)

Three major systems outside the brain—gastrointestinal (carcinoid, malabsorption, acute gastroenteritis, intestinal obstruction and congenital anomalies of the gastrointestinal tract), vascular (collagen–vascular disease, migraine, [following] myocardial infarction) and thyroid (hypothyroid [infants], hyperthyroid)—can cause abnormalities in serotonin levels in blood. Stress, drugs and even body rhythms can affect the level of serotonin in an individual. Diet has very little effect; in an extraordinary experiment where a child consumed 1.6mg/kg of exogenous serotonin in a food very high in serotonin (bananas), there was only a temporary change of 3ng/mL of whole blood serotonin level per banana (Coleman 1973*a,b*). Most meals have no effect on whole blood levels of serotonin (Anderson *et al.* 1985), although it is known from rat experiments that the ingestion of food containing tryptophan or stimulating insulin may have some effect on serotonin levels in the CNS (Fernstrom and Wurtman 1971). Serotonin levels are also affected by many drugs prescribed for patients with autism (see Chapter 22).

In patients with autism, once it is clear that the abnormal value is not due to drugs or systemic problems, then the disease entities of the autistic syndromes which have CNS correlations with unusual serotonin values (Table 10.2) should be investigated in those patients who have test values out of the normal range. Whether patients who suffer from either autism or mental retardation (or both) with these diseases are more likely to have hyperserotoninaemia than those who do not is a highly relevant question worthy of further statistical investigation in each of these disease entities (Kuperman *et al.* 1987, August and Realmuto 1989). Undoubtedly, new disease entities will be added to this list as the underlying diseases involved in autism unfold. Most patients with hyperserotoninaemia do not have one of the underlying diseases listed in the table; the hard work of diagnosing most of the hyperserotoninergic patients with autism lies ahead.

It has been known for some time, at least in mentally retarded patients, that blood serotonin levels in pathological states are not fixed and that abnormalities of whole blood serotonin may be able to be changed if the underlying biochemical disorder is identified and treated. For example, in a published case of hyperserotoninaemia associated with infant hypothyroidism, the excessively high level of blood serotonin appeared to be diminished by treatment of the underlying condition with thyroid therapy (Coleman 1970). Conversely, the hyposerotoninaemia of phenylketonuria (a disease entity which includes a subgroup of patients with autism—see Chapter 17) may be improved, even elevated into the normal range, by dietary therapy (Pare *et al.* 1958, Baldridge *et al.* 1959, McKean 1971). McKean reported a simultaneous 'abrupt increase in blood serotonin and improved behavior' at phenylalanine levels of 10 to 12mg/dL in three patients and at levels of 5mg/dL in a fourth child. In this study there appeared to be a close relationship between blood serotonin and behaviour.

One interesting aspect of monoamine metabolism in human beings is that often there is a familial factor in the levels of the amines and their enzymes (Ebstein *et al.* 1974). To take one example, in the case of blood serotonin, a non-autistic severely retarded patient with extremely high levels was described in the literature (Coleman *et al.* 1970) and later had a sibling born with moderately elevated levels of blood serotonin. Although this laboratory finding provoked concern in both the medical staff and the parents, the infant developed into a bright, normal child.

In the case of serotonin levels in children with autism, a number of studies have found familial factors (Kuperman *et al.* 1985, Leventhal *et al.* 1990, Piven *et al.* 1991). Kuperman *et al.* reported that platelet-rich plasma was significantly correlated between parents and children within families with a proband with autism. Specifically, the presence of hyperserotoninaemia has been documented as familial between patients with autism and their first-degree relatives (Abramson *et al.* 1989, Cook *et al.* 1990, Leventhal *et al.* 1990). The latter study found first-degree relatives were 2.4 times more likely to be hyperserotoninaemic if the child with autism was hyperserotoninaemic than if s/he was not. Piven *et al.*(1991) noted that the serotonin levels of subjects with autism who had affected siblings were significantly higher than those of probands without affected siblings and suggested that serotonin levels in subjects with autism may be associated with genetic factors or a predisposition to autism.

Serotonin has a special relevance to developmental disorders, including autism, because it is specifically involved in early neurogenesis (Lauder and Krebs 1978, Whitaker-Azmitia *et al.* 1987, Zhou *et al.* 1987, Azmitia *et al.* 1990). One question that the consistent finding of blood serotonin abnormalities in a number of children with autism raises is whether these findings reflect biochemical aberrations also present during fetal life. If that were so, it might be relevant to the developmental cortical malformations, particularly polymicrogyria, that have been described in patients with autism (see Chapter 19).

Studies of catecholamine metabolism

Another area where a great deal of work has been done with patients with autism is that of catecholamine metabolism (Fig. 10.2). As in the serotonin studies, often some of the patients in these studies were on medication that could affect monoamine values. Catecholamine studies are further complicated by the factor of stress, even of the test itself, which can be reflected in these measured values.

The catecholamine pathway is a metabolic pathway where enzyme errors are known to occur that can cause CNS diseases. An error in the first enzyme in the pathway, phenylalanine hydroxylase, which converts phenylalanine to tyrosine, causes the disease phenylketonuria. A significant number of these patients have autistic symptoms (see Chapter 17) if they are not adequately treated for this metabolic disease. Late maturation of the enzyme in the second step of the pathway can cause a neonatal tyrosinaemia whose symptoms include later learning disabilities and other brain dysfunction (Menkes *et al.* 1972). The third amino acid

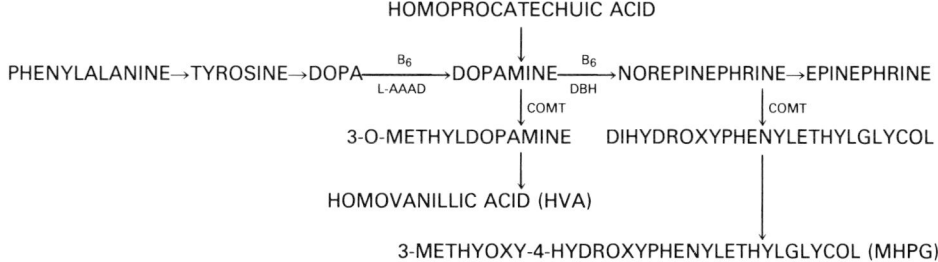

HOMOPROCATECHUIC ACID

PHENYLALANINE→TYROSINE→DOPA $\xrightarrow[\text{L-AAAD}]{\text{B}_6}$ DOPAMINE $\xrightarrow[\text{DBH}]{\text{B}_6}$ NOREPINEPHRINE→EPINEPHRINE

3-O-METHYLDOPAMINE   DIHYDROXYPHENYLETHYLGLYCOL

HOMOVANILLIC ACID (HVA)

3-METHYOXY-4-HYDROXYPHENYLETHYLGLYCOL (MHPG)

Fig. 10.2. Metabolic pathway of catecholamines.

in the pathway, dioxyphenylalanine (dopa), can be used to affect the level of the following amine, dopamine. Dopa, in its levo-form L-dopa, is used therapeutically in brain diseases with evidence of decreased levels of the amines of the catecholamine pathway (Parkinson disease, dystonia). Dopamine, norepinephrine and epinephrine are the active amines of the pathway; the first two amines are particularly vital for CNS function.

There is only a tiny amount of dopamine in human plasma, which makes it difficult to measure—one study of children with autism found a normal amount (Launay *et al.* 1987), while another found an elevated amount (Israngkun *et al.* 1986). Platelet dopamine levels were decreased in the former study. Regarding studies on the brain itself, increased dopamine presynaptic uptake carrier sites have been found in post-mortem studies on three adults with Tourette syndrome (a syndrome where autistic symptoms are found in some children) (Singer *et al.* 1991). These findings suggest enhanced dopamine uptake within the striatum of these patients with Tourette syndrome.

Dopamine is the neurotransmitter of a brain system especially vulnerable to the effects of cocaine. Infants exposed to the cocaine derivative crack *in utero* (so-called 'crack babies') have been reported to have autistic symptoms such as tactile hypersensitivity and not liking to be held, major attentional disorders and a problem of easily being overwhelmed by stimulation, inability to form close human relationships and poor attachment to caregivers, disinterest in toys, etc. Microcephaly is now documented in a number of these infants, possibly induced by impaired maternal nutrition and/or vasoconstriction in the placenta (Fulroth *et al.* 1989). However, the complexity of the real life factors affecting these children makes any generalization about dopamine systems premature. In fact, a prospective study by Chasnoff *et al.* (1992) suggests that if intervention occurs (maintenance of maternal prenatal care and nutrition and support for the mother after birth), the overwhelming majority of babies do not show the autistic-like symptoms.

Plasma norepinephrine and epinephrine have been measured in patients with autism, though it is possible that the stress of the mere insertion of the catheter to perform these studies may affect the results. The studies to date suggest that plasma norepinephrine (Lake *et al.* 1977, Cook *et al.* 1990, Leventhal *et al.* 1990) or both plasma norepinephrine and epinephrine (Israngkun *et al.* 1986, Launay *et al.* 1987) appear to be elevated in patients with autism. One interpretation of these findings is that they are relevant to brain function in autism, since plasma and CSF norepinephrine are closely correlated; another interpretation suggests that patients with autism handle stress less well than the controls. A platelet study found decreased levels of platelet norepinephrine and epinephrine in subjects with autism (Launay *et al.* 1987).

Dopamine-β-hydroxylase is an enzyme stored with norepinephrine in the granular vesicles of nerve endings of the sympathetic nervous system as well as the chromaffin granules of the adrenal medulla. It is released into the blood with norepinephrine and epinephrine after sympathetic nervous system stimulation of the adrenal gland. Low levels (Goldstein *et al.* 1976, Lake *et al.* 1977), normal levels (Young *et al.* 1980) and elevated levels in a subgroup (Garnier *et al.* 1986) and in children with functional psychoses (Belmaker *et al.* 1978) are all reported in the literature.

The end-product of dopamine metabolism is homovanillic acid (HVA), while the final metabolite of norepinephrine is 3-methoxy-4-hydroxyphenylethylglycol (MHPG). As can be seen in Table 10.3, HVA has been studied in both CSF and urine. The CSF studies have been contradictory, with some showing normal ranges and others demonstrating higher values. The urine studies have also shown both elevated and normal values. A recent study of plasma HVA levels in persons with autism showed results not significantly different from normal controls (Minderaa *et al.* 1989). Of course, in none of these studies is HVA exclusively from the brain being examined; even in CSF studies, much of the result comes from an ultrafiltrate of blood. A recent study reported that the urinary increase of HVA in children with autism appears to be in the free (unconjugated) portion, while an increase which is also noted in retarded children comes from the conjugated portion (Garreau *et al.* 1988).

A series of studies of MHPG in autism by Young *et al.* (1979, 1981) reported decreased urinary levels but plasma and CSF values within normal limits. A study by Gillberg *et al.* (1983) also found CSF values within the normal range.

Catecholamines are inactivated by O-methylation via the enzyme catechol-O-methyltransferase. The enzyme measured in the red cells (O'Brien *et al.* 1976, Belmaker *et al.* 1978, Giller *et al.* 1980) and the fibroblasts (Giller *et al.* 1980) of individuals with autism has been reported to be in the normal range. Monoamine oxidase, another degradation enzyme in both the catecholamine and serotonin pathways, has also been extensively studied and found to be within the normal range in plasma, platelets and fibroblasts.

Cyclic AMP

Cyclic AMP (adenosine monophosphate) is believed to act as the 'second

TABLE 10.3

Homovanillic acid (HVA) levels reported in persons with autism

Study	Patients/Controls*	Medium tested	Results
Cohen *et al.* (1974)	9A/11At/15Neu	CSF	Levels in patients with autism higher than in patients with epilepsy
Cohen *et al.* (1977)	10A/33Neu	CSF	Levels in patients not significantly different from controls
Lelord *et al.* (1978)	37A/11	Urine	Levels higher in patients (p<0.01)
Garreau *et al.* (1980)	44A/20	Urine	Levels higher in patients (p<0.01)
Winsberg *et al.* (1980)	8A/0	CSF	With no controls, hard to interpret
Martineau *et al.* (1981)	12A/11	Urine	Levels higher in patients (p<0.01)
Gillberg *et al.* (1983)	13A/22	CSF	Levels higher in patients (p<0.02)
Garnier *et al.* (1986)	19A/15	Urine	Levels higher in patients (p<0.02)
Gillberg and Svennerholm (1987)	25A/20	CSF	Levels higher in patients (p<0.001)
Barthélémy *et al.* (1988)	8A/8	Urine	Levels of free (unconjugated) HVA higher in patients (p<0.05)
Garreau *et al.* (1988)	34A/34	Urine	Increased HVA in autism is in the free (unconjugated) portion (p<0.05)
Minderaa *et al.* (1989)	40A/20	Urine	Levels in patients not significantly different from controls
		Plasma	Levels in patients not significantly different from controls

*A = patients with autism; At = patients with atypical 'autistic-like' conditions; Neu = patients with other neurological impairments. Where unspecified, controls were normal individuals.

messenger' inside the cell for neurotransmitters such as serotonin and the catecholamines; thus it could be considered as a possible reflector of post-synaptic receptor activity for some active amines in the CNS. It also affects calcium release in platelets (Moos and Goldberg 1988).

Belmaker *et al.* (1978) studied plasma cyclic AMP in eight children with autism compared to children with other types of psychiatric diagnoses and found no statistical difference between the levels; however, these were all elevated compared to adult control values. The following year, Hoshino *et al.* (1979) found elevated levels in 20 children with autism compared to both normal children and adults. The authors also reported a positive relationship between plasma cyclic AMP and serum serotonin. Another study by this group, carefully repeated with subjects with autism not on any medication, again found elevated levels compared to controls but also found that hyperkinetic mentally retarded children also had elevated levels (Hoshino *et al.* 1980). Goldberg *et al.* (1984) compared adolescents with autism and 'pervasive developmental disorder' to normal adolescents and again confirmed an elevation of plasma cyclic AMP in the patient group. (An additional interesting finding was that plasma cyclic GMP (guanine monophosphate), a nucleotide stimulated by different neurotransmitters, such as acetylcholine, was not elevated.)

These studies suggest that plasma cyclic AMP may be elevated in psychiatrically disturbed children, including those with autism.

Glial fibrillary acidic protein (GFA)
The CSF of 47 children with autism, contrasted to that of children with other neuropsychiatric disorders and of normal controls, was studied for GFA, a marker for the degree of gliosis and an indicator of neuronal density (Ahlsén, personal communication). GFA is elevated in both acute and chronic states of brain degeneration; glial S-100, a soluble marker for neurons, is elevated only in the acute state. GFA in autism and autistic-like conditions was at a level almost three times that in the normal group, putting autism into a category with other chronic neurological diseases; S-100 was unchanged. This very large study of CSF is an important first step in defining this area of research in the autistic syndromes.

Amino acids/organic acids
It is now well established that one error in amino acid metabolism (phenylketo-nuria) can produce autistic-like symptoms (see Chapter 17). To date, no other metabolic errors have been described in relation to amino acid metabolism in children with autistic symptoms. A study by Perry *et al.* (1978) of amino acid levels in plasma, urine and CSF of 34 children with childhood psychoses (28 having infantile autism) showed no known disease entities. In this CSF study, ethanol-amine appeared to be elevated in some autistic patients. Another study of CSF amino acids in children with autism (Winsberg *et al.* 1980) found them normal as a group, although two children did have an elevation of arginine.

The 34 children in the Perry *et al.* (1978) study also had organic acid levels in plasma, urine and CSF tested by gas chromatography. None of the known diseases of organic acid metabolism was found, although unidentified peaks were noted.

Peptides
Many individuals with autism are relatively insensitive to pain or are self-injurious, and this has led to an interest in studying opiate activity in this patient group. The endogenous opioids, or endorphins, constitute a chemically complex family of peptides which serve as so-called neuroregulators of the human CNS. Decreased levels of humoral endorphins (plasma opiates) have been reported in patients with autism (Weizman *et al.* 1984, 1988). Plasma beta-endorphin levels in children with autism have also been reported as lower (Sandman *et al.* 1991). Urinary peptide patterns have been reported as both abnormal (Trygstad *et al.* 1980, Israngkun *et al.* 1986, Reichelt *et al.* 1986) and normal (Le Couteur *et al.* 1988).

Gillberg *et al.* (1985) reported elevated CSF endorphin fraction II in 20 children with autism, 11 of whom had both decreased pain sensitivity and CSF fraction II levels above the highest control value. Both abnormally high (Ross *et al.* 1987) and abnormally low (Gillberg *et al.* 1990) levels of CSF beta-endorphin have been reported.

Mineral and ion studies

Levels of several ions have been reported as abnormal in children with autism. The most consistent finding has been reports of lower levels of magnesium. Saladino and Sankar (1973) reported that magnesium levels were lower in the erythrocytes of a child psychiatric patient group compared to normal controls. This finding led to serum magnesium being included in a large biochemical study of 59 children with autism (Coleman *et al.* 1976); levels in these children were significantly lower than in normal controls (p<0.001). Another study (Hayek 1991) also showed lower values of magnesium in erythrocytes in children with autism; Rett syndrome children were studied separately and did not have a significantly lower value.

Magnesium, the second most abundant intracellular cation, is an important ion in brain function; low levels are known to predispose to apathy, irritability and seizures. In animal experiments, magnesium deficiency in the presence of high thiamine levels can result in significant elevations of blood serotonin (Itokawa *et al.* 1972). Magnesium is involved in several of the metabolic systems already identified as working abnormally in one or more children with autism (see Chapters 17 and 23). Since magnesium is lost in the processing of many modern foods, evaluation of magnesium levels in a patient with autistic symptoms, particularly if they are accompanied by seizures, is indicated.

Magnesium is a mimic/antagonist of calcium. One study has been done of serum and 24-hour urinary levels of calcium in children with autism (Coleman *et al.* 1976). No statistically significant differences were found in the serum or urine calcium levels, although the results were highly skewed, 22 per cent of the patients having urinary levels >2 SD below the mean. At the time of the study, 10 per cent of the patients had received a diagnosis of coeliac disease from their paediatricians; later follow-up studies indicated that these children in fact did not have coeliac disease (McCarthy and Coleman 1979).

Potassium levels have been tested in patients with autism; a depression of red blood cell potassium was reported in patients compared to controls (Saladino and Sankar 1973).

In contrast to the other minerals discussed in this section, lead has no known enzymatic function in the human body: it is a contaminant. Several studies have shown that lead levels tend to be higher in some patients with autism, a worrisome finding (Cohen *et al.* 1976, Accardo *et al.* 1988).

Conclusion

A more complete understanding of the biochemistry patterns seen in patients with autism may help in the future to develop a more specific pharmacology for this syndrome. A start has been made in this direction.

REFERENCES

Abramson, R.K., Wright, H.H., Carpenter, R., Brennan, W., Lumpuy, O., Cole, E., Young, S.R. (1989) 'Elevated serotonin in autistic probands and their first-degree relatives.' *Journal of Autism and Developmental Disorders*, **19**, 397–407.

Accardo, P., Whitman, B., Caul, J., Rolfe, U. (1988) 'Autism and plumbism.' *Clinical Pediatrics*, **27**, 41–44.

Anderson, G.M., Horne, W.C., Chatterjee, D., Cohen, D.J. (1990) 'The hyperserotonemia of autism.' *Annals of the New York Academy of Sciences*, **600**, 331–340.

—— Feibel, F.C., Wetlaufer, L.A., Schlicht, K.R., Ort, S.M., Cohen, D.J. (1985) 'Effect of a meal on human whole blood serotonin.' *Gastroenterology*, **88**, 86–89.

—— Freedman, D.X., Cohen, D.J., Volkmar, F.R., Hoder, E.L., McPhedran, P., Minderaa, R.B., Hansen, C.R., Young, J.G. (1987) 'Whole blood serotonin in autistic and normal subjects.' *Journal of Child Psychology and Psychiatry*, **28**, 885–900.

—— Minderaa, R.B., Cho, S.C., Volkmar, F.R., Cohen, D.J. (1989) 'The issue of hyperserotonemia and platelet serotonin exposure: a preliminary study.' *Journal of Autism and Developmental Disorders*, **19**, 349–351. *(Letter.)*

August, G.J., Realmuto, G.M. (1989) 'Williams syndrome: serotonin's association with developmental disabilities.' *Journal of Autism and Developmental Disorders*, **19**, 137–141.

Azmitia, E.C., Frankfurt, M., Davila, M., Whitaker-Azmitia, P.M., Zhou, F.C. (1990) 'Plasticity of fetal and adult CNS serotonergic neurons: role of growth-regulatory factors.' *Annals of the New York Academy of Sciences*, **600**, 343–363.

Badcock, N.R., Spence, J.G., Stern, L.M. (1987) 'Blood serotonin levels in adults, autistic and non-autistic children, with a comparison of different methodologies.' *Annals of Clinical Biochemistry*, **24**, 625–634.

Baldridge, R.C., Borofsky, L., Baird, H., Reichle, F., Bullock, D. (1959) 'Relationship of serum phenylalanine levels and ability of phenylketonurics to hydroxylate tryptophan.' *Proceedings of the Society of Experimental Biology*, **100**, 529–531.

Barthélémy, C., Bruneau, N., Cottet-Eymard, J.M., Domenech-Jouve, J., Garreau, B., Lelord, G., Muh, J.P., Peyrin, L. (1988) 'Urinary free and conjugated catecholamines and metabolites in autistic children.' *Journal of Autism and Developmental Disorders*, **18**, 583–591.

Belendiuk, K., Belendiuk, G.W., Freedman, D.X. (1980) 'Blood monoamine metabolism in Huntington's disease.' *Archives of General Psychiatry*, **37**, 325–332.

—— —— —— Antel, J.P. (1981) 'Neurotransmitter abnormalities in patients with motor neuron disease.' *Archives of Neurology*, **38**, 415–417.

Belmaker, R.H., Hattab, J., Ebstein, R.P. (1978) 'Plasma dopamine-beta-hydroxylase in childhood psychosis.' *Journal of Autism and Childhood Schizophrenia*, **8**, 293–298.

Bertaccini, G. (1960) 'Tissue 5-hydroxytryptamine and urinary 5-HIAA after partial or total removal of the gastroinestinal tract in the rat.' *Journal of Physiology*, **153**, 239–249.

Campbell, M., Friedman, E., DeVito, E., Greenspan, L., Collins, P. (1974) 'Blood serotonin in psychotic and brain damaged children.' *Journal of Autism and Childhood Schizophrenia*, **4**, 33–41.

Chasnoff, I.J., Griffith, D.R., Freier, C., Murray, J. (1992) 'Cocaine/polydrug use in pregnancy: two-year follow-up. *Pediatrics*, **89**, 284–289.

Cohen, D.J., Shaywitz, B.A., Johnson, W.T., Bowers, M.B. (1974) 'Biogenic amines in autistic and atypical children: cerebrospinal fluid measures of homovanillic acid and 5-hydroxyindoleacetic acid.' *Archives of General Psychiatry*, **31**, 845–853.

—— Johnson, W.T., Caparulo, B.K. (1976) 'Pica and elevated blood lead level in autistic and atypical children.' *American Journal of Diseases of Children*, **130**, 47–48.

—— Caparulo, B.K., Shaywitz, B.A., Bowers, M.B. (1977) 'Dopamine and serotonin metabolism in neuropsychiatrically disturbed children: CSF homovanillic acid and 5-hydroxyindoleacetic acid.' *Archives of General Psychiatry*, **34**, 545–550.

Coleman, M. (1970) 'Serotonin levels in infant hypothyroidism.' *Lancet*, **2**, 365. *(Letter.)*

—— (1973*a*) 'Appendix IX-1' *In:* Coleman, M. (Ed.) *Serotonin in Down's Syndrome.* Amsterdam: North Holland; New York: Elsevier, pp. 213–216.

—— (1973*b*) 'Appendix IX-2' *In:* Coleman, M. (Ed.) *Serotonin in Down's Syndrome.* Amsterdam: North Holland; New York: Elsevier, p. 217.

—— Barnet, A., Boullin, D. (1970) 'Parachlorophenylalanine administration to a retarded patient with high blood serotonin levels.' *Transactions of the American Neurological Association*, **95**, 224–226.

—— Landgrebe, M.A., Landgrebe, A.R. (1976) 'Celiac autism: calcium studies and their relationship to celiac disease in autistic patients.' *In:* Coleman, M. (Ed.) *The Autistic Syndromes.* Amsterdam:

North Holland; New York: Elsevier, pp. 197–205.

—— Hart, P.N., Randall, J., Lee, J., Hijada, D., Bratendahl, C.G. (1977) 'Serotonin levels in the blood and central nervous system of a patient with sudanophilic leukodystrophy.' *Neuropädiatrie*, **8**, 459–466.

Cook, E.H. (1990) 'Autism: review of neurochemical investigation.' *Synapse*, **6**, 292–308.

—— Leventhal, B.L., Freedman, D.X. (1988) 'Free serotonin in plasma: autistic children and their first-degree relatives.' *Biological Psychiatry*, **24**, 488–491.

—— —— Heller, W., Metz, J., Wainwright, M., Freedman, D.X. (1990) 'Autistic children and their first-degree relatives: relationships between peripheral neurotransmitter levels and measured intelligence.' *Journal of Neuropsychiatry and Clinical Neurosciences*, **2**, 268–274.

Douay, O., Debray-Ritzen, P., Kamoun, P. (1980) 'Sérotonine et tryptophane sanguin dans l'autisme.' *Annales de Biologie Clinique*, **38**, 243.

Down, J.H.L. (1866) 'Observations on an ethnic classification of idiots.' *London Hospital Reports*, **3**, 259–262. (*Reprinted 1990 in* Down, J.L. *Mental Affections of Childhood and Youth. Classics in Developmental Medicine No. 5.* London: MacKeith Press with Blackwell Scientific; Philadelphia: J.B. Lippincott, pp. 127–131.)

Ebstein, R.P., Freedman, L.S., Lieberman, A., Park, D., Pasternack, B., Goldstein, M., Coleman, M. (1974) 'A familial study of serum dopamine-beta-hydroxylase levels in torsion dystonia.' *Neurology*, **24**, 684–687.

Fernstrom, J.D., Wurtman, R.J. (1971) 'Brain serotonin content: increase following ingestion of carbohydrate diet.' *Science*, **174**, 1023–1025.

Ferrari, P., Bursztejn, C., Launay, J.M., Haimart, M., Braconnier, A., Lancrenon, S., Bondoux, D., Tabuteau, F., Luong, C.L., Fermanian, J., *et al.* (1987) 'Bioamines et autisme infantile.' *In:* Gremy, F., Tomkiewicz, S., Ferrari, P., Lelord, G. (Eds) *Autisme Infantile, Vol. 146.* Paris: INSERM, pp. 121–128.

Freedman, D.X., Belendiuk, K., Belendiuk, G.W., Crayton, J.W. (1981) 'Blood tryptophan metabolism in chronic schizophrenics.' *Archives of General Psychiatry*, **38**, 655–659.

Fulroth, R., Phillips, B, Durand, D.J. (1989) 'Perinatal outcome of infants exposed to cocaine and/or heroin in utero.' *American Journal of Diseases of Children*, **143**, 905–910.

Garnier, C., Comoy, E., Barthélémy, C., Leddet, I., Garreau, B., Muh, J.P., Lelord, G. (1986) 'Dopamine-beta-hydroxylase (DBH) and homovanillic acid (HVA) in autistic children.' *Journal of Autism and Developmental Disorders*, **16**, 23–29.

Garreau, B., Barthélémy, C., Sauvage, D., Muh, J.P., Lelord, G., Calloway, E. (1980) 'Troubles du métabolisme de la dopamine chez des enfants ayant un comportement autistique. Resultats des examens cliniques et des dosages urinaires de l'acide homovanilique.' *Acta Psychiatrica Belgica*, **80**, 249–265.

—— —— Jouve, J., Bruneau, N., Muh, J.P., Lelord, G. (1988) 'Urinary homovanillic acid levels of autistic children.' *Developmental Medicine and Child Neurology*, **30**, 93–98.

Geller, E., Yuwiler, A., Freeman, B.J., Ritvo, E.R. (1988) 'Platelet size, number and serotonin content in blood of autistic, childhood schizophrenic and normal children.' *Journal of Autism and Developmental Disorders*, **18**, 119–126.

Gillberg, C., Svennerholm, L. (1987) 'CSF monoamines in autistic syndromes and other pervasive developmental disorders of early childhood.' *British Journal of Psychiatry*, **151**, 89–94.

—— —— Hamilton-Hellberg, C. (1983) 'Childhood psychosis and monoamine metabolism in spinal fluid.' *Journal of Autism and Developmental Disorders*, **13**, 383–396.

—— Terenius, L., Lonnerholm, G. (1985) 'Endorphin activity in childhood psychosis.' *Archives of General Psychiatry*, **42**, 780–783.

—— —— Hagberg, B., Witt-Engerström, I., Eriksson, I. (1990) 'CSF beta-endorphin in childhood neuropsychiatric disorders.' *Brain and Development*, **12**, 88–92.

Giller, E.L., Young, J.G., Breakefield, X.O., Carbonari, C., Braverman, M., Cohen, D.J. (1980) 'Monoamine oxidase and catechol-O-methyltransferase activites in cultured fibroblasts and blood cells from children with autism and the Gilles de la Tourette syndrome.' *Psychiatry Research*, **2**, 187–197.

Goldberg, M., Hattab, J., Meir, D., Ebstein, L., Belmaker, R. (1984) 'Plasma cyclic AMP and cyclic GMP in childhood-onset psychoses.' *Journal of Autism and Developmental Disorders*, **14**, 159–164.

Goldstein, M., Mahanand, D., Lee, J., Coleman, M. (1976) 'Dopamine-beta-hydroxylase and endogenous total 5-hydroxyindole levels in autistic patients and controls.' *In:* Coleman, M. (Ed.) *The Autistic Syndromes.* Amsterdam: North Holland; New York: Elsevier, pp. 57–63.

Hanley, H.G., Stahl, S.M., Freeman, D. (1977) 'Hyperserotonemia and amine metabolites in autistic and retarded children.' *Archives of General Psychiatry*, **34**, 521–531.

Haverback, B.J., Davidson, J.D. (1958) 'Serotonin and the gastrointestinal tract.' *Gastroenterology*, **35**, 570–578.

Hayek, J. (1991) 'Intracellular magnesium in autistic subjects.' *Brain Dysfunction. (In press.)*

Hoshino, Y., Kumashiro, H., Kaneko, M., Numata, Y., Honda, K., Yashima, Y., Tachibana, R., Watanabe, M. (1979) 'Serum serotonin, free tryptophan and plasma cyclic AMP levels in autistic children—with special reference to their relation to hyperkinesia.' *Fukushima Journal of Medical Science*, **26**, 79–91.

—— Ohno, Y., Murata, S., Yokoyama, F., Kaneko, M., Kumashiro, H. (1980) 'Plasma cyclic AMP level in psychiatric diseases of childhood.' *Folia Psychiatrica et Neurologica Japonica*, **34**, 9–16.

—— Yamamoto, T., Kaneko, M., Tachibana, R., Watanabe, M., Ono, Y., Kumashiro, H. (1984) 'Blood serotonin and free tryptophan concentration in autistic children.' *Neuropsychobiology*, **11**, 22–27.

Israngkun, P.P., Newman, H.A.I., Patel, S.T., Duruibe, V.A., Abou-Issa, H. (1986) 'Potential biochemical markers for infantile autism.' *Neurochemical Pathology*, **5**, 51–70.

Itokawa, Y., Tanaka, C., Kimura, M. (1972) 'Effect of thiamine on serotonin levels in magnesium-deficient animals.' *Metabolism*, **21**, 375–379.

Jouve, J., Martineau, J., Mariotte, N., Barthélémy, C., Muh, J.P., Lelord, G. (1986) 'Determination of urinary serotonin using liquid chromatography with electrochemical detection.' *Journal of Chromatography*, **378**, 437–443.

Kuperman, A., Beeghly, J.H.L., Burns, T.L., Tsai, L.Y. (1985) 'Serotonin relationships of autistic probands and their first-degree relatives.' *Journal of the American Academy of Child and Adolescent Psychiatry*, **24**, 186–190.

—— —— —— —— (1987) 'Association of serotonin concentration to behavior and IQ in autistic children.' *Journal of Autism and Developmental Disorders*, **17**, 133–140.

Lake, C.R., Ziegler, M.G., Murphy, D.L. (1977) 'Increased norepinephrine levels and decreased dopamine-beta-hydroxylase activity in primary autism.' *Archives of General Psychiatry*, **34**, 553–556.

Lauder, J.M., Krebs, H. (1978) 'Serotonin as a differentiation signal in early neurogenesis.' *Developmental Neuroscience*, **1**, 15–30.

Launay, J.M., Bursztejn, C., Ferrari, P., Dreux, C., Braconnier, A., Zarifian, E., Lancrenon, S., Fermanian, J. (1987) 'Catecholamine metabolism in infantile autism—a controlled study of 22 autistic children.' *Journal of Autism and Developmental Disorders*, **17**, 333–348.

—— Ferrari, P., Haimart, M., Bursztejn, C., Tabuteau, F., Braconnier, A., Pasques-Bondoux, D., Luong, C., Dreux, C. (1988) 'Serotonin metabolism and other biochemical parameters in infantile autism.' *Neuropsychobiology*, **20**, 1–11.

Le Couteur, A., Trygstad, O., Evered, C., Gillberg, C., Rutter, M. (1988) 'Infantile autism and urinary excretion of peptides and protein-associated peptide complexes.' *Journal of Autism and Developmental Disorders*, **18**, 181–190.

Leckman, J.F., Cohen, D.J., Shaywitz, B.A., Caparulo, B.K., Heninger, G.R., Bowers, M.B. (1980) 'CSF monoamine metabolites in child and adult psychiatric patients: a developmental perspective.' *Archives of General Psychiatry*, **37**, 677–681.

Lelord, G., Callaway, E., Muh, J.P., Arlot, J.C., Sauvage, D., Garreau, B., Domenech, J. (1978) 'L'acide homovanilique urinaire et ses modifications par ingestion de vitamine B6: exploration fonctionnelle dans l'autisme de l'enfant.' *Revue Neurologique*, **134**, 797–801.

Leventhal, B.L., Cook, E.H., Morford, M., Ravitz, A., Freedman, D.X. (1990) 'Relationships of whole blood serotonin and plasma norepinephrine within families.' *Journal of Autism and Developmental Disorders*, **20**, 499–512.

Leysen, J.E., de Chaffoy de Courcelles, D., de Clerck, F., Niemegeevs, C.J.E., Van Nueten, J.M. (1984) 'Serotonin-S_2 receptor binding sites and functional correlates.' *Neuropharmacology*, **23**, 1493–1501.

Martineau, J., Garreau, B., Barthélémy, C., Callaway, E., Lelord, G. (1981) 'Effects of vitamin B6 on averaged evoked potentials in infantile autism.' *Biological Psychiatry*, **16**, 627–641.

128

McBride, P.A., Anderson, G.M., Hertzig, M.E., Sweeney, J.A., Kream, J., Cohen, D.J., Mann, J.J. (1989a) 'Serotonergic responsivity in male young adults with autistic disorder.' *Archives of General Psychiatry*, **46**, 213–221.

—— —— Mann, J.J. (1989b) 'Serotonin-mediated responses in autism.' *Biological Psychiatry*, **25**, 183A.

McCarthy, D.M., Coleman, M. (1979) 'Response of intestinal mucosa to gluten challenge in autistic subjects.' *Lancet*, **2**, 877–878.

McKean, C.M. (1971) 'Effects of totally synthetic low phenylalanine diet on adolescent phenylketonuria patients.' *Archives of Disease in Childhood*, **46**, 608–615.

Menkes, J.H., Welcher, D.W., Levi, H.S., Dallas, J., Gretsky, N.E. (1972) 'Relationship of elevated blood tyrosine to the ultimate intellectual performance of premature infants.' *Pediatrics*, **49**, 218–224.

Minderaa, R.B., Anderson, G.M., Volkmar, F.R., Akkerhuis, G.W., Cohen, D.J. (1987) 'Urinary 5-hydroxyindoleacetic acid and whole blood serotonin and tryptophan in autistic and normal subjects.' *Biological Psychiatry*, **22**, 933–940.

—— —— —— —— —— (1989) 'Neurochemical study of dopamine functioning in autistic and normal subjects.' *Journal of the American Academy of Child and Adolescent Psychiatry*, **28**, 190–194.

Moos, M., Goldberg, N.D. (1988) 'Cyclic AMP opposes IP_3-induced calcium release from permeabilized platelets.' *Second Messengers and Phosphoproteins*, **12**, 163–170.

O'Brien, R.A., Semenuk, G., Coleman, M., Spector, S. (1976) 'Catechol-O-methyltransferase activity in erythrocytes of children with autism,' *In:* Coleman, M. (Ed.) *The Autistic Syndromes*. Amsterdam: North Holland; New York: Elsevier, pp. 43–50.

Paasonen, M.K. (1968) 'Platelet 5-hydroxytryptamine as a model in pharmacology.' *Annales Medicinae Experimentalis et Biologiae Fenniae*, **46**, 416–422.

Pare, C.M.B., Sandler, M., Stacey, R.S. (1958) 'Decreased 5-hydroxytryptophan decarboxylase activity in phenylketonuria.' *Lancet*, **2**, 1099–1101.

Peroutka, S.J., Schmidt, A.W., Sleight, A.J., Harrington, M.A. (1990) 'Serotonin receptor "families" in the central nervous system: an overview.' *Annals of the New York Academy of Sciences*, **600**, 104–110.

Perry, B.D., Cook, E.H., Leventhal, B.L., Wainwright, M.S., Freedman, D.X. (1991) 'Platelet 5-HT_2 serotonin receptor binding sites in autistic children and their first-degree relatives.' *Biological Psychiatry*, **30**, 121–130.

Perry, T., Hansen, S., Christie, R.G. (1978) 'Amino compounds and organic acids in the CSF, plasma and urine in autistic children.' *Biological Psychiatry*, **13**, 575–586.

Piven, J., Tsai, G., Nehme, E., Coyle, J.T., Chase, G.A., Folstein, S.E. (1991) 'Platelet serotonin, a possible marker for familial autism.' *Journal of Autism and Developmental Disorders*, **21**, 51–60.

Pletscher, A. (1968) 'Metabolism, transfer and storage of 5-hydroxytryptamine in blood platelets.' *British Journal of Pharmacology*, **32**, 1–16.

Plioplys, A.V., Hemmens, S.E., Regan, C.M. (1990) 'Expression of a NCAM serum fragment is depressed in autism.' *Journal of Neuropsychiatry and Clinical Neuroscience*, **2**, 413–417.

Reichelt, K.L., Saelid, G., Lindback, T., Boler, J.B. (1986) 'Childhood autism: a complex disorder.' *Biological Psychiatry*, **21**, 1279–1290.

Ritvo, E.R., Yuwiler, A., Geller, E., Ornitz, E.M., Saeger, K., Plotkin, S. (1970) 'Increased blood serotonin and platelets in early infantile autism.' *Archives of General Psychiatry*, **23**, 566–572.

Ross, D., Pickar, D., DeJong, J., Karoum, F., Linnoila, M. (1987) 'Reduction of elevated CSF beta-endorphin by fenfluramine in infantile autism.' *Pediatric Neurology*, **3**, 83–86.

Saladino, C.F., Sankar, D.V. (1973) 'Studies on erthyrocyte magnesium and potassium levels in children, schizophrenia and growth.' *Physician's Drug Manual*, **4–5**, 107–110.

Sandman, C.A., Barron, J.L., Chicz-DeMet, A., DeMet, E.M. (1991) 'Brief report: plasma beta-endorphin and cortisol levels in autistic patients.' *Journal of Autism and Developmental Disorders*, **21**, 83–87.

Schain, R.J., Freedman, D.X. (1961) 'Studies on 5-hydroxyindole metabolism in autistic and other mentally retarded children.' *Journal of Pediatrics*, **58**, 315–320.

Singer, H.S., Hahn, I-H., Moran, T.H. (1991) 'Abnormal dopamine uptake sites in postmortem striatum from patients with Tourette's syndrome.' *Annals of Neurology*, **30**, 558–562.

Suemitsu, S., Yoshikawa, T., Egusa, Y., Akiyama, Y., Akiyama, Y., Yoshimoto, J., Fujimara, J.,

Otsuki, S. (1974) 'Serum serotonin levels in infantile autism.' *Psychiatria et Neurologia Paediatrica Japonica*, **14**, 105–109.

Takahashi, S., Kanai, H., Miyamoto, Y. (1976) 'Reassessment of elevated serotonin levels in blood platelets in early infantile autism.' *Journal of Autism and Childhood Schizophrenia*, **6**, 317–326.

Todd, R.D., Ciaranello, R.D. (1985) 'Demonstration of inter- and intraspecies differences in serotonin binding sites by antibodies from an autistic child.' *Proceedings of the National Academy of Sciences of the USA*, **82**, 612–616.

Trygstad, O.E., Reichelt, K.L., Foss, I., Edminson, P.D., Saelid, G., Bremer, J., Hole, K., Orbeck, H., Johansen, J.H., Boler, J.B., *et al.* (1980) 'Patterns of peptides and protein-associated peptide complexes in psychiatric disorders.' *British Journal of Psychiatry*, **136**, 59–72.

Weizman, R., Weizman, A., Tyano, S., Szekely, B.A., Sarne, Y.H. (1984) 'Humoral-endorphin blood levels in autistic, schizophrenic and healthy subjects.' *Psychopharmacology*, **82**, 363–370.

—— Gil-Ad, I., Dick, J., Tyano, S., Szekely, G., Laron, Z. (1988) 'Low plasma immunoreactive beta-endorphin.' *Journal of the American Academy of Child and Adolescent Psychiatry*, **27**, 430–433.

Whitaker-Azmitia, P.M., Lauder, J.M., Shemmer, A., Azmitia, E.C. (1987) 'Postnatal changes in serotonin receptors following prenatal alterations in serotonin levels: further evidence for functional fetal serotonin receptors.' *Brain Research*, **430**, 285–289.

Winsberg, B.G., Sverd, J., Castells, S., Hurwic, M., Perel, J.M. (1980) 'Estimation of monoamine and cyclic-AMP turnover and amino acid concentrations in spinal fluid of autistic children.' *Neuropediatrics*, **11**, 250–255.

Young, J.G., Cohen, D.J., Caparulo, B.K., Brown, S.L., Maas, J.W. (1979) 'Decreased 24-hour urinary MHPG in childhood autism.' *American Journal of Psychiatry*, **136**, 1055–1057.

—— Kypri, R.M., Ross, N.T., Cohen, D.J. (1980) 'Serum dopamine-beta-hydroxylase activity: clinical applications in child psychiatry.' *Journal of Autism and Developmental Disorders*, **10**, 13.

—— Cohen, D.J., Kavanagh, M.E., Landis, H.D., Shaywitz, B.A., Maas, J.W. (1981) 'Cerebrospinal fluid, plasma, and urinary MHPG in children.' *Life Sciences*, **28**, 2837–2845.

Yuwiler, A., Ritvo, E.R., Bald, D., Kipper, D., Koper, A. (1971) 'Examination of circadian rhythmicity of blood serotonin and platelets in autistic and non-autistic children.' *Journal of Autism and Childhood Schizophrenia*, **1**, 421–435.

—— —— Geller, E., Glousman, R., Schneiderman, G., Matsuno, D. (1975) 'Uptake and efflux of serotonin from platelets of autistic and nonautistic children.' *Journal of Autism and Childhood Schizophrenia*, **5**, 83–98.

Zhou, F.C., Auerbach, S., Azmitia, E.C. (1987) 'Denervation of serotonergic fibers in the hippocampus induced a trophic factor which enhances the maturation of transplanted serotonergic neurons but not norepinephrine neurons.' *Journal of Neuroscience Research*, **17**, 235–246.

11
ENDOCRINE AND IMMUNOLOGICAL STUDIES

The CNS has many similarities to the immune system. Examples of shared characteristics are the large repertoire of recognition, memory and the high rate of developmental cell death. In syndromes presenting with neurodevelopmental abnormalities, such as the autistic syndromes, the search for immunological and endocrinological abnormalities is a reasonable approach to studying this patient group.

Endocrine studies

Endocrine studies have been conducted with groups of children with autism in a number of areas related to pituitary and hypothalamic function. Those relating to neurotransmitters were discussed in the previous chapter. In this chapter, studies of the hormones themselves are reviewed.

Thyroid studies

The thyroid hormone is critical to the programming of the developing nervous system and in the maintenance of CNS function in the perinatal and postnatal periods. Since autistic symptoms can present as early as the newborn period, the finding that the mothers of such infants can have thyroid difficulties during gestation is of interest; in fact, there is an increased incidence of hypothyroidism in both fathers and mothers of children with autism (see Chapter 9). Autoimmune dysfunction may be a factor in this small subgroup of parents.

Do autistic syndromes ever develop in infants with congenital hypothyroidism? Unfortunately, the answer is yes, and the cases known so far are those in which the congenital hypothyroidism was diagnosed after the critical first three months of life when with treatment the intelligence of the child can often be kept in the normal range. Diagnosed at the ages of 6 months and 7 months (Ritvo *et al.* 1990) and 9 months (M.C., personal case), these children all have IQs below the normal range and meet DMS-III-R criteria for autism.

Looking at the problem the other way around, studies of thyroid function in other patients with autism have not shown much abnormality. In fact, there are several studies where thyroid was administered to children with autism even though they were euthyroid.

Sherwin *et al.* (1958) studied thyroid function in two children with autism and found them to be euthyroid. Nevertheless, they decided to administer T_3 to the

131

children and reported an apparent clinical improvement. Subsequently, Khan (1970) reported diminished T_3 uptake values in 45 of 62 children with autism.

Following these early reports, a group of investigators at New York University conducted five studies (Campbell *et al.* 1972, 1973, 1978*a,b*; Campbell and Fish 1974). In the 1973 study, tri-iodothyronine, administered to 14 preschool children with psychosis, resulted in improved social and stereotypic behaviour. However, in their second 1978 study, Campbell *et al.* were unable to support their previous findings of the beneficial effects, except in the case of a few symptoms. The 1978 studies were performed on 30 young, clinically euthyroid children and used a careful, placebo-controlled, double-blind, crossover methodology. One interesting detail of this study was the improvement in bone age in three of the children by more than two standard deviations, reaching the normal range by the end of the treatment.

Also in 1978, Abbassi *et al.* evaluated T_3, T_4 and thyroid-stimulating hormone (TSH) levels in 13 children with autism; all patients were euthyroid. Two of the patients had retarded bone ages; they were treated with tri-iodothyronine for six months. However, clinical signs of hyperthyroidism developed when T_3 levels exceeded physiological concentrations in these two patients.

Another study (Cohen *et al.* 1980) of thyroid function (T_4, TSH, total thyroxine binding capacity, present binding saturation, and estimated free thyroxine) in 20 randomly selected children with autism again found no statistical difference between patients and controls in these parameters of thyroid function.

Besides studying baseline levels, another approach to evaluation of thyroid function is to measure the effects of thyrotropin-releasing hormone (TRH) loading tests. Three such studies have been conducted (Campbell *et al.* 1978*a*, Hoshino *et al.* 1985, Hashimoto *et al.* 1991). The study by Hoshino *et al.* reported accelerated plasma TSH after TRH loading in children with autism compared to normal controls: this study used the smallest TRH dose and the controls were not age-matched. (Previously, Hoshino *et al.* (1984) had reported a suppressed response to prolactin when the precursor of serotonin, L-5HTP, was used for a provocative test.)

The other two studies found the opposite result: in subjects with autism the TSH response to TRH was lower than in controls, and in the Hashimoto *et al.* study the TRH secretion was different from that of mentally retarded children and children with minimal brain dysfunction (although no difference was found in prolactin levels). Hashimoto *et al.* checked their results in two separate groups of children with autism (IQs above and below 80) and found the lower TSH results consistently in both groups compared to the three control groups. These latter two studies may be indicative of a brain lesion (?hypothalamic dysfunction), selectively found in children with autism, which is different from the lesions of mental retardation or minimal brain dysfunction.

If, in spite of normal baseline TSH levels in most patients with autism, it is further substantiated that TRH loading tests result in diminished TSH response, this could be considered evidence of subtle hypothyroidism in this patient group. Of course, the autistic syndromes have multiple aetiologies and there may only be a subgroup who have the abnormal TRH response. The past medical literature tells us that T_3 supplementation is generally not effective (Abbassi *et al.* 1978, Campbell *et al.* 1978*b*), but the patients given these therapeutic trials were not selected in advance by TRH loading tests; perhaps this needs to be the next research approach.

The implication of the TRH studies to an understanding of neurotransmitters (see Chapter 10) is especially interesting. The administration of the precursor of dopamine is known to antagonize the ability of TRH to release TSH (Burrow *et al.* 1977); also the administration of a neuroleptic, haloperidol, with strong anti-dopaminergic properties has been reported to have a therapeutic effect in children with autism (see Chapter 22). Could these thyroid studies be further evidence of a neurotransmitter balance in the hypothalamic–infundibular system that has the functional effect of enhanced dopaminergic activity?

There is one case of clear-cut hypopituitarism in a child with autism; the pituitary deficiency was diagnosed shortly after birth (Ritvo *et al.* 1990). This boy also had septal dysplasia that caused a lack of development of the optic nerve with resulting blindness, which complicates the interpretation of his autistic symptoms.

Human growth hormone has been tested by three methods in patients with autism. Loading with L-5HTP produced a normal response (Hoshino *et al.* 1984). However, loading with both insulin and L-dopa resulted in abnormal responses in a subgroup of children with autism (Deutsch *et al.* 1985, 1986).

Studies of corticosteroids
Yamazaki *et al.* (1975) first studied corticosteroids in children with autism. They can be tested in very young children by reactivity to pyrogen, a pattern established in the early months or years of life, or by marking the circadian rhythm of plasma steroid hormones, which is established slightly later (with 4 years as the outside limit). These two tests were performed on seven children with autism ranging from 6 to 10 years of age. The authors reported that for the most part reactivity was sufficient in the pyrogen test, although a normal circadian rhythm could scarcely be observed. They interpreted their findings as evidence of hypothalamic dysfunction related to basal ACTH secretion in children with autism. In the same year, Maher *et al.* found that 11 children with autism hypersecreted cortisol in response to insulin-induced hypoglycaemia.

Jensen *et al.* (1985) performed a dexamethasone suppression test on 13 children with autism. If dexamethasone fails to suppress cortisol secretion in an individual, a dysregulation of the hypothalamic–pituitary–adrenal hormone production is thought to be responsible. (The test is non-specific: it can be positive in depression, bulimia, anorexia nervosa, alcoholism, opiate addiction and Alzheimer disease.) Jensen *et al.* found it positive in 11 of the 13 children with autism.

Precocious puberty

Idiopathic precocious puberty is a rare syndrome that has been reported in a few children with autistic features (Gillberg 1984, Mouridsen 1989). In the Gillberg study, the frequency was found to be 1:2500 for childhood psychosis. In the girl reported by Mouridsen, extensive neuroradiological and endocrinological testing was uninformative.

If one looks at the studies so far reported in this chapter, the evidence appears to be building for dysfunction of the hypothalamic/pituitary axis in many children with autism. The problem appears to be central rather than at the end-organ.

Immunological studies

Several infectious illnesses of the CNS have been described in children with autism or autistic-like conditions (see Chapter 18). In most reported cases it is not known whether (1) these infections occurred by chance, (2) the patients were predisposed to develop an infectious illness due to an already altered immune system in themselves or their mothers, or (3) prenatal or perinatal infections altered the later immune responses of some of the children with autism.

Because congenital or perinatal infections sometimes persist for years, active infections with rubella or cytomegalovirus were tested for in a study of 78 children with autism aged over 3 years, but with negative results (Peterson and Torrey 1976).

In regard to infections *in utero*, prenatal rubella is the best documented of these among children with autistic symptoms. Rubella *in utero* has been shown to cause an altered immune response in some infants owing to the prenatal viral insult (South and Alford 1973, Fuccillo *et al.* 1974). Lack of an antibody response to a previous vaccination is helpful in diagnosing retrospectively an episode of prenatal rubella. Stubbs (1976) checked rubella titres in 13 children with autism who had had a previous rubella vaccination. In contrast to controls, five of the 13 children with autism had undetectable titres in spite of a previous vaccination. However, in the same study, a rubella vaccine challenge did not differentiate children with autism from the control subjects.

Stubbs *et al.* (1977) did a follow-up immunological study of 12 children with autism using phytohaemagglutinin-P (PHA) to check T-cell stimulation and pokeweed mitogen (PWM) as a measure of B lymphocyte responsiveness. Results of this study were the first to suggest that children with autism may have a relative T-cell deficiency. This study raised the question of whether children with autism have a genetic predisposition to relative T-cell deficiency or whether some viruses have a predilection for interfering with the thymus (which differentiates T-cells). Stubbs *et al.* (1982) also noted that inherited enzyme deficiencies in purine nucleotide degradation have been associated with immune deficiencies.

Immunoglobulins in both serum (Peterson and Torrey 1976) and CSF (Young *et al.* 1977) have been studied in children with autism and no abnormalities have been found.

Weizman *et al.* (1982) studied cell mediated immune response to human myelin basic protein by the macrophage inhibition factor test. They compared the results in 17 patients with autism to those in a control group of 11 patients with other mental disorders. 13 of the 17 patients with autism demonstrated inhibition of macrophage migration, whereas none of the control group showed such a response. This study suggested that there may exist a cell-mediated immune response to brain tissue.

Warren *et al.* (1986) studied 31 patients with autism and found several immune-system abnormalities in the blood. These authors confirmed an earlier finding by Stubbs (1977) that lymphocytes of patients with autism have a defective response to T-cell mitogen PHA and also found that the lymphocytes had reduced responses to the T-cell mitogen con A and the B-cell mitogen PWM. There appeared to be a reduced number of T cells. In a later study, this research group was able to identify the T-cells that had a lower percentage and number—CD4+ (helper) cells—and reported a diminution in CD2+ and CD20+ cells as well as a lower percentage and number of total lymphocytes compared to siblings and normal controls (Yonk *et al.* 1990).

Another problem regarding immunity in some patients with autism is the possibility of autoimmune deficiency. This is suggested by several findings. The increased incidence of hypothyroid disease in the parents (as described in Chapter 9) is one such factor. Money *et al.* (1971) reported on a family suffering from both autoimmune disorder and autism. These authors raised the possibility of auto-antibodies against the CNS in this family. Another study unexpectedly found 12.5 per cent of mothers of children with autism suffering from rheumatoid arthritis (Raiten and Massaro 1986).

A recent study of immunological factors associated with autoimmune disease in this patient group has shown that subjects with autism and their mothers had a significantly increased phenotypic frequency of the C4B null allele (Warren *et al.* 1991). This finding was not present in the fathers. The authors questioned whether this partial deficiency of C4 complement proteins would allow an infectious agent or immune complex to persist, resulting in prolonged immunological stimulus and triggering of an autoimmune reaction. The authors speculate as follows: perhaps, during her pregnancy, the mother did not clear a viral infection in an immunocompetent manner, resulting in an intrauterine fetal infection that damaged the developing nervous system or triggered an autoimmune response. These interesting and provocative results should lead to follow-up research studies.

A great deal more work is needed before it is fully understood how the immunological factors in patients or families could predispose to the infectious aetiology of autism; a start has been made.

REFERENCES

Abbassi, V., Linscheid, T., Coleman, M. (1978) 'Triiodothyronine (T$_3$) concentration and therapy in autistic children.' *Journal of Autism and Childhood Schizophrenia*, **8**, 383–388.

Burrow, G.N., May, P.B., Spaulding, S.W., Donabedian, R.K. (1977) 'TRH and dopamine interactions affecting pituitary hormone secretion.' *Journal of Clinical Endocrinology and Metabolism*, **45**, 65–72.

Campbell, M., Fish, B. (1974) 'Triiodothyronine in schizophrenic children.' *In:* Prange, A.J. (Ed.) *The Thyroid Axis, Drugs and Behavior.* New York: Raven Press, pp. 87–102.

—— —— David, R., Shapiro, T., Collins, P., Koh, C. (1972) 'Response to triiodothyronine and dextroamphetamine: a study of preschool schizophrenic children.' *Journal of Autism and Childhood Schizophrenia*, **2**, 343–358.

—— —— —— —— —— (1973) 'Liothyronine treatment in psychotic and nonpsychotic children under 6 years of age.' *Archives of General Psychiatry*, **29**, 602–608.

—— Hollander, C.S., Ferris, S., Greene, L.W. (1978a) 'Response to thyrotropin-releasing hormone stimulation in young psychotic children: a pilot study.' *Psychoneuroendocrinology*, **3**, 195–201.

—— Small, A.M., Hollander, C.S., Korein, J., Cohen, I.L., Kalmijn, M., Ferris, S. (1978b) 'A controlled crossover study of triiodothyronine in autistic children.' *Journal of Autism and Childhood Schizophrenia*, **8**, 371–381.

Cohen, D.J., Young, J.G., Lowe, T.L., Harcherik, D. (1980) 'Thyroid hormone in autistic children.' *Journal of Autism and Developmental Disorders*, **10**, 445–450.

Deutsch, S., Campbell, M., Sachar, E., Green, W.H., David, R. (1985) 'Plasma growth hormone response to oral L-DOPA in infantile autism.' *Journal of Autism and Developmental Disorders*, **15**, 205–212.

—— —— Perry, R., Green, W.H., Poland, R.E., Rubin, R.T. (1986) 'Plasma growth hormone response to insulin-induced hypoglycemia in infantile autism: a pilot study.' *Journal of Autism and Developmental Disorders*, **16**, 59–68.

Fuccillo, D.A., Steele, R.W., Hensen, S.A., Vincent, M.M., Hardy, J.B., Bellanti, J.A. (1974) 'Impaired cellular immunity to rubella virus in congenital rubella.' *Infection and Immunity*, **9**, 81–84.

Gillberg, C. (1984) 'Infantile autism and other childhood psychoses in a Swedish region: epidemiological aspects.' *Journal of Child Psychology and Psychiatry*, **25**, 35–43.

Hashimoto, T., Aihara, R., Tayama, M., Miyazaki, M., Shirakawa, Y., Kuroda, Y. (1991) 'Reduced thyroid-stimulating hormone response to thyrotropin-releasing hormone in autistic boys.' *Developmental Medicine and Child Neurology*, **33**, 313–319.

Hoshino, Y., Watanabe, M., Tachibana, R., Kaneko, M., Kumashiro, H. (1984) 'The hypothalamo-pituitary function in autistic children.' *Neurosciences*, **10**, 285–291.

—— —— —— —— —— (1985) 'The TRH and LH-RH loading test in autistic children.' *Fukushima Journal of Medical Science*, **31**, 55–61.

Jensen, J.B., Realmuto, G.M., Garfinkel, B.D. (1985) 'The dexamethasone suppression test in infantile autism.' *Journal of the American Academy of Child Psychiatry*, **24**, 263–265.

Khan, A.A. (1970) 'Thyroid dysfunction.' *British Medical Journal*, **4**, 495.

Maher, K.R., Harper, J.F., Macleay, A., King, M.G. (1975) 'Peculiarities in the endocrine response to insulin stress in early infantile autism.' *Journal of Nervous and Mental Disorders*, **161**, 180–184.

Money, J., Bobrow, N.A., Clarke, F.C. (1971) 'Autism and autoimmune disease: a family study.' *Journal of Autism and Childhood Schizophrenia*, **1**, 146–160.

Mouridsen, S.E. (1989) 'Pervasive developmental disorder and idiopathic precocious puberty in a 5-year-old girl.' *Journal of Autism and Developmental Disorders*, **19**, 351–353. *(Letter.)*

Peterson, M.R., Torrey, E.F. (1976) 'Viruses and other infectious agents as behavioral teratogens.' *In:* Coleman, M. (Ed.) *The Autistic Syndromes.* Amsterdam: North Holland; New York: Elsevier, pp. 23–42.

Raiten, D.J., Massaro, T. (1986) 'Perspectives on the nutritional ecology of autistic children.' *Journal of Autism and Developmental Disorders*, **16**, 133–144.

Ritvo, E.R., Mason-Brothers, A., Freeman, B.J., Pingree, C., Jenson, W.R., McMahon, W.M., Petersen, P.B., Jorde, L.B., Mo, A., Ritvo, A. (1990) 'The UCLA–University of Utah epidemiologic survey of autism: the etiologic role of rare diseases.' *American Journal of Psychiatry*, **147**, 1614–1621.

Sherwin, A.C., Flach, F.F., Stokes, P.E. (1958) 'Treatment of psychoses in early childhood with triiodothyronine.' *American Journal of Psychiatry*, **115**, 166–167.

South, M.A., Alford, C.A. (1973) 'Congenital intrauterine infections.' *In:* Stiehm, E.R., Fulginiti,

V.A. (Eds) *Immunologic Disorders in Infants and Children.* Philadelphia: W.B. Saunders, pp. 566–576.

Stubbs, E.G. (1976) 'Autistic children exhibit undetectable hemagglutination-inhibition antibody titers despite previous rubella vaccination.' *Journal of Autism and Childhood Schizophrenia*, **6**, 269–274.

—— Crawford, M.L., Burger, D.R., Vandenbark, A.A. (1977) 'Depressed lymphocyte responsiveness in autistic children.' *Journal of Autism and Childhood Schizophrenia*, **7**, 49–55.

—— Litt, M., Lis, F., Jackson, R., Voth, W., Lindberg, A., Litt, R. (1982) 'Adenosine deaminase activity decreased in autism.' *Journal of the American Academy of Child Psychiatry*, **21**, 71–74.

Warren, R.P., Margaretten, N.C., Pace, N.C., Foster, A. (1986) 'Immune abnormalities in patients with autism.' *Journal of Autism and Developmental Disorders*, **16**, 189–197.

—— Singh, V.K., Cole, P., Odell, J.D., Pingree, C.B., Warren, W.L., White, E. (1991) 'Increased frequency of the null allele at the complement C4b locus in autism.' *Clinical and Experimental Immunology*, **83**, 438–440.

Weizman, A., Weizman, R., Szekely, G.A., Wijsenbeek, H., Livni, E. (1982) 'Abnormal immune response to brain tissue antigen in the syndrome of autism.' *American Journal of Psychiatry*, **139**, 1462–1465.

Yamazaki, K., Saito, Y., Okada, F., Fujieda, T., Yamashita, I. (1975) 'An application of neuroendocrinological studies in autistic children and Heller's syndrome.' *Journal of Autism and Childhood Schizophrenia*, **5**, 323–332.

Yonk, L.J., Warren, R.P., Burger, R.A., Cole, P., Odell, J.D., Warren, W.L., White, E., Singh, V.K. (1990) 'CD4+ helper T cell depression in autism.' *Immunology Letters*, **25**, 341–346.

Young, J.G., Caparulo, B.K., Shaywitz, B.A., Johnson, W.T., Cohen, D.J. (1977) 'Childhood autism: cerebrospinal fluid examination and immunoglobulin levels.' *Journal of the American Academy of Child Psychiatry*, **16**, 174–179.

12
ELECTROPHYSIOLOGICAL STUDIES

The neurophysiology of persons with autism has been extensively studied. Perhaps because of the multiple aetiologies involved, the results from excellent laboratories sometimes give the impression that they must be working with different subsets of patients because of the conflicting results reported. But there certainly have been a number of thought-provoking studies performed on individuals with autism.

Standard electroencephalograms (EEGs)

One of the first tools to look at children with autism from a neurological point of view was the EEG. A sizeable proportion of patients have been found to have definite EEG abnormalities, although it varies from study to study (White *et al.* 1964, Creak and Pampiglione 1969, Kolvin *et al.* 1971). No EEG pattern unique to autism was found in any study. The EEG has been used to try to find clinical correlations, *e.g.* with language patterns (Dorenbaum *et al.* 1987). When a computerized EEG technique was applied to 11 low-functioning children with autism from a developmental centre, the pattern resembled one from toddlers or much younger children, supporting a model of maturational lag (Cantor *et al.* 1986).

Can the EEG be a useful tool for prognosis? It is a limited tool; however, in one study by Small (1975), 42 per cent of the children with autism and a normal EEG were found to be either educable or within normal or borderline range on follow-up, whereas more than 75 per cent of those with EEG abnormalities on admission were in the lower trainable or subtrainable categories. In a study of 100 patients, Tsai *et al.* (1985) found that the group with normal EEGs had a much higher boy:girl ratio than the group with abnormal EEGs, reinforcing what had been known from a variety of other studies, that females with autism tend, on average, to be more severely affected than males.

Most of the EEG abnormalities described in the literature are bilateral or comprise both diffuse and localized abnormalities (Tsai and Stewart 1982), although occasional focal lesions are reported (Rutter and Bartak 1971). In patients with autism, the main clinical value of the EEG is in relation to seizure disorders, where the EEG can be helpful (see Chapter 6).

Brainstem auditory evoked responses

There is a great deal of evidence from the clinical literature that suggests that autistic behaviours might result, in part, from distortions in the sensation or perception of environmental signals. This has led many investigators to study patients with autism using the brainstem auditory evoked response (BAER), which is a measure of the activity of the auditory pathway from the acoustic nerve to higher midbrain structures (Ornitz and Walter 1975; Student and Sohmer 1978, 1979; Novick *et al*. 1980; Ornitz *et al*. 1980; Rosenblum *et al*. 1980; Skoff *et al*. 1980; Fein *et al*. 1981; Arick 1982; Ross 1982; Tanguay *et al*. 1982; Taylor *et al*. 1982; Gillberg *et al*. 1983; Rumsey *et al*. 1984; Grillon *et al*. 1989; Sersen *et al*. 1990; Thivièrge and Côté 1990; Thivièrge *et al*. 1990).

This long list of studies is remarkable in its lack of a coherent result. In fact, some studies contradict others in spite of the fact that many groups were using quite credible diagnostic and electrophysiological techniques. Prolonged Wave I latencies (implying peripheral hearing impairment) were found by some studies; prolonged Wave III latencies (suggesting pathology at midbrain levels of the auditory pathway) was a frequent finding; prolonged latencies between waves have been inconsistently reported. On the other hand, normal or shorter Wave III and even shorter interpeak latencies have also been reported, as have completely normal BAER readings.

This inconsistent and contradictory literature is particularly disappointing because of the greater consistency of BAER results found in developmental syndromes which have specifically defined aetiologies, such as Down syndrome. If nothing else has been learned, it is becoming clearer that autism is not as easily studied as a disease entity with a consistent single chromosome error. The one finding that recent authors seem to agree on is that BAER abnormalities are not present in all children with autism—therefore, under current testing conditions, the BAER abnormalities which have been recorded in the literature are not indicative of a universal finding of abnormal sensory processing in the brainstem in persons with autism (Grillon *et al*. 1989, Sersen *et al*. 1990, Thivièrge *et al*. 1990). That a subgroup of children with autism have sensory hearing loss is, of course, already well established (see Chapter 21).

In the earlier studies, the number of patients examined ranged from five to 26. Recently, a very large BAER study of 48 patients with autism (Sersen *et al*. 1990) tried to eliminate or control for several potentially important variables. This study was limited to males. Children in whom autism was associated with a gross neurological disorder or systemic disease were excluded, and patients were only accepted into the study if their BAER thresholds were known to be within normal limits. The authors also carefully compared sedated and unsedated patients. The results showed that the unsedated group did not differ from controls and, in fact, had somewhat shorter latencies for most components. On the other hand, the sedated group showed longer latencies for all components following Wave III. Since the patients who were sedated were somewhat younger and of lower levels of functioning, the statistics were reexamined with covariance for age and functional level. The adjusted measures revealed only an increase in the differences between the sedated and unsedated groups. (In contrast, in the same study a much more homogeneous group of Down syndrome patients showed no difference between

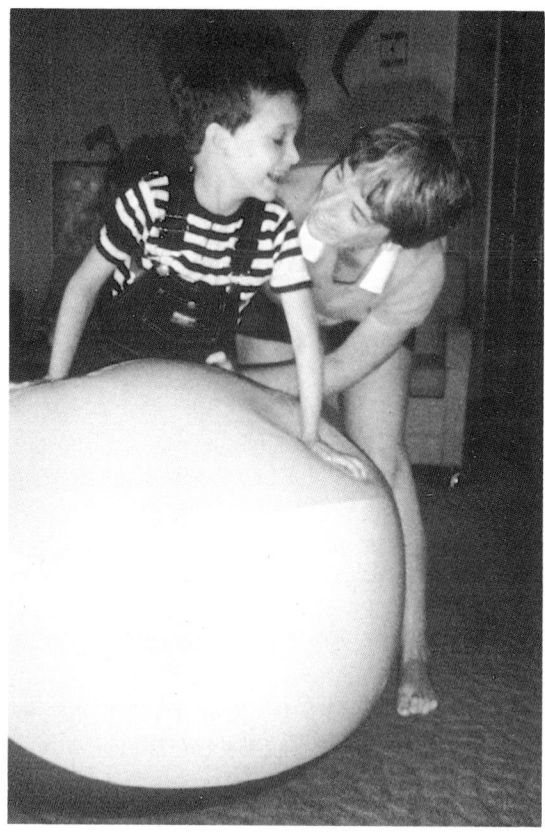

Fig. 12.1. Vestibular therapy can be a fun experience for both child and mother.

sedated and unsedated groups.) In an attempt to explain the results in the autism patients, the authors wondered about the effects of sedation but also raised the question of whether those individuals who needed sedation comprised a different group of patients who had different, subtle neurological dysfunction including abnormalities of the brainstem.

Thivièrge *et al.* (1990), after reviewing the literature and noting the contradictory results in different BAER studies of autism, suggested that calcium abnormalities in the brainstem might explain the disparate results, since calcium is important in synaptic transmission and calcium levels appear to influence BAER results. (A study of dialysis patients has shown that the lower the calcium level, the greater the BAER absolute latency and interpeak latency values—Pratt *et al.* 1986.) The Thivièrge *et al.* BAER study of 20 patients with autism found that 16 had an abnormality of interpeak latencies. They did not attempt to measure calcium levels in their patients. (A study reporting hypocalcinuria in 22 per cent of children with autism has been referred to in Chapter 10.)

A BAER study was recently performed in conjunction with oculomotor testing in 11 children with infantile autism or autistic-like conditions (Rosenhall *et al.* 1988). In six of the children, measurement of voluntary horizontal non-predictable saccades showed eye motor function to be abnormal, while five had abnormal brainstem potentials. Looking at the study as a whole, eight of the 11 children had either pathological saccades, abnormal brainstem potentials or both. This dual approach study using both electrophysiological and clinical modalities suggested that one subset of these children in fact had brainstem–cerebellar dysfunction. Such studies have lent additional support to the importance of vestibular therapies for children with autism (Fig. 12.1).

Somatosensory evoked potentials (SSEPs)

Short-latency SSEPs can also be used to measure brainstem function but have received less attention than BAERs. One study described a larger brainwave latency in this patient group, raising the question of whether the stimuli took an unusually long time to be transmitted (Hashimoto *et al.* 1986). This study adds additional support to the concept that there is brainstem dysfunction in autism in some patients.

Cortical evoked potentials and event-related potentials

Cortical evoked potentials (CEPs) and cortical event-related potentials (ERPs) are used to study stimulation evaluation modalities above the brainstem level (Small *et al.* 1971; Walter *et al.* 1971; Ornitz *et al.* 1972; Lelord *et al.* 1973; Barnet 1979; Novick *et al.* 1979, 1980; Niwa *et al.* 1983; August *et al.* 1984; Courchesne *et al.* 1984, 1985*a,b*, 1989; Pritchard *et al.* 1987; Dawson *et al.* 1988; Ciesielski *et al.* 1990; Erwin *et al.* 1992).

Barnet (1979), in an excellent review of the early work in this field, pointed out that there were extraordinary difficulties in obtaining reliable results in protocols that require children with autism to cooperate actively. These early studies found that CEPs were not elicited as frequently (Walter *et al.* 1971, Lelord *et al.* 1973), that they were smaller in amplitude (Small *et al.* 1971, Ornitz *et al.* 1972), or that they appeared only when stimuli were paired (Lelord *et al.* 1973). Later studies began to look at interesting phenomena such as evoked potentials to missing stimuli (Novick *et al.* 1979, Nakkamura *et al.* 1986), or to focus on special patient subgroups (all non-retarded) (Courchesne *et al.* 1985*a*) or special laboratory conditions designed to measure the patient's ability to focus attention on incoming stimuli (Ciesielski *et al.* 1990).

Nakamura *et al.* (1986) studied adults with autism and reported that the MSPs (missing stimulus potentials) partially resembled those of normal adults, describing them as having mature patterns with specific laterality. They indicated that this was a positive sign regarding cognitive function (which, of course, is no surprise to educators working with children with autism).

141

From the beginning of this work, it has often been reported that P3 amplitude of the CEP was smaller in children with autism than in normal children (Small *et al.* 1971; Novick *et al.* 1979, 1980). P3 is a complex long-latency wave which appears to be influenced by processes related to attention, arousal and cognition. It has been shown that the various components of the P3 complex vary independently with stimulus, as well as perceptual and cognitive demands placed by the experimental paradigm. The 'cognitive P300' (P3b) component is a positive wave that peaks at approximately 300ms post-stimulus and reaches maximal amplitude over the parietal area of the scalp. It is a potential that is acutely sensitive to the ability of the patient to attend. Several P3b studies have been performed with non-retarded subjects with autism in an attempt to limit the variables being studied. In contrast to the BAER studies, many of these studies consistently reported the abnormally small auditory P3b responses in patients with autism elicited by a variety of verbal, phonemic, non-verbal and non-sensory (*i.e.* omitted) targets (see Courchesne *et al.* 1989). However, visual P3b responses are less likely to be attenuated and may even be normal (Pritchard *et al.* 1987).

In a study of the P3 amplitude of the auditory evoked potentials produced from phonetic and tone stimuli, Dawson *et al.* (1988) again noted the smaller amplitude, but raised the possibility that in autism the failure to allocate an appropriate amount of attention to linguistic stimuli may result from an increased allocation of attentional resources to other stimuli. Recent research by Erwin *et al.* (1992) focused primarily on getting adequate auditory attention from the 11 adult men with autism (ages 17 to 39) being studied. In this study, where the important and difficult to control variable of attention was fairly well controlled, normal P3 amplitudes were recorded to phonemic stimuli. Contrary to the investigator's hypothesis, emotional–prosodic stimuli appeared to be particularly effective in activating the neural substrate of the P3 generator system.

Although Pritchard *et al.* (1987), who studied visual P3b responses, found many similarities between patients with autism and controls, they did note a significant increase in amplitude as the flash intensity increased in individuals with autism. This could be interpreted as suggesting that children with autism experience a degree of stimulus overload in the visual modality, particularly as the intensity of the stimulus increases. However, this same phenomenon can be seen in normal persons too. Martineau *et al.* (1987) studied auditory–visual cross-modal associations and conditioning phenomena. They reported that children with autism are significantly differentiated from both normal and mentally retarded children on the basis of smaller amplitudes. In their conditioning experiments, they found that the patterns of responses in normal children and in those with autism were similar, but that those of mentally retarded children were different. Although conditioning did not reach fully normal levels in the children with autism, the authors remark that the finding suggests a slow but real learning ability.

Abnormalities in other ERP responses (Nd, N270, Nc) have also been reported in individuals with autism. Combined with possible P3b abnormalities, these findings have led to an interesting hypothesis about the possibility of different selective attentional processing mechanisms in patients with autism (Ciesielski *et al.* 1990).

A recent approach to studying arousal/attentional mechanisms involves looking at a series of potentials preceding the longer-latency ERPs. Buchwald *et al.* (1992) report that a mid-latency AER—the P1 potential, its generator substrate closely linked to cholinergic components of the ascending reticular activator system and their thalamic target cells—was abnormal in 11 high functioning adults with autism.

A lot of work with possible theoretical implications lies ahead in this field, including designing series with larger numbers and well-defined subsets of patients with autistic symptoms, and using experimental paradigms that control for the confounding variables and apply more sophisticated techniques to the analysis of evoked potential data. Evoked potential mapping combined with physiological imaging techniques such as PET (position emission tomography) also hold promise for extending knowledge and understanding of brain function in patients with autism. The ability to focus the attention of the participant with autism in these studies remains a continuing problem.

Electroretinograms (ERGs)

There is one paper in the literature where ERGs were performed on 27 patients with autism (Ritvo *et al.* 1988). Cooperation is involved in this test, so the patients were selected by the criteria of ability to participate actively in the testing procedure. In this first study there was evidence of abnormal retinal function, as demonstrated by a subnormal b-wave amplitude, in nearly half the patients as compared to age- and sex-matched controls. This provocative result needs replication.

Sleep studies

Some patients with autism have a sleep disturbance, although many sleep for a normal number of hours. Abnormalities of the sleep–wakefulness cycle in some patients with autism may be related to an abnormal circadian rhythm (Segawa 1985).

In the 1960s and '70s, the UCLA research group addressed itself to the problem of sleep in children with autism and published a series of careful studies, evaluating normal rapid eye movement (REM) and non-REM sleep cycle patterns (Ornitz *et al.* 1965, 1968, 1969, 1971, 1972, 1973; Tanguay *et al.* 1976). In the earliest studies, the overall REM/non-REM sleep cycle patterns appeared to be comparable to those of control children (Ornitz *et al.* 1965, 1969). However, when attention was directed to some of the phasic activities occurring during the REM portion of the cycle, it was found that children with autism differed from age-matched, normal controls in several ways. Children with autism have failed to show a phasic inhibition of the AER during the eye movement/burst phase of REM sleep

(Ornitz *et al.* 1968). They also showed significantly fewer single eye movements and a decreased percentage of time of eye movements/burst activity (Ornitz *et al.* 1969). These authors reported that in children with autism the tonic aspects of REM sleep appeared to be within the normal range, while the phasic aspects were reported as abnormal compared with age- and sex-matched controls.

This work also raised the question of whether eye movement during REM sleep actually resembles the pattern of much younger, normal children (Ornitz *et al.* 1971). Tanguay *et al.* (1976) found no significant differences between the patterns of school-age children with autism and those of normal children under 18 months of age in both tonic and phasic REM activities. A recent study by Bergonzi *et al.* (1991) of institutionalized children with autism supports this concept—in fact, these authors relate the REM sleep patterns of some of these children to patterns seen in preterm infants.

EEG studies and cerebral lateralization
An increased incidence of left- and mixed handedness has been documented in a number of population studies of people with autism (reviewed by Gillberg *et al.* 1983, Bishop 1990) and is also seen in other developmental disability syndromes. Small (1975) suggested that a failure of cerebral lateralization might underlie the autistic syndrome. She found that normal children have higher EEG voltages over the left hemisphere than over the right during a standard EEG, whereas children with autism do not show this hemispheric difference.

AERs have also been used to compare right/left differences in autism. Tanguay *et al.* (1976) found no consistent hemispheric differences in autism compared with the usual larger evoked response seen over the right hemisphere in REM sleep in normal children.

Ogawa *et al.* (1982) studied the EEG in 21 right-handed children with autism compared with 28 normal children in the same age range. The children were studied during stage 2 sleep. Using analytic techniques including autoregressive analysis and component analysis, the authors found that there was significant hemispheric lateralization in the EEG of normal children but not in children with autism, supporting Small's thesis.

Tsai and Stewart (1982) and Tsai (1984) thoughtfully studied the correlation of handedness and EEG in general. They were unable to confirm a relationship between handedness and EEG patterns, and indicated that there are a number of factors that contribute to the discrepant finding in a normal population. They found no EEG pattern unique to autism, and they noted that the finding of bilateral abnormalities in a number of patients adds weight to the idea that autism results from dysfunction in both sides of the brain.

Fein *et al.* (1985) studied 62 children diagnosed as having 'pervasive developmental disorder' and found that left-handers tended to do better than right-handers on cognitive measures, while mixed-preference children tended to be the lowest on cognitive measures.

Physiological curiosity

As the theoretical discussion in autism focuses more and more on the presence or absence of empathy in this patient group, neurophysiology has an important and long neglected contribution to make (Heuyer *et al.* 1957; Lelord 1957, 1966). When normal children and adults, attached to EEG equipment, are watching a movie sequence of motor activity in human actors, an electrocortical modification in the motor area of the spectator occurs. Lelord *et al.* (1991) have shown that this phenomenon requires physiological curiosity. This EEG 'motor imitation' of another human being's action indicates focus on, and possibly identification with, the person on the movie screen. In contrast to normal children, children with autism pay attention to everything on the movie screen but do not focus on the people in the movie and do not exhibit EEG 'motor imitation', as physiological curiosity is scattered. If anything, they appear to be overwhelmed by the stimuli, even closing their eyes.

Other uses of electrophysiological studies

Electrophysiological data have started to be used as variables to measure the effects of pharmacological agents on patients with autism. This information is reviewed in Chapter 22.

REFERENCES

Arick, J.R. (1982) 'Auditory brainstem evoked response: comparative analysis of autistic, mentally retarded, normal children and normal toddlers.' *Dissertation Abstracts International*, **42**, 4764-A.

August, G.J., Raz, N., Papanicolaou, A.C., Baird, T.D., Hirsch, S.L., Hsu, L.L. (1984) 'Fenfluramine treatment in infantile autism: neurochemical, electrophysiological and behavioral effects.' *Journal of Nervous and Mental Disease*, **172**, 604–612.

Barnet, A.B. (1979) 'Sensory evoked potentials in autism.' *In:* Lockman, L.A., Swaiman, K.F., Drage, J.S., Nelson, K.B., Marsden, H.M. (Eds) *Workshop on the Neurobiological Basis of Autism. National Institutes of Health Monograph No. 23.* Bethesda, MD: NIH.

Bergonzi, P., Elia, M., Ferri, R., Musumeci, S.A. (1991) 'REM modulation in the night sleep of autistic institutionalized children.' *Brain Dysfunction. (In press.)*

Bishop, D.V.M. (1990) 'Autism and Rett syndrome.' *In: Handedness and Developmental Disorder. Clinics in Developmental Medicine No. 110.* London: MacKeith Press with Blackwell Scientific Publications; Philadelphia: J.B. Lippincott, pp. 110–116.

Buchwald, J.S., Erwin, R., Van Lancker, D., Guthrie, D., Schwafel, J., Tanguay, P. (1992) 'Midlatency auditory evoked responses: P1 abnormalities in adult autistic subjects.' *Electroencephalography and Clinical Neurophysiology*, **84**, 164–171.

Cantor, D.S., Thatcher, R.W., Hrybyk, M., Kaye, H. (1986) 'Computerized EEG analysis of autistic children.' *Journal of Autism and Developmental Disorders*, **16**, 169–187.

Ciesielski, K.T., Courchesne, E., Elmasian, R. (1990) 'Effects of focused selective attention tasks on event-related potentials in autistic and normal individuals.' *Electroencephalography and Clinical Neurophysiology*, **75**, 207–220.

Courchesne, E., Kilman, B.A., Galambos, R., Lincoln, A.J. (1984) 'Autism: cognitive processing of novel information measured by event-related potentials.' *Electroencephalography and Clinical Neurophysiology*, **59**, 238–248.

—— Courchesne, R., Hicks, G., Lincoln, A.J. (1985*a*) 'Functioning of the brain-stem auditory pathway in non-retarded autistic individuals.' *Electroencephalography and Clinical Neurophysiology*, **61**, 491–501.

—— Lincoln, A.J., Kilman, B.A., Galambos, R. (1985*b*) 'Event-related brain potential correlates of the processing of novel and auditory information in autism.' *Journal of Autism and Developmental Disorders*, **15**, 55–76.

—— —— Yeung-Courchesne, R., Elmasian, R., Grillon, C. (1989) 'Pathophysiologic findings in nonretarded autism and receptive developmental language disorder.' *Journal of Autism and Developmental Disorders*, **19**, 1–17.

Creak, M., Pampiglione, G. (1969) 'Clinical and EEG studies on a group of 35 psychotic children.' *Developmental Medicine and Child Neurology*, **11**, 218–227.

Dawson, G., Finley, C., Phillips, S., Galpert, L., Lewy, A. (1988) 'Reduced P3 amplitude of the event-related brain potential: its relationship to language ability in autism.' *Journal of Autism and Developmental Disorders*, **18**, 493–504.

Dorenbaum, D., Mencel, E., Blume, W.T., Fisman, S. (1987) 'EEG findings and language patterns in autistic children: clinical correlations.' *Canadian Journal of Psychiatry*, **32**, 31–34.

Erwin, R., Van Lancker, D., Guthrie, D., Schwafel, J., Tanguay, R., Buchwald, J.S. (1992) 'P3 responses to prosodic stimuli in adult autistic subjects.' *Electroencephalography and Clinical Neurophysiology*, **80**, 561–571.

Fein, D., Skoff, B., Mirsky, A.F. (1981) 'Clinical correlates of brainstem dysfunction in autistic children.' *Journal of Autism and Developmental Disorders*, **11**, 303–315.

—— Waterhouse, L., Lucci, D., Pennington, B., Hume, S.M. (1985) 'Handedness and cognitive functions in pervasive developmental disorder.' *Journal of Autism and Developmental Disorders*, **15**, 323–334.

Gillberg, C., Rosenhall, U., Johansson, E. (1983) 'Auditory brainstem responses in childhood psychosis.' *Journal of Autism and Developmental Disorders*, **13**, 181–195.

Grillon, C., Courchesne, E., Akshoofmoff, N. (1989) 'Brainstem and middle latency auditory evoked potentials in autism and developmental language disorder.' *Journal of Autism and Developmental Disorders*, **19**, 255–269.

Hashimoto, T., Tayama, M., Miyao, M. (1986) 'Short latency somatosensory evoked potentials in children with autism.' *Brain and Development*, **8**, 428–432.

Heuyer, G., Cohen-Seat, G., Lelord, G., Rebeillard, M. (1957) 'Etudes EEG d'enfants inadaptés soumis à la stimulation filmique.' *Neuropsychiatrie Infantile et d'Hygiene Mentale de l'Enfance*, **9–10**, 494–511.

Kolvin, I., Ounsted, C., Roth, M. (1971) 'Studies in the childhood psychoses. 5: Cerebral dysfunction and childhood psychoses.' *British Journal of Psychiatry*, **118**, 407–414.

Lelord, G. (1957) 'Modalités réactionnelles différentes de rythmes moyens et antérieurs autour de 10 c/s.' *Revue Neurologique*, **96**, 524–526.

—— (1966) 'Intérêt des méthodes electrophysiologiques: dans l'étude de l'action du film cinématographique chez l'enfant et l'adolescent.' *Pédo-psychiatrie*, **1**, 159–166.

—— Laffont, F., Jusseaume, P., Stephant, J.L. (1973) 'Comparative study of conditioning of average evoked responses by coupling sound and light in normal and autistic children.' *Psychophysiology*, **10**, 415–425.

—— Barthélémy, C., Martineau, J., Bruneau, N., Garreau, B. (1991) 'Physiological bases of exchange and developmental therapies in infantile autism.' *Brain and Development. (In press.)*

Martineau, J., Garreau, B., Roux, S., Lelord, G. (1987) 'Auditory evoked responses and their modification during conditioning paradigm in autistic children.' *Journal of Autism and Developmental Disorders*, **17**, 525–540.

Nakamura, K., Toshima, T., Takemura, I. (1986) 'The comparative and developmental study of auditory information processing in autistic adults.' *Journal of Autism and Developmental Disorders*, **16**, 105–118.

Niwa, S., Ohta, M., Yamazaki, K. (1983) 'P300 and stimulus evaluation process in autistic subjects.' *Journal of Autism and Developmental Disorders*, **13**, 33–42.

Novick, B., Kurtzberg, D., Vaughan, H.G. (1979) 'An electrophysiologic indication of defective information storage in childhood autism.' *Psychiatry Research*, **1**, 101–108.

—— Vaughan, H.G., Kurtzberg, D., Simon, R. (1980) 'An electrophysiologic indication of auditory processing defects in autism.' *Psychiatry Research*, **3**, 107–114.

Ogawa, T., Sugiyama, A., Suzuki, M., Nakashita, Y., Ishiwa, S. (1982) 'Hemispheric lateralization of EEG in early infantile autism.' *Noto Shinkei*, **34**, 981–988. *(Japanese.)*

Ornitz, E.M., Walter, D.O. (1975) 'The effect of sound pressure waveform on human brainstem auditory evoked responses.' *Brain Research*, **92**, 490–498.

—— Ritvo, E.R., Walter, R.D. (1965) 'Dreaming sleep in autistic and schizophrenic children.' *American Journal of Psychiatry*, **122**, 419–424.

—— —— Pahman, L.M., Lee, Y.H., Carr, E.M., Walter, R.D. (1968) 'The auditory evoked response in normal and autistic children during sleep.' *Electroencephalography and Clinical Neurophysiology*, **25**, 221–230.

—— —— Brown, M.B., LaFranchi, S., Parmelee, T., Walter, R.D. (1969) 'The EEG and rapid eye movements during REM sleep in normal and autistic children.' *Electroencephalography and Clinical Neurophysiology*, **26**, 167–175.

—— Wechter, V., Hartman, D., Tanguay, P.E., Lee, J.C.M., Ritvo, E.R., Walter, R.D. (1971) 'The EEG and rapid eye movements during REM sleep in babies.' *Electroencephalography and Clinical Neurophysiology*, **30**, 350–353.

—— Tanguay, P.E., Lee, J.C.M., Ritvo, E.R., Silvertsen, B., Wilson, C. (1972) 'The effect of stimulus interval on the auditory evoked response during sleep in autistic children.' *Journal of Autism and Childhood Schizophrenia*, **2**, 140–150.

—— Forsythe, A.B., de la Pena, A. (1973) 'The effect of vestibular and auditory stimulation on the rapid eye movements of REM sleep in autistic children.' *Archives of General Psychiatry*, **29**, 786–791.

—— Mo, A., Olson, S.T., Walter, D.O. (1980) 'Influence of click sound pressure direction on brainstem responses in children.' *Audiology*, **19**, 245–254.

Pratt, H., Brodsky, G., Goldsher, M., Ben-David, Y., Harari, R., Podoshin, L., Eliachar, I., Grushka, E., Better, O., Garty, J., (1986) 'Auditory brain stem evoked potentials in patients undergoing dialysis.' *Electroencephalography and Clinical Neurophysiology*, **63**, 18–24.

Pritchard, W.S., Raz, N., August, G.J. (1987) 'Visual augmenting/reducing and P300 in autistic children.' *Journal of Autism and Developmental Disorders*, **17**, 231–242.

Ritvo, E.R., Creel, D., Realmuto, G., Crandall, A.S., Freeman, B.J., Bateman, B., Barr, R., Pingree, C., Coleman, M., Purple, R. (1988) 'Electroretinograms in autism: a pilot study of b-wave amplitudes.' *American Journal of Psychiatry*, **145**, 229–232.

Rosenblum, S.M., Arick, J.R., Krug, D.A., Stubbs, E.G., Young, N.B., Pelson, R.O. (1980) 'Auditory brainstem evoked responses in autistic children.' *Journal of Autism and Developmental Disorders*, **10**, 215–225.

Rosenhall, U., Johansson, E., Gillberg, C. (1988) 'Oculomotor findings in autistic children.' *Journal of Laryngology and Otology*, **102**, 435–439.

Ross, K.P. (1982) 'A comparison of the brainstem auditory evoked potentials of children.' *Dissertation Abstracts International*, **43**, 2001-B.

Rumsey, J.M., Grimes, A.M., Pikus, A.M., Duara, R., Ismond, D.R. (1984) 'Auditory brainstem responses in pervasive developmental disorders.' *Biological Psychiatry*, **19**, 1403–1417.

Rutter, M., Bartak, L. (1971) 'Causes of infantile autism: some considerations from recent research.' *Journal of Autism and Childhood Schizophrenia*, **1**, 20–32.

Segawa, M. (1985) 'Circadian rhythm in early infantile autism.' *Advances in Neurological Sciences*, **29**, 140–153.

Sersen, E.A., Heaney, G., Clausen, J., Belser, R., Rainbow, S. (1990) 'Brainstem auditory-evoked responses with and without sedation in autism and Down's syndrome.' *Biological Psychiatry*, **27**, 834–840.

Skoff, B.F., Mirsky, A.F., Turner, D. (1980) 'Prolonged brainstem transmission time in autism.' *Psychiatry Research*, **2**, 157–166.

Small, J.G. (1976) 'EEG and neurophysiological studies of early infantile autism.' *Biological Psychiatry*, **10**, 385–397.

—— DeMyer, M.K., Milstein, V. (1971) 'CNV responses of autistic and normal children.' *Journal of Autism and Childhood Schizophrenia*, **1**, 215–231.

Student, M., Sohmer, H. (1978) 'Evidence from auditory nerve and brainstem evoked responses for an organic brain lesion in children with autistic traits.' *Journal of Autism and Childhood Schizophrenia*, **8**, 13–20.

—— —— (1979) 'Erratum.' *Journal of Autism and Developmental Disorders*, **9**, 309.

Tanguay, P.E., Ornitz, E.M., Forsythe, A.B., Ritvo, E.R. (1976) 'Rapid eye movement (REM) activity in normal and autistic children during REM sleep.' *Journal of Autism and Childhood*

Schizophrenia, **6**, 275–288.

—— Edwards, R.M., Buchwald, J., Schwafel, J., Allen, V. (1982) 'Auditory brainstem evoked responses in autistic children.' *Archives of General Psychiatry*, **39**, 174–180.

Taylor, M.J., Rosenblatt, B., Linschoten, L. (1982) 'Auditory brainstem response abnormalities in autistic children.' *Canadian Journal of Neurological Sciences*, **9**, 429–434.

Thivièrge, J., Côté, R. (1990) 'Brain-stem auditory evoked response: normative values in children.' *Electroencephalography and Clinical Neurophysiology*, **77**, 309–313.

—— Bedard, C., Côté, R., Maziade, M. (1990) 'Brainstem auditory evoked response and subcortical abnormalities in autism.' *American Journal of Psychiatry*, **147**, 1609–1613.

Tsai, L.Y. (1984) 'The development of hand laterality in infantile autism.' *Journal of Autism and Developmental Disorders*, **14**, 447–450.

—— Stewart, M.A. (1982) 'Handedness and EEG correlation in autistic children.' *Biological Psychiatry*, **17**, 595–598.

—— Tsai, M.C., August, G.J. (1985) 'Brief report: implication of EEG diagnoses in the subclassification of infantile autism.' *Journal of Autism and Developmental Disorders*, **15**, 339–344.

Walter, W.G., Aldridge, V.J., Cooper, R., O'Gorman, G., McCallum, C., Winter, A.L. (1971) 'Neurophysiological correlates of apparent defects of sensori-motor integration in autistic children.' *In:* Churchill, D.W., Alpern, G.D., DeMyer, M. (Eds) *Infantile Autism: Proceedings of the Indiana University Colloquium.* Springfield: IL: C.C. Thomas, pp. 265–276.

White, P.T., DeMyer, W., DeMyer, M. (1964) 'EEG abnormalities in early childhood schizophrenia.' *American Journal of Psychiatry*, **120**, 950–958.

13
BRAIN IMAGING

Studies of the brain using imaging techniques have been performed on patients with autistic symptoms by a number of research groups in an effort to delineate any evidence of structural brain damage. These techniques have included pneumo-encephalography (PEG), computerized tomography (CT), magnetic resonance imaging (MRI), positron emission tomography (PET) and single photon emission computerized tomography (SPECT). As might be expected in the study of a disorder of multiple aetiologies, these surveys have shown no consistent pattern, no consistent evidence of any of type of lesion, and no single location of any lesion.

Pneumoencephalographic studies

A review of PEG studies in the older medical literature (Schönfelder 1964, Melchior *et al.* 1965, Boesen and Aarkrog 1967) discloses that when abnormalities were reported, mild or moderate ventricular dilatation was the most common finding. In a detailed study by Aarkrog (1968) of 46 children with infantile autism or 'borderline autism', 25 were reported to have abnormalities that could be detected by PEG. It should be noted, however, that PEG tends to yield more pathological results with regard to widening of the ventricles than more modern imaging methods because of some disturbance of the anatomical state of the brain by PEG methodology.

Hauser *et al.* (1975) reported on the results of PEG studies of 18 developmentally delayed children who had autistic symptoms. The PEGs showed enlargement of the left ventricular system and especially of the left temporal horns in 13 cases; in two other cases the widening was isolated to the left temporal horn only. There was no association between the severity of the clinically assessed symptoms and the degree to which the left temporal horns were enlarged, or between the severity of PEG findings. DeLong *et al.* (1981) discussed these same patients in greater detail; five had definite focal findings on neurological examination. This study probably included a specific cohort of children, some of whom may have had a reversible encephalopathy syndrome as described by DeLong *et al.* Thus, there may have been more uniformity in its findings than has been found in other studies.

PEG is an invasive procedure with morbidity in some cases and has been largely supplanted by imaging techniques such as CT and MRI.

Studies by computerized tomography

CT was developed in the 1970s and the first study on patients with autism was

TABLE 13.1

TABLE 13.1

CT studies in persons with autism

Study	Patients/controls*	Findings
Hier *et al.* (1979)	16A/44MR, 100Neu	Majority had left/right asymmetry of parieto-occipital region
Damasio *et al.* (1980)	17A/49Nor	Ventricular enlargement; right frontal lobe lesions in 2 patients; occult communicating hydrocephalus in 1
Caparulo *et al.* (1981)	22A/30Neu	Ventricular enlargement in 4 patients
Campbell *et al.* (1982)	45A/19Neu	Subgroup with ventricular enlargement
Tsai *et al.* (1982, 1983)	18A/18Neu	No evidence of asymmetry
Gillberg and Svendsen (1983)	27A/23MR, 16Nor	No evidence of ventricular enlargement
Hoshino *et al.* (1984)	24A/179Neu	Gradual increase in width of 3rd ventricle with age
Prior *et al.* (1984)	9A/—	No evidence of asymmetry
Rosenbloom *et al.* (1984)	13A/10Neu	Structural substrate heterogeneous; small proportion had ventricular enlargement
Creasey *et al.* (1986)	12A/16Nor	No statistically significant abnormalities
Gillberg *et al.* (1987)	17A, 3AS/—	Atrophy in region of fissura interhemispherica; periventricular calcification (tuberous sclerosis); right lateral geniculate body defect; moderate left frontal horn atrophy
Rumsey *et al.* (1988)	15A/20Nor (male only)	No asymmetry or posterior fossa abnormalities
Jacobsen *et al.* (1988)	9A/13Nor (adults)	3rd ventricular enlargement; caudate nuclei—signal change
Ballottin *et al.* (1989)	45A/19Neu	Left temporal porencephaly; septum pellucidum cyst; cerebellar hypoplasia, microcephaly
Steffenburg (1990)	46A/46Neu	Ventricular hypertrophy; periventricular calcification; general atrophy; porencephaly (sign of intracerebral haemorrhage)

*A = patients with autism, AS = patients with Asperger syndrome, MR = mentally retarded controls, Neu = neurologically impaired controls, Nor = normal controls.

performed by Hier *et al.* in 1979. Since then at least 16 studies have been published (Table 13.1), and the presence of ventricular enlargement in a subgroup of patients with autism originally identified by PEG has also been reported by CT methods.

The study by Hier *et al.* evaluated 16 patients with autism and compared them with many mentally or neurologically impaired patients. Although none of the patients with autism had evidence of focal or diffuse brain injury, the authors found morphologic asymmetry in more than half, the right parieto-occipital region being wider than the left. Although such asymmetry has been described in up to 25 per cent of other neurologically impaired patients, the higher proportion in this first CT study raised the question of whether the reversal of the asymmetry may have some significance for autism. However, in the second published study, Damasio *et al.* (1980) examined 17 patients with autistic behaviour and found the reverse asymmetry described by Hier *et al.* in only three of this group. They also reported that five patients had evidence of bilateral ventricular enlargement; one patient had a diagnosis of hydrocephalus; and another had lesions in the right frontal lobe.

Caparulo *et al.* (1981) found ventricular enlargement (occipital horn dilatation, left ventricles) in only two of 22 males examined by CT scan, but this patient group included a mix of diagnoses including autism, language disorders, attention deficit disorders and Tourette syndrome. The following year, a larger study was performed of 45 carefully diagnosed and clinically homogeneous children with autism compared to control children hospitalized with neurological problems such as seizures, headaches, tumours or trauma (Campbell *et al.* 1982). The patients with autism were selected to be as free as possible from primary neurological abnormalities. 11 of the 45 patients in this group had mild or moderately prominent enlargement of the ventricular system, a finding compatible with the Damasio *et al.* study.

Tsai *et al.* (1982, 1983) published a two-part study of 18 children with autism compared to control children examined for headache, seizures and linear skull fractures. Left-handed children were excluded from the study. None of the CT scans of either the children with autism or the controls showed evidence of focal or diffuse brain pathology. This study looked closely at the issue of cerebral asymmetries and found that the CT pattern of cerebral asymmetries in children with autism was the same as that observed in patients with neurological disorders. One of the striking findings of the study was that the brains of the children with autism appeared, if anything, to be more symmetrical than those of normal controls. (A similar lack of the unusual prevalence of left parieto-occipital preponderance has also been reported in individuals with dyslexia—Haslam *et al.* 1981.)

Gillberg and Svendsen (1983) compared 27 children with autism against normal and mentally retarded control groups. When matched against the mentally retarded children, findings of ventricular widening were no longer apparent.

In 1984 several issues regarding CT studies were clearly defined. Rosenbloom *et al.* used CT scanning for special studies of linear and volumetric measurements of ventricles, subarachnoid cisterns and cranial size. The population with autism was carefully preselected by omitting those with neurological signs or symptoms. The detailed measurements of this study confirmed that a small proportion of children with autism do have ventricular enlargement, but otherwise they did not reveal any consistent differences in comparison to controls. The authors made a significant contribution by pointing out that the structural substrate in autism was clearly a heterogeneous one. That year Prior *et al.* also did a special study, in this case limited to nine boys with autism who had borderline or normal intelligence. All scans were judged normal with no evidence of unusual asymmetry. This study raised the question of whether there may be a difference in the CT findings of retarded and non-retarded individuals with autism. A third study done in 1984 focused on the question of age-related abnormalities in autism: Hoshino *et al.* investigated evolving abnormalities in CT scans with age. They detected a gradual increase in the width of the third ventricle, interpreting their findings as possibly suggesting a progressive disorder of the thalamus, hypothalamus or midbrain (the structures surrounding the third ventricle).

The Prior *et al.* study suggested the possibility that high-functioning children with autism were less likely to have documented CT abnormalities. Gillberg *et al.* (1987) performed a comprehensive neurobiological assessment, including CT scans, of 17 children with classical Kanner autism and three children with Asperger syndrome, all of whom had full-scale IQs >65. The CT scans on boys with autism showed periventricular calcification (tuberous sclerosis) in one case, a defect in the region of the right lateral geniculate body in a second case, and moderate atrophy in the region of the left frontal horn in a third patient. Another boy with autism had conspicuously narrow frontal horns. A boy with Asperger syndrome showed atrophy in the region of the frontoparietal fissura interhemispherica. [Other cases of Asperger syndrome with structural abnormalities noted by imaging techniques have also been reported in the literature—a case of low density in the left temporal region with atrophy of the left temporal lobe revealed by CT (Jones and Kerwin 1990), and two or more cases of developmental cortical anomalies and opercular dysplasia evinced by MRI (Berthier *et al.* 1990, Piven *et al.* 1990*b*).]

The Hoshino *et al.* (1984) study had raised questions about the possibility of progressive widening of the third ventricle in older individuals with autism. Subsequently, adults with autism were scanned in studies using detailed methods of measurement. Creasey *et al.* (1986) compared 12 adults with autism with age- and sex-matched controls, measuring intracranial volumes, white matter, grey matter, CSF volumes and ventricular volumes, plus the caudate, lenticular nuclei and thalamus. No anatomical abnormalities were statistically significant, although there were trends toward increased third ventricular and left lateral ventricular volumes in the subjects with autism. A second study (Rumsey *et al.* 1988) focused on the possibility of hemispheric asymmetries, fourth ventricular size and cerebellar morphology in 15 adults with autism compared to controls. This study failed to support the hypothesis of unusual hemispheric asymmetry or macroscopic abnormalities of the posterior fossa in the men with autism they were studying.

However, Jacobson *et al.* (1988) compared the CT scans of nine adult males with autism with those of healthy controls and reported significantly greater third ventricular widths and indices in their small patient population. They also noted that regional brain densities were significantly lower in the right and left caudate

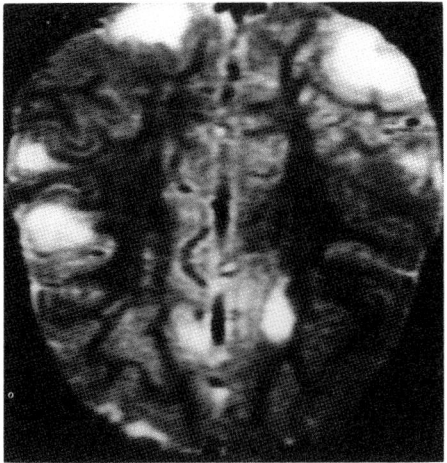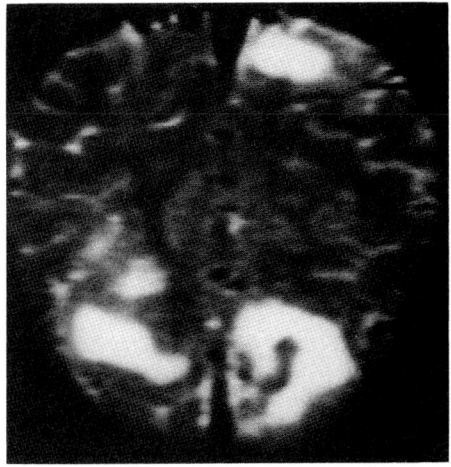

Fig. 13.1. Axial MRI showing multiple, large bifrontal *(left)* and posterior *(right)* tubers in a child with tuberous sclerosis and autism.

nuclei but not in other brain regions. A detailed mathematical study of the CT scans of 45 children with autism and 19 controls was carried out by Balottin *et al.* (1989). The population of children with autism was unusual in that the ratio of boys to girls was 5:4. The authors reported two cases of left temporal porencephaly, one cyst of the septum pellucidum, a cerebellar hypoplasia, and one child with microcephaly. Their elaborate measurements showed a trend toward enlargement of the right lateral ventricle, particularly in patients with severe language impairment.

In a study of 46 children with autism and autistic-like conditions, Steffenburg (1990) found 10 children with CT abnormalities, including five patients with widening of the ventricular system (three at the pontine/brainstem level and two in the temporal lobes), three with signs of intracerebral haemorrhage/porencephaly, and one each with general atrophy and periventricular calcification.

Studies by magnetic resonance imaging

A new development in imaging techniques, MRI was first applied to patients with autism in 1987. Regarding the brain, this method is particularly helpful. For example, in the evaluation of posterior fossa structures, MRI has excellent multiplanar visualization without the beam-hardening artifact seen with CT scanning. Also, because the methodology does not involve any exposure to radiation, it is particularly suitable for children and for exploratory studies involving a large number of slices in any single patient (Fig. 13.1).

Published studies employing MRI in persons with autism are listed in Table 13.2. In the first of these Gaffney and Tsai (1987) found six out of 14 patients with

TABLE 13.2

MRI studies in persons with autism

Study	Patients/controls*	Findings
Courchesne et al. (1987)	1A/—	Underdevelopment of cerebellum
Gaffney and Tsai (1987)	14A/—	Interpeduncular cistern epidermoid cyst; enlarged fourth ventricle; signal change bilaterally in globus pallidi; dilated lateral ventricles; left occipital heterotopic grey matter; right parietal signal change; temporal lobe ganglioglioma
Gaffney et al. (1987a,b)	13A/35Neu	Statistically significant posterior fossa enlargement
Courchesne et al. (1988)	18A/12Neu	Diminished size of cerebellar lobules VI and VII in 14/18
Ritvo and Garber (1988)	15A/15Nor	No significant difference in cerebellar size
Reiss et al. (1988)	4AFRAX/4Nor	Diminished size of cerebellar lobules VI and VII
Gaffney et al. (1988, 1989)	13A/35Neu	Diminished size of pons; enlarged anterior horns and lateral ventricles; smaller lenticular nuclei on right
Murakami et al. (1989)	10A/8Nor	Diminished size of cerebellar lobules VI and VII; smaller than normal cerebellar hemispheres
Hashimoto et al. (1989)	18A/11Neu/18Nor	Brain asymmetry
Nowell et al. (1990)	53A/32Neu	Atrophy of cerebellar vermis in subgroup of 8%; pineal cyst; small white matter lesions—uncal, periatrial, temporal lobe
Piven et al. (1990)	13A/13Nor (male only)	Cerebral cortical malformations (polymicrogyria, macrogyria, schizencephaly) in 54%

*AFRAX = patients with autism and fragile X; other abbreviations as for Table 13.1.

detectable lesions. These included basal ganglia abnormalities, heterotopic grey matter, a right posterior temporal lobe cystic mass (later proven on biopsy to be a ganglioglioma) and dilatation of lateral and fourth ventricles. In two subsequent papers in 1987, Gaffney et al. reported on fourth ventricular and cerebellar size in patients with autism using MRI. In one study, they performed sagittal slices and did not find any significant difference in cerebellar size compared to controls (Gaffney et al. 1987a). In the other, they performed coronal and axial images; this time they found the cerebellum significantly smaller and the fourth ventricle significantly larger on the coronal images (Gaffney et al. 1987b). This second study was performed on 13 'high level' children and adolescents with autism (mean IQ = 55) compared to 35 controls. In the same year, Courchesne et al. reported underdevelopment of part of the cerebellum in a non-retarded man with autism.

As a result of these preliminary findings, the question of whether there was a diminution of the fourth ventricular structures in patients with autism had been raised and a number of studies addressed this question. Courchesne et al. (1988) studied 18 'high level' subjects with autism (mean IQ = 88; mean age = 21 years) and compared them to 12 controls. They carefully excluded patients with known neurological disease and those on antiepileptic or antipsychotic medication. 14 out of the 18 patients had a 25 per cent decrease in the size of cerebellar lobules VI and VII. A follow-up study reevaluated nine of the original patients (plus one new one) with MRI and added the finding that, in addition to having abnormally small cerebellar vermal lobules VI and VII, the subjects had smaller than normal cerebellar hemispheres (Murakami et al. 1989). They postulated that developmental failure rather than atrophy was responsible for the diminished size of the cerebellar lobules.

At this point, the possible finding of a consistent structural defect in patients with autism caused a great deal of comment, including an editorial in the *New England Journal of Medicine* (Volkmar and Cohen 1988). Other psychiatric diseases also began to be studied. For example, in an MRI study of 30 schizophrenic males, cerebellar vermal lobules VI and VII were found to be statistically significantly smaller in patients with perinatal complications compared to those without such complications while the other cerebellar lobules in these patients were unchanged (Nasrallah et al. 1989). Another example was the catatonic syndrome, within schizophrenia, which was reported to have increased cerebellar atrophy by another investigator (Wilcox 1991).

Meanwhile, Ritvo and Garber (1988) responded to the papers of the Courchesne group with an MRI reevaluation of 15 patients with autism, specifically aimed at the question of focal atrophy of cerebellar lobules VI and VII. They reported no significant difference between patients and controls regarding cerebellar size. On the other hand, Reiss et al. (1988) studied four patients with the fragile X syndrome and found the size of vermal lobules VI and VII decreased in this patient group, a number of whom have autistic symptoms. Reiss and his research group continued to write extensively about the role of the cerebellum in autistic symptoms (Reiss 1988, Reiss et al. 1991), including describing such symptoms in two patients with Joubert syndrome—a syndrome specifically characterized by cerebellar agenesis (Holroyd et al. 1991). Gaffney et al. (1988) reentered the discussion describing 13 high-functioning patients, but reporting that a different abnormality accounted for the enlargement of the fourth ventricle: in their studies, it was the pons rather than the cerebellum that was significantly smaller.

In 1990, a paper was published which tried to sort out the problems presented by the earlier studies; an attempt was made to compensate for the relatively small number of patients in previous studies and the fact that the investigators were often not blind as to the patient's diagnosis. Nowell et al. studied the MRIs of 53 unselected patients from a clinic specializing in autism, using neuroradiologists blind as to whether the MRI was from a patient or a control. One of the evaluating neuroradiologists did not even know that the disease entity being studied was autism. In this study, the overwhelming majority of subjects had normal fourth ventricular size (92 per cent of the children with autism and 90 per cent of controls). However, four of the children with autism (7.5 per cent) were noted to have significant vermian atrophy, representing a small subgroup within the whole. Small white matter lesions were also seen in three patients at the left uncal, periatrial and temporal lobes; none were seen in the controls. The exact meaning of these particular lesions was not clear but delayed myelination is known to exist in several conditions which have been associated with autistic syndromes, *e.g.* phenylketonuria, congenital rubella.

New findings were published when MRI studies were focused on the cortex. Piven *et al.* (1990*a*) reported finding cerebral cortical malformations in seven of 13 high-functioning male subjects with autism. These lesions included polymicrogyria, macrogyria and schizencephaly; the lesions were clearly visible in the photographs published in the paper. The concept that these abnormalities resulted from a defect in the migration of neurons during the first six months of gestation led the authors to reinterpret papers by others. They suggested that the temporal lobe atrophy reported by Jones and Kerwin (1990) in a patient with Asperger syndrome was more likely an open operculum, a defect from abnormal neuronal migration (Piven *et al.* 1990*b*). The same investigators also published evidence of developmental cortical anomalies in two subjects with Asperger syndrome.

The fourth ventricle is not the only ventricle being closely examined in patients with autism' using MRI techniques. Gaffney *et al.* (1989) have focused a study on the lateral ventricles and anterior horns and reported them enlarged in their patient group. They interpret the enlarged anterior horns to indicate defects in the nearby fornix and generally relate the enlarged ventricles to possible limbic dysfunction. They also recorded a smaller lenticular nucleus on the right. (The caudate nuclei, reported to have diminished densities bilaterally in a CT study by Jacobson *et al.* (1988), are part of the lenticular nuclei.)

The question of asymmetry of the brain, originally described by Hier *et al.* (1979) with CT methodology, has also resurfaced with MRI studies. Hashimoto *et al.* (1989) evaluated 18 individuals with autism and reported a reversal of brain asymmetry. These authors contrasted the results in autism with those found in mental retardation in general, suggesting that early structural impairment may differ in subjects with autism.

Positron emission tomography and single photon emission computerized tomography
PET is a relatively new imaging technique that offers a means to assess parameters of brain function regionally and quantitatively. PET displays physiological data in a way analogous to a conventional CT image. Techniques have been developed for measuring cerebral blood flow and the consumption of oxygen and glucose, the two

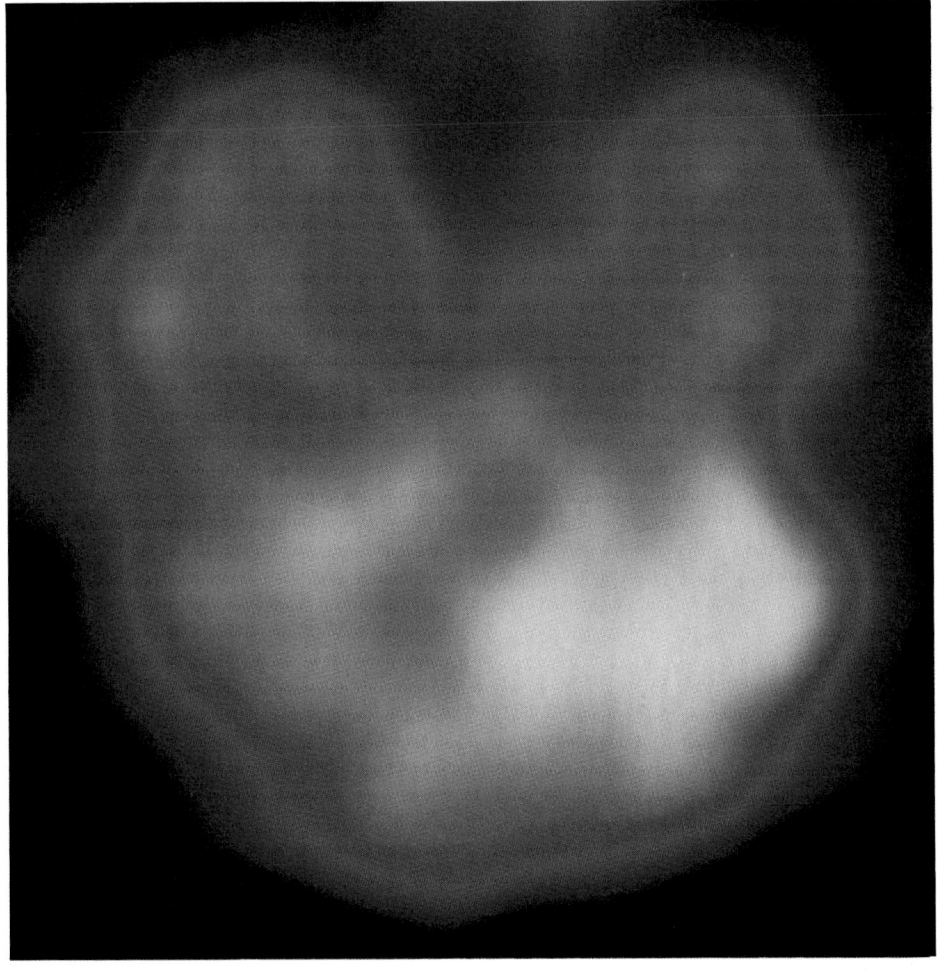

Fig. 13.2. Cerebral SPECT of 22-year-old man with autism.

virtually exclusive substrates of cerebral energy metabolism. The test is sensitive to factors such as anxiety and distraction, making the results difficult to interpret. It is also invasive with brief dosages of ionizing radiation.

Using glucose as the tracer, adult males with autism with well-documented diagnoses of infantile autism have been evaluated in comparison with controls (Rapoport *et al.* 1983, Rumsey *et al.* 1985). Although the results showed no deficiencies in the resting cerebral metabolic rates for glucose, diffusely elevated metabolic rates were seen in the autism group taken as a whole, with a large degree of overlap with the control groups. In these studies, no specific brain regions demonstrated lowered glucose metabolism. A similar study found no difference at all between male subjects with autism and their controls; even the borderline glucose hypermetabolism was not substantiated (Herold *et al.* 1988). In addition, regional blood flow and oxygen consumption were not significantly different from control levels.

A study of the cerebellar area in patients with autism vs. controls also found equal (or possibly slightly greater) rates of glucose metabolism (Heh *et al.* 1989). There was no evidence of diminished function in this study, a possibility raised by MRI studies.

PET techniques have also been used to provide a measure of functional association between brain regions. This relatively new work is quite difficult to interpret and needs careful duplication. The first published results by Horwitz *et al.* (1988) showed the possibility of fewer positive correlations between the frontal/parietal regions and thalamic, neostriatal areas in individuals with autism.

SPECT has also been tried with individuals with autism (Fig. 13.2). No regional abnormality has been demonstrated in published studies (Sherman *et al.* 1984, Chiron *et al.* 1992), but preliminary data from Göteborg suggest that the temporal lobes may be affected, with reduced blood flow (usually bilaterally) (C.G., personal data).

Ultrasonography

A transcranial Doppler study of 13 children with autism compared to non-autistic children with psychiatric disorders and normal controls was performed with and without auditory stimulation (Bruneau *et al.* 1992). The 'activating' pattern to auditory stimulation found on the left side in the other two groups was not seen in the children with autism. Further studies are needed to determine whether the haemodynamic modifications observed are a consequence of cardiac effects or if they are part of defective central processing of sensory events.

Discussion

What is one to make of this imaging literature, which is full of contradictions and disputes? If autism is a single disease with homogeneous patients, this wide spectrum of findings performed by reliable investigators using imaging methodology makes little sense. The original hopes that imaging techniques would discover a specific location in the CNS for the symptoms of autism is no longer viable.

What we can learn from these many studies is that there may be some subgroups among patients with autism who can be defined by imaging techniques. It seems possible that there is a subgroup with non-specific ventricular hypertrophy; it is interesting that one of the first descriptions of a patient with autism and neurological deficit was of a child with arrested hydrocephalus (head circumference 54cm) (Schain and Yannet 1960). It is also possible that there is another subgroup with cerebellar atrophy (?related to perinatal problems, the chromosomal syndromes or a long history of medication), and another small subgroup with left temporal damage (?viral or traumatic in origin).

However, at this stage of the development of imaging techniques, this information is of limited clinical use. At this time, the main clinical reason for performing an imaging study on an individual with an autistic syndrome is either (1) to rule in or out the space-occupying lesions very occasionally found in this patient group, *e.g.* subarachnoid cysts (Segawa *et al.* 1986, see Chapter 19), or (2) to confirm the presence of a congenital lesion, such as heterotopy, porencephaly, developmental cortical anomaly, etc. for diagnostic purposes.

REFERENCES

Aarkrog, T. (1968) 'Organic factors in infantile psychoses and borderline psychoses.' *Danish Medical Bulletin*, **15**, 283–288.
Balottin, U., Bejor, M., Cecchini, A., Martelli, A., Palazzi, S., Lanzi, G. (1989) 'Infantile autism and computerized tomography brain-scan findings: specific versus non-specific abnormalities.' *Journal of Autism and Developmental Disorders*, **19**, 109–118.
Berthier, M.L., Starkstein, S.E., Leiguarda, R. (1990) 'Developmental anomalies in Asperger's syndrome: neuroradiological findings in two patients.' *Journal of Neuropsychiatry*, **2**, 197–201.
Boesen, U., Aarkrog, T. (1967) 'Pneumoencephalography of patients in a child psychiatric department.' *Danish Medical Bulletin*, **14**, 210–218.
Bruneau, N., Dourneau, M-C., Garreau, B., Arbeille, P., Pourcelot, L., Lelord, G. (1992) 'Modifications of cerebral blood flow with auditory stimulations in children with autistic behavior: a transcranial doppler ultrasonography study.' *Biological Psychiatry. (In press.)*
Campbell, M., Rosenbloom, S., Perry, R., George, A.E., Kricheff, I.I., Anderson, L., Small, A.M., Jennings, S.J. (1982) 'Computerized axial tomography in young autistic children.' *American Journal of Psychiatry*, **139**, 510–512.
Caparulo, B.K., Cohen, D.J., Rothman, S.L., Young, J.G., Katz, J.D., Shaywitz, S.E., Shaywitz, B.A. (1981) 'Computed tomographic brain scanning in children with developmental neuro-psychiatric disorders.' *Journal of the American Academy of Child Psychiatry*, **20**, 338–357.
Chiron, C., Raynaud, C., Maziere, B., Zilbovicius, M., Laflamme, L., Masure, M., Dulac, O., Bourgllignon, M., Syrota, A. (1992) 'Changes in regional cerebral blood flow during brain maturation in children and adolescents.' *Nuclear Medicine*, **33**, 696–703.
Courchesne, E., Hesselink, J., Jernigan, T.L., Yeung-Courchesne, R. (1987) 'Abnormal neuroanatomy in a non-retarded person with autism.' *Archives of Neurology*, **44**, 335–341.
—— Yeung-Courchesne, R., Press, G.A., Hesselink, J.R., Jernigan, T.L. (1988) 'Hypoplasia of cerebellar vermal VI and VII in autism.' *New England Journal of Medicine*, **318**, 1349–1354.
Creasey, H., Rumsey, J., Schwartz, M., Duara, R., Rapoport, J., Rapoport, S.I. (1986) 'Brain morphometry in autistic men as measured by volumetric computed tomography.' *Archives of Neurology*, **43**, 669–672.
Damasio, H., Maurer, R.G., Damasio, A.R., Chui, H.C. (1980) 'Computerized tomographic scan findings in patients with autistic behavior.' *Archives of Neurology*, **37**, 504–510.
DeLong, G.R., Beau, S.C., Brown, F.R. (1981) 'Acquired reversible autistic syndrome in an acute encephalopathic illness in children.' *Archives of Neurology*, **38**, 191–194.
Gaffney, G., Tsai, L. (1987) 'Brief report: magnetic resonance imaging of high-level autism.' *Journal of Autism and Developmental Disorders*, **17**, 433–438.
—— Kuperman, S., Tsai, L.Y., Minchin, S., Hassanein, K.M. (1987*a*) 'Midsagittal magnetic resonance imaging of autism.' *British Journal of Psychiatry*, **151**, 831–833.
—— Tsai, L.Y., Kuperman, S., Minchin, S. (1987*b*) 'Cerebellar structure in autism.' *American Journal of Diseases of Children*, **141**, 1330–1332.
—— Kuperman, S., Tsai, L., Minchin, S. (1988) 'Morphologic evidence for brainstem involvement in infantile autism.' *Biological Psychiatry*, **24**, 578–586.
—— —— Tsai, L., Minchin, S. (1989) 'Forebrain structure in infantile autism.' *Journal of the American Academy of Child and Adolescent Psychiatry*, **28**, 534–537.
Gillberg, C., Svendsen, P. (1983) 'Childhood psychosis and computed tomographic brain scan findings.'

159

Journal of Autism and Developmental Disorders, **13**, 19–32.

—— Steffenburg, S., Jakobsson, G. (1987) 'Neurobiological findings in 20 relatively gifted children with Kanner-type autism or Asperger syndrome.' *Developmental Medicine and Child Neurology*, **29**, 641–649.

Hashimoto, T., Tayama, M., Mori, K., Fujnio, K., Miyazaki, M., Kuroda, Y. (1989) 'Magnetic resonance imaging in autism; preliminary report.' *Neuropediatrics*, **20**, 142–146.

Haslam, R.H.A., Dalby, J.T., Johns, R.D., Rademaker, A.W. (1981) 'Cerebral asymmetry in developmental dyslexia.' *Archives of Neurology*, **38**, 679–682.

Hauser, S.L., DeLong, G.R., Rosman, N.P. (1975) 'Pneumographic findings in the infantile autism syndrome: a correlation with temporal lobe disease.' *Brain*, **98**, 667–688.

Heh, C.W., Smith, R., Wu, J., Hazlett, E., Russel, A., Asarnow, R., Tanguay, P., Buchsbaum, M.S. (1989) 'Positron emission tomography of the cerebellum in autism.' *American Journal of Psychiatry*, **146**, 242–245.

Herold, S., Frackowiak, R.S.J., Le Couteur, A., Rutter, M., Howlin, P. (1988) 'Cerebral blood flow and metabolism of oxygen and glucose in young autistic adults.' *Psychological Medicine*, **18**, 823–831.

Hier, D.E., LeMay, M., Rosenberger, P.B. (1979) 'Autism and unfavourable left-right asymmetries of the brain.' *Journal of Autism and Developmental Disorders*, **9**, 153–159.

Holroyd, S., Reiss, A.L., Bryan, R.N. (1991) 'Autistic features in Joubert syndrome: a genetic disorder with agenesis of the cerebellar vermis.' *Biological Psychiatry*, **29**, 287–294.

Horwitz, B., Rumsey, J.M., Grady, C.L., Rapoport, S.I. (1988) 'The cerebral metabolic landscape in autism: intercorrelations of regional glucose utilization.' *Archives of Neurology*, **45**, 749–755.

Hoshino, Y., Manome, T., Kaneko, M., Yashima, Y., Kumashiro, H. (1984) 'Computed tomography of the brain in children with early infantile autism.' *Folia Psychiatrica et Neurologica Japonica*, **38**, 33–43.

Jacobson, R., Le Couteur, A., Howlin, P., Rutter, M. (1988) 'Selective subcortical abnormalities in autism.' *Psychological Medicine*, **18**, 39–48.

Jones, P.B., Kerwin, R.W. (1990) 'Left temporal lobe damage in Asperger's syndrome.' *British Journal of Psychiatry*, **156**, 570–572.

Melchior, J.C., Dyggve, H.V., Gylstorff, H. (1965) 'Pneumoencephalographic examination of 207 mentally retarded patients.' *Danish Medical Bulletin*, **12**, 38–42.

Murakami, J.W., Courchesne, E., Press, G.A., Yeung-Courchesne, R., Hesselink, J.R. (1989) 'Reduced cerebellar hemisphere size and its relationship to vermal hypoplasia in autism.' *Archives of Neurology*, **46**, 689–694.

Nasrallah, H.A., Schwarzkopf, S.B., Coffman, J.A., Olson, S.C. (1989) 'Perinatal complications and superior posterior vermian hypoplasia in schizophrenia on MRI scans.' *Biological Psychiatry*, **25** (Suppl.) 14A. *(Abstract.)*

Nowell, M.A., Hackney, D.B., Muraki, A.S., Coleman, M. (1990) 'Varied MR appearance of autism: fifty-three pediatric patients have the full autistic syndrome.' *Magnetic Resonance Imaging*, **8**, 811–816.

Piven, J., Berthier, M.L., Starkstein, S.E., Nehme, E., Pearlson, G., Folstein, S. (1990a) 'Magnetic resonance imaging evidence for a defect of cerebral cortical development in autism.' *American Journal of Psychiatry*, **147**, 734–739.

—— Starkstein, S., Berthier, M.L. (1990b) 'Temporal lobe atrophy versus open operculum in Asperger's syndrome.' *British Journal of Psychiatry*, **157**, 457–458. *(Letter.)*

Prior, M.R., Tress, B., Hoffman, W.L., Boldt, D. (1984) 'Computed tomographic study of children with classic autism.' *Archives of Neurology*, **431**, 482–484.

Rapoport, J.L., Rumsey, J., Duavas, R., Schwartz, M., Kessler, R., Culten, N., Rapoport, S.I. (1983) 'Cerebral metabolic rate for glucose in adult autism as measured by positron emission tomography.' *Journal of Cerebral Blood Flow Metabolism*, **3** (Suppl. 1), 264–265.

Reiss, A.L. (1988) 'Cerebellar hypoplasia and autism.' *New England Journal of Medicine*, **319**, 1152–1153.

—— Patel, S., Kumar, A.J., Freund, L. (1988) 'Preliminary communication: neuroanatomical variations of the posterior fossa in men with fragile X (Martin-Bell) syndrome.' *American Journal of Medical Genetics*, **31**, 407–414.

—— Aylward, E., Freund, L.S., Joshi, P.K., Bryan, R.N. (1991) 'Neuroanatomy of fragile X syndrome: the posterior fossa.' *Annals of Neurology*, **29**, 26–32.

Ritvo, E.R., Garber, H.J. (1988) 'Cerebellar hypoplasia and autism.' *New England Journal of Medicine*, **319**, 1152. *(Letter.)*

Rosenbloom, S., Campbell, M., George, A., Kricheff, I., Taleporos, E., Anderson, L., Reuben, R., Korein, J. (1984) 'High-resolution CT scanning in infantile autism: a quantitative approach.' *Journal of the American Academy of Child Psychiatry*, **23**, 72–77.

Rumsey, J., Duara, R., Grady, C., Rapoport, J., Margolin, R.A., Rapoport, S.I., Cutler, N.R. (1985) 'Brain metabolism in autism: resting cerebral glucose utilization rates as measured with positron emission tomography.' *Archives of General Psychiatry*, **42**, 448–455.

—— Creasey, H., Stepanek, J., Dorwart, R., Patronas, N., Hamburger, S.D., Duara, R. (1988) 'Hemispheric asymmetries, fourth ventricular size and cerebellar morphology in autism.' *Journal of Autism and Developmental Disorders*, **18**, 127–137.

Schain, R.J., Yannet, H. (1960) 'Infantile autism: an analysis of 50 cases and a consideration of certain relevant neurophysiologic concepts.' *Journal of Pediatrics*, **57**, 560–567.

Schönfelder, T. (1964) 'Uber frühkindliche Antriebsstörungen.' *Acta Paedopsychiatrica*, **31**, 112–129.

Segawa, M., Nomura, Y., Nagata, E., Hata, K., Saitoh, S. (1986) 'Autism with middle fossa arachnoid cyst.' *Journal of Child Neurology*, **1**, 276.

Sherman, M., Nass, R., Shapiro, T. (1984) 'Regional cerebral blood flow in autism.' *Journal of Autism and Developmental Disorders*, **14**, 439–446.

Steffenburg, S. (1990) *Neurobiological Correlates of Autism*. M.D. thesis, University of Göteborg.

Tsai, L.Y., Jacoby, C.G., Stewart, M.A., Beisler, J.M. (1982) 'Unfavorable left-right asymmetries of the brain and autism: a question of methodology.' *British Journal of Psychiatry*, **140**, 312–319.

—— —— —— (1983) 'Morphological cerebral asymmetries in autistic children.' *Biiological Psychiatry*, **18**, 317–327.

Volkmar, F.R., Cohen, D.J. (1988) 'Neurobiologic aspects of autism.' *New England Journal of Medicine*, **318**, 1390–1391. *(Editorial.)*

Wilcox, J.A. (1991) 'Cerebellar atrophy and catatonia.' *Biological Psychiatry*, **29**, 733. *(Letter.)*

14
NEUROPATHOLOGICAL STUDIES

One of the scandals in the field of autism is that there are so few accurate neuropathological data available even now, almost 50 years after Kanner first described the condition. The lack of clinicopathological correlation studies is a major hindrance to rapid progress toward accurate diagnosis and treatment. In 1976, the association of parents of children with autism in the USA (National Society for Autistic Children—NSAC) started a national autopsy research committee in association with a major university (UCLA). This approach, extended to other countries, will eventually correct this lacuna in the field of autism research.

In the few studies now available where competent neuropathological techniques have been applied, often the clinical diagnosis and/or medical work-up of the patient during life was inadequate. In a disorder of multiple aetiologies, the significance of any single pathological study to other patients with the condition is limited. In any event, to date such studies have not revealed any unique neuropathological findings associated with autism.

A generation after Kanner's first description, a string of individual case studies with widely diverging clinical criteria and diagnostic confusion were reviewed by Darby (1976). He had searched the literature to find all possible neuropathological cases that could be related to autism. Because of the lack of consistent clinical criteria, the information is of limited value except historically to demonstrate what confusion existed about this patient group in the decades after it was first described. For example, there was the slowly deteriorating girl who received psychotherapy three times a week until her death at 11 years of age because most of her physicians believed that her mother's rejection caused the child's problems (Ross 1959). Autopsy revealed a diffuse encephalopathy of the brain which included cortical atrophy, diffuse gliosis of the white matter as well as lesions in the hypothalamus, mammillary bodies, hypophyseal eminence, reticular formation, anterior nuclei of the thalamus and cerebellum. In an unpublished DeMyer case reported by Darby (1976), a microcephalic child with autistic features had a brain biopsy which indicated non-specific histological and ultrastructural abnormalities. Abnormal but non-specific neuropathological findings were frequent in the Darby survey.

Williams *et al.* (1980) performed a careful neuropathological examination limited primarily to the cerebral cortex in four individuals who exhibited prominent autistic features throughout life. It is not clear that all of their patients would meet current diagnostic criteria for autism. They studied the hippocampus, parahippocampal gyrus, thalamus, hypothalamus, striatum and midbrain tectum. The brainstem was not examined. The methodology included neurons impregnated with the rapid Golgi method and electron microscopic analyses. Two patients (one male and one female) had many classic autistic symptoms combined with normal motor milestones: no abnormalities were found in these two brains. A third case was a boy who was severely retarded and did not walk until 2 years of age, then developed grand mal seizures at age 5; he had a sister with similar problems. Another was a child with phenylketonuria. In the last two cases, subtle changes limited to the dendrites and spines of layer V pyramidal neurons of the mid-frontal gyrus were found. In both brains, although the pyramidal neurons from layer V were oriented normally and had richly branched dendritic arbors, there was a subtle diminution of dendritic calibre and spine density. (The development of dendritic spines begins around the 30th gestational week and continues until the age of 1 year or older.) In the familial case, the actual density of the Purkinje cells also seemed generally reduced but no cell count was done.

In 1984, a very detailed autopsy was performed on the brain of a man with autism who died by drowning (Bauman and Kemper 1985). As a child, he had displayed classical features of autism. At 4 years of age, he began intensive individual psychotherapy and attended a special therapeutic nursery school, but it resulted in no appreciable progress. Language never progressed beyond two-word phrases. Starting in adolescence, he was treated with psychotropic drugs because of self-injurious behaviour and temper outbursts; these included chlorpromazine, trifluoperazine, diazepam and up to 300mg/day of thioridazine as an adult. Seizures started at 21 years of age and he took anticonvulsant drugs, varying among primidone, phenobarbitone and phenytoin, until his death at 29 years. After the seizure disorder began, he had an EEG which showed a photoconvulsive pattern and a PEG which revealed mild ventricular dilation. It was not known if he had ever been tested for any specific aetiology of the autistic syndrome.

In this detailed study, serial sections of the brain (Fig. 14.1) were compared with those of a sex-matched control. In the patient's brain there was a clear zone, deep to the superficial layer, which was not present in the control. This clear zone (lamina desicans) normally disappears by 15 months of age. Atrophy of the neocerebellar cortex was present in the biventer, gracile, tonsil and semilunar lobules. There was no atrophy of the vermis. There was a marked loss of Purkinje cells and, to a lesser extent, the granule cells in the neocerebellum; also small neurons which were reduced in number were described in the emboliform, globose and fastigial nuclei. Part of the inferior olive showed abnormally small, pale neurons (rather than the expected retrograde cell loss from the neocerebellum). Also reported was reduced cell size with increased cell packing density in the hippocampal complex, the entorhinal cortex, selected nuclei of the amygdala, the mammillary bodies and septal nuclei which project to the hippocampus. The cytoarchitectonic abnormalities noted in the forebrain included reduced neuronal size and increased cell-packing, both features of an immature brain. This study showed abnormalities concentrated in the forebrain and the cerebellum.

Coleman *et al.* (1985) compared a careful count of the neurons and glia in the

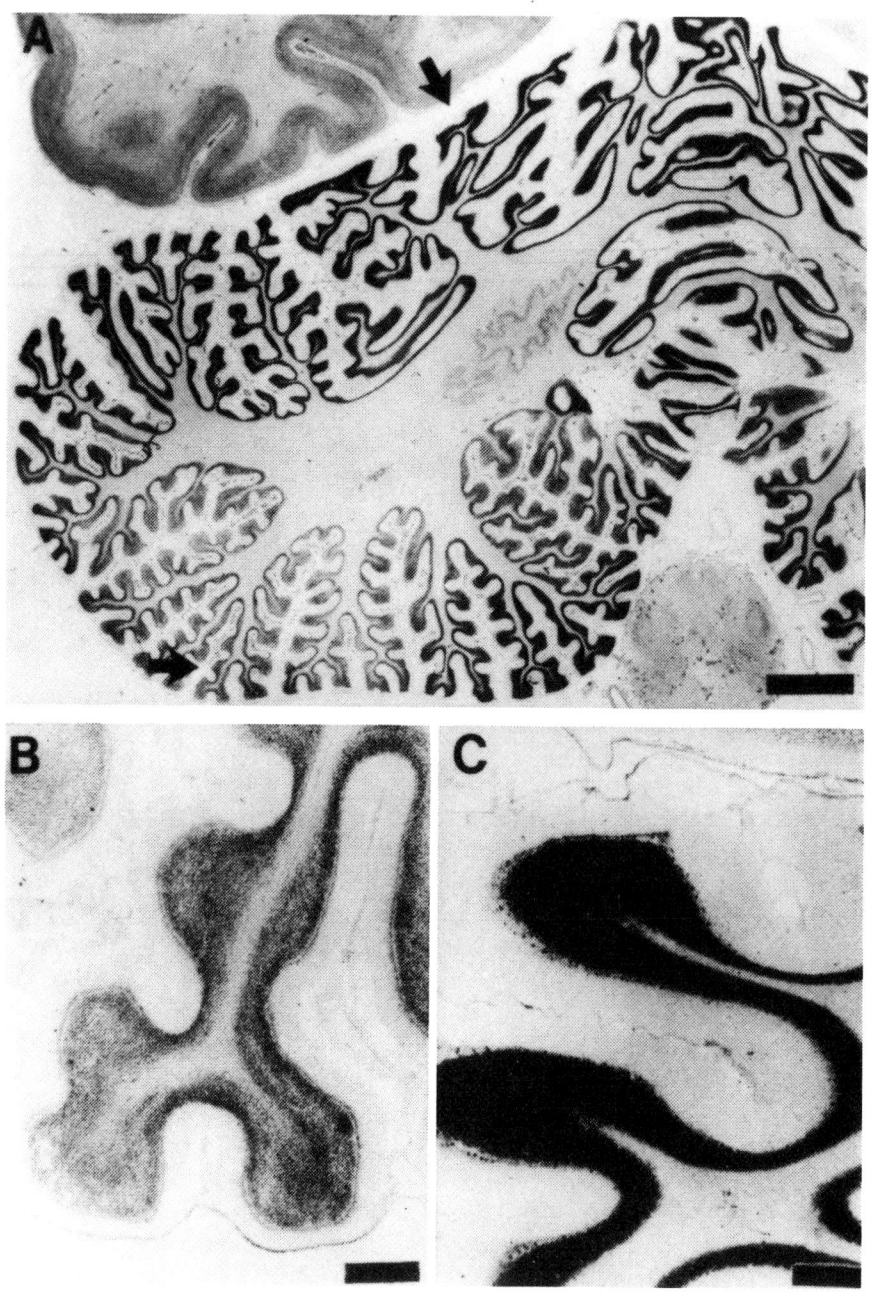

Fig. 14.1. Nissl-stained section of the cerebellum of a 29-year-old man with autism never specifically diagnosed during his lifetime. He received antipsychotic and anticonvulsant medications. Note atrophy of cerebellar cortex of lateral and inferior parts of hemisphere (A, *lower arrow*) and normal-appearing cortex of anterior lobe and vermis (A, *upper arrow*). In atrophic area (B) there is a striking loss of Purkinje cells compared to an unaffected area (C). (Bar in A = 5mm; in B and C = 500μm.)

cortex of a patient with autism and two age/sex-matched controls. In this detailed study, 17,689 cells were manually counted and categorized. This study included the primary auditory cortex, Broca's speech area and the auditory association cortex. No consistent differences in brain cell density were found between the subject and the control individuals.

A selective study of the cerebellum was conducted on the brains of four males aged 10 to 22 years by Ritvo *et al.* (1986). All four patients met DSM-III criteria for the diagnosis of autism. Three were low-functioning patients (IQs 20–40) while the fourth had an IQ of 103. This last patient committed suicide at 15 years of age. No patient had a seizure disorder, although the three low-functioning patients all had abnormal EEGs (type unspecified). Two of the patients were on no medication; one was on haloperidol, the other on chlordiazepoxide. The low-functioning patient on haloperidol had received a CT scan which showed bilateral ventricular enlargement. There is no medical work-up mentioned for the other three individuals.

Pathology results demonstrated that one patient had microgyria of the occipital and temporal lobes. Total Purkinje cell counts were significantly lower in the cerebellar hemisphere and vermis of each of the four patients compared to comparison cases. Purkinje cells are the largest and quite important cells in cerebellar functioning and help process incoming sensory information.

These results make a contribution that fits with other data obtained by imaging studies. Microgyria have also been demonstrated in patients with autism by MRI (see Chapter 13).

Diminution of the number of cerebellar cells in neuropathological studies were also reported in one of the Williams *et al.* (1980) cases and and in the Bauman and Kemper (1985) case, although exact counts were not performed in these earlier studies. There appears to be a subgroup of patients with autism with reduction in the size of the cerebellum demonstrable by MRI studies (see Chapter 13).

However, since there were findings of diminished counts of cerebellar neurons, it would be extremely relevant to know what neuronal counts were like elsewhere in the same brains. Also, the patients' work-ups were so limited that there is not even a description of the type of EEG abnormalities in the records.

Summary

Autistic syndromes have multiple aetiologies; so clinico-pathological correlations are especially difficult to interpret. First, there have to be adequately worked-up case histories matched to modern neuropathological techniques. Then the debates can begin.

REFERENCES

Bauman, M., Kemper, T.L. (1985) 'Histoanatomic observations of the brain in early infantile autism.' *Neurology*, **35**, 866–874.
Coleman, P.D., Romano, J., Lapham, L., Simon, W. (1985) 'Cell counts in cerebral cortex of an

autistic patient.' *Journal of Autism and Developmental Disorders*, **15**, 245–255.

Darby, J.C. (1976) 'Neuropathologic aspects of psychosis in children.' *Journal of Autism and Childhood Schizophrenia*, **6**, 339–352.

Ritvo, E.R., Freeman, B.J., Scheibel, A.B., Duong, T., Robinson, H., Guthrie, D., Ritvo, A. (1986) 'Lower Purkinje cell counts in the cerebella of four autistic subjects: initial findings of the UCLA-NSAC autopsy research report.' *American Journal of Psychiatry*, **143**, 862–866.

Ross, I.S. (1959) 'An autistic child.' *Pediatric Conferences (Babies Hospital Units, United Hospital of Newark, NJ)*, **2**, 1–13.

Williams, R.S., Hauser, S.L., Purpura, D.P., DeLong, G.R., Swisher, C.N. (1980) 'Autism and mental retardation. Neuropathologic studies performed in four retarded persons with autistic behavior.' *Archives of Neurology*, **37**, 749–753.

15
NEUROPSYCHOLOGY

The notion that children with autism cannot be reliably tested—or indeed tested at all—with conventional psychometric cognitive measures has strongly restricted empirical study in the field. This has led to a situation in which the neuropsychology of autism has become a fairly small branch on the now rather healthy tree of autism research. However, recent years have witnessed an increasing interest in the basic psychology of autism, and some of the most interesting developments in all of autism research have emerged from neuropsychologically inclined studies of young children with autism and of adult high-functioning men with autism. During the 1980s there were basically four seats of innovative research studies in the neuropsychological domain which have had a profound influence on the way we now think about autism. Uta Frith and her colleagues (Baron-Cohen et al. 1985, Leslie and Frith 1988, Baron-Cohen 1989a) have studied the 'theory of mind' concept; Deborah Fein and Lynn Waterhouse have focused on the neuropsychological heterogeneity in groups of patients diagnosed as autistic or autistic-like (Waterhouse and Fein 1989); Peter Hobson (1984, 1986a,b, 1987) has studied various aspects of egocentricity and perception along Piagetian lines; and Judith Rumsey and her co-workers (Rumsey et al. 1988) have expanded the field of study of cognitive abilities in high-functioning adult males with autism. These studies, and a handful of other more 'isolated' attempts at finding core neuropsychological features in autism (Dawson and McKissick 1984, Whitehouse and Harris 1984), have considerably changed our whole conceptual framework in autism research. The pioneering work of Hermelin and O'Connor (1970) is still influential and has inspired some of the most important recent studies by the Frith group, for instance. This chapter reviews selectively the work done to date in an attempt to summarize what is currently known concerning the neuropsychology of autism.

Cognition and cognitive strategies in autism

In spite of assertions to the contrary, it has been documented for decades that many children with autism are also mentally retarded (i.e. they test reliably below IQ 70 on conventional IQ tests—Clark and Rutter 1979). The proportion of children with autism who also show mental retardation has varied somewhat between studies, but most authors agree that the figure is somewhere in the range of 65 to 85 per cent (Lotter 1967, Wing and Gould 1979, Bohman et al. 1983, Gillberg 1984, Gillberg and Steffenburg 1987). Recent studies suggesting a much higher prevalence rate for Asperger synrome (usually with IQ >70)—possibly equivalent with high functioning autism—than for autism 'proper' (Gillberg and Gillberg 1989; Wing, personal communication) could imply that the rate of clear mental retardation in autism, although much higher than in the general population, might be in the 10 to 25 per cent range instead. At any rate, most authorities agree that even within the range of so-called normal intellectual functioning, children with autism (and Asperger syndrome) all show cognitive problems.

Defining features of autism (notably social, language and symbolic play deficits) make it clear that various cognitive functions associated with these deficits are likely to be particularly affected. The long standing debate as to whether autism is *either* cognitive or social tends to miss the point. The issue really is not *whether* it is cognitive or social but rather *how* the social and cognitive deficits can be conceptualized as emerging from one common 'primary' dysfunction. However, with regard to neuropsychological views of autism, the semantic squabble over 'cognitive' on the one hand and 'social' on the other still has far-reaching consequences in that the former is being regarded as 'cortical' (new brain) and the latter 'subcortical' (old brain) dysfunction. The overall point in this connection is that there is danger that the way we use words ('cognitive', 'language', and 'social', for instance) might substantially influence the way in which we conceptualize autism as *primarily* this or the other, when in fact it may be neither. For example, much emphasis has been put on language (supposedly more 'cognitive' than 'social') as a 'primary' deficit in autism, even though there is now good evidence that people with autism can have excellent (at least formal expressive) language skills (Wing 1980, Gillberg *et al.* 1987, Rumsey *et al.* 1988), and that language deficits often associated with autism (e.g. pronominal reversal) might be conceptualized as delay rather than deviance (Oshima-Takana and Benaroya 1989). This emphasis has led to expectations that neuroimaging techniques aimed at visualizing cerebral cortical areas would show much promise in the disclosure of the common neurobiological denominator in autism. So far such studies have by and large been disappointing.

Cognitive impairment is usually thought of as a global phenomenon: all cognitive functions in a child with cognitive impairment are expected to be affected. This is a gross oversimplification even in children who are mentally retarded but do not show autism (cf. Down syndrome and Williams syndrome, two mental retardation syndromes with clearly different cognitive profiles). In autism it is essential that the cognitive impairment be recognized as showing in (sometimes extremely) uneven cognitive profiles (Frith 1989*a*). Verbal abilities are usually poorer than performance skills, comprehension is quite often much more impaired than word production, fine motor skills may be better than gross motor skills, and a variety of measures reflecting rote memory skills demonstrate good or even superior results (Wing 1980, Ohta 1987). The typical profile on the WISC is one with relatively good results on Block Design and good results in Picture Assembly, but poor or very poor results on Comprehension and Picture Arrangement (Lockyer and Rutter 1970, Ohta 1987, Rumsey and Hamburger 1988, Frith 1989*a*). It has recently been suggested (Frith 1989*a*) that a 'cognitive profile' of this kind might be diagnostic of autism or at least highly suggestive of autism or autism spectrum disorders.

In a number of children, adolescents and adults with autism there is, in addition, an 'islet of special ability' (Shah and Frith 1983). Something like every 1:2 have an area of functioning which stands out as exceptionally good compared with other areas. In a very few cases (c. 5 per cent according to O'Connor and Hermelin 1988; fewer still according to the present authors) there may exist extraordinary 'savant skills' (Treffert 1989), such as shown by Raymond (Dustin Hoffman) in the Barry Levinson film *Rain Man*. Such individuals ('idiots savants' or 'autistic savants') usually show extremely superior rote memory abilities, musical giftedness or mathematical skills. Similar, though not quite such striking giftedness (not so striking because of the overall better cognitive level) is also seen in cases with autism spectrum disorders (*e.g.* Asperger syndrome—Wing 1981).

It appears that many children with autism rely on visuospatial rather than temporal processing (Hermelin and O'Connor 1970) and that meaningful information tends to be less often correctly identified (Aurnhammer-Frith 1969). Many children with autism show excellent skills with jigsaw puzzles but cannot conceive of the notion of time. This is unlike normal children who tend to extract as many meaningful clues as possible in trying to solve problems. Also, whereas normal children will make use of several clues, children with autism will often depend on one single piece of information when attending to a task.

Recent developments in the field of cognitive neuropsychology and autism
In the 1980s, the focus of neuropsychological studies in autism shifted gradually from language and other conservative measures of cognition to the description and delineation of social and pragmatic deficits. Two relatively distinct theories have emerged which have been subjected to systematic scientific study. For the purpose of brevity, they will here be referred to as the *affective theory* (Hobson 1986a) and the *meta representation theory* (Baron-Cohen 1988). Because both, particularly the latter, are currently influential both in guiding research and in clinical concepts of autism, they will be described in this context.

The affective theory goes back to Kanner's original assertions that children with autism have 'inborn disturbances of *affective* contact' [our italics] and to the theories of Piaget. In the affective theory, autism is seen as stemming from an affective deficit which is primary and irreducible and involves a dysfuncion in the ability to perceive other people's mental states as reflected in their bodily expressions. This primary affective dysfunction underlies the social and communication problems. Support for the theory has been generated by a number of interesting experiments concerned with various aspects of emotion recognition in children with autism (see review by Hobson *et al.* 1988). However, the studies by Marian Sigman and her group (Sigman and Ungerer 1984, Sigman *et al.* 1986) have demonstrated convincingly that some attachment behaviours, eye contact and reaching after tickling are usually preserved in autism. Such behaviours can all be seen as primarily 'affective' variables. Also, most authorities agree that children with autism may have well developed primary emotions such as anger and gladness.

The meta representation theory—sometimes also referred to as the 'cognitive theory' (to distinguish it from the affective theory)—argues rather differently that mental states with content (such as 'invisible' knowing and believing and not 'obvious' happiness and anger) are not directly observable but have to be inferred.

The ability to impute mental states with content to other people has been referred to as a 'theory of mind' (Premack and Woodruff 1978). This 'theory' is present in normal children from at least 4 years of age (Hogrefe *et al.* 1986) but could be in operation much earlier, perhaps even before age 1 year (Leslie 1987). The specific cognitive peaks and troughs encountered in autism (low scores on comprehension and picture arrangement and high on block design on the WISC; low scores on hearing and speech and practical reasoning and high on motor and performance on the Griffiths) could be taken to indicate the lack of a core capacity for coherence in autism. Uta Frith (1989*a*) and her collaborators (Baron-Cohen *et al.* 1985, Baron-Cohen 1990) have proposed a theory to account for the basic psychological features of autism. They hypothesize that underlying the behavioural symptoms of autism is a central disorder of empathy characterized by inability or decreased capacity to conceive of other people's mental states (such as knowing and believing). If a deficit of this kind exists, then it could explain the lack of coherence and need for coherence in autism. If you do not understand that behind people's actions are thought-out purposes and wilful planning, much of what people do will stand out as incomprehensible. What they say will be even more 'uncommunicative': not understanding that the spoken words are a 'message from the mind' makes spoken language something you may learn to imitate but not a tool for communication. Not having a well-developed theory of mind will lead to extreme deficits in reciprocal social interaction, in communication and 'creative' imagination. However, not having a theory of mind does not necessarily affect memory or visuospatial skills, areas in which many people with autism excel. Feats of rote memory and jigsaw puzzle solving are fairly common in autism. These are skills that are not dependent on having a theory of mind. Such skills are reflected in high scores on block design and performance. The theory predicts that only specific social capacities should be constantly restricted in autism (namely those that require a concept of other people's wishes, beliefs and thoughts, *e.g.* reciprocal social interactions or 'empathy'), whereas other social capacities might be spared (viz, those that require only perception of the observable world, *e.g.* face recognition). The theory further predicts that the pragmatics of existing language skills in a child with autism will be specifically impaired. A number of simple, yet thought provoking experiments have been performed to test this theory (see Baron-Cohen 1990 for a review). In one of these, two dolls, Sally and Anne, were presented to normal children, children with Down syndrome and children with autism. In Sally's basket was a marble, but in Anne's box was nothing. Sally then 'left the room', meaning that she could no longer see what was going on. In the meantime, Anne moved the marble to her box. When Sally 'came back', the children participating in the study were asked: 'Where will Sally look for the marble?' Children with Down syndrome and normal children said she looked where it was when she left the room (a false but reasonable belief), whereas most of the children with autism said she would look in the box, where it actually is (a true but unreasonable belief). Children with autism under age 11 years and with a mental age under 6 years constantly fail this task according to Baron-Cohen (1990). One way to account for this finding—and similar findings from other experiments —would be the lack of a theory of mind; if the child cannot understand that Sally has a mind (a belief/thought about the marble being where it once was), s/he will believe only what s/he sees or hears. There is now considerable support for its validity, not only from Frith's group, but also from past research (reviewed by Baron-Cohen 1988) and from independent experimenters (*e.g.* Dawson and Fernald 1987, and indirectly from van Bourgondien and Mesibov 1987).

Even though there have been experimental studies that have challenged the theory of mind theory of autism (Prior *et al*. 1990), the accumulating evidence is such that it is hard to dismiss. The theory provides a plausible account for the developmental changes in the clinical picture of autism across time and IQ levels. Impairments in 'first order belief attribution' (*e.g.* 'I think he thinks') may be typical of the most severely affected people with autism, whereas impairments of 'second order belief attribution' (*e.g.* 'I think he thinks she thinks') may typify high-functioning cases diagnosed as Asperger syndrome (see also Baron-Cohen 1989*b*). A proposed deficient theory of mind in autism has the merit of making comprehensible to parents and professionals alike some of the mystifying features of autism. A theory of this kind has the great merit of being testable at several levels and also of providing a clinically relevant model for the development of autism.

The affective and meta representation theories are not necessarily mutually exclusive and there may be potential in trying to examine to what extent they can be reconciled. Both provide excellent possibilities for empirical study and have fuelled the previously speculation-loaded area of autism psychology with a number of interesting experiments which have already yielded important theoretical and clinical insights.

Is psychological testing in autism useful?
It is often, though by no means always, problematic to test a young child with autism using conventional IQ tests. Problems are most likely to occur, of course, if the tester is not very well acquainted with the underlying deficits and clinical manifestations of autism. In order for it to be worthwhile testing a child with autism, testing and results on tests must have some meaning. So what are IQ tests and other tests in autism good for?

IQ tests in childhood have been shown to be the best available single instrument for roughly predicting outcome in autism (Rutter 1983). A very low IQ

(<50) in childhood usually predicts a similar IQ and relatively poor social outcome in adult age. As has already been pointed out above, some IQ tests yield a typical 'profile' in autism. On the WISC (for school-age children), peaks in block design (and picture assembly) and troughs in word comprehension and picture arrangement are typical. On the Griffiths developmental scale (Griffiths 1970), children with autism peak in motor and daily life activities but score very poorly on the hearing/language scales (Nydén, personal communication). For these, and other, reasons it is clear that IQ testing is essential in the work-up of any child and for predicting outcome in a reasonable way.

Results on specific tests of language performed in childhood can also help establish a fairly accurate prognosis. Useful speech at age 5 years is one of the best predictors of outcome (Gillberg 1991). In particular, it is helpful to try to pinpoint the receptive deficits (which, contrary to earlier assertions, are often even more pronounced than the expressive skill deficits) and to find out to what extent there might be added problems of 'pure' dysphasia over and above any language–communication deficits that could be accounted for by autism alone.

Finally, psychometric assessment is required because children with autism are unique individuals: though they share some core deficits, they are quite different from each other. A detailed test of various functional capacities will help provide a fuller picture of assets and deficits, such that a better understanding of what will be the most useful coping strategies can be achieved.

The psychometric work-up in autism and autistic-like conditions: some suggestions
Any child who is being examined for the first time under the suspicion that s/he might be suffering from autism must have a proper psychometric assessment, or, if examined in the first 10 years of life, be scheduled for such assessment some years later.

Exactly which test to choose depends on a number of variables, such as the age of the child, the tests available, and the psychologist's familiarity with certain tests. Also, some tests are more appropriate when evaluating autism because they have been used extensively in the scientific study of autism.

In the very young child (<5 years) with autism, the assessment by an experienced clinician often yields as much information about the child's developmental level as any developmental test. In Sweden, the Griffiths developmental scales are often used in the assessment of young children with autism. However, this test (as most other tests used with this age group) yields little detail and has very low discriminative capacity in the groups with mild, low-normal, normal and high intelligence. Nevertheless, it can be a valuable aid in the evaluation of the severely impaired group. Another test which may be useful in this age group is the Raven's Coloured Progressive Matrices (Raven 1960). The Leiter International Performance Scale (Shah and Holmes 1985) is sometimes a very good instrument for evaluating non-verbal IQ in preschool children with autism. One must keep in mind the typical peaks in visual performance skills shown by children with autism, which infer that superior results on the Leiter need not necessarily be a reflection of overall superior IQ.

The Vineland Social Maturity Scale can also be helpful, particularly when evaluating overall/adaptive skills. The Vineland social quotient has been shown to correlate fairly strongly with measures of IQ (Freeman 1976).

In the school-age period, the WISC-R is definitely the best documented of all tests currently available for the evaluation of cognition in autism. Every child with autism or an autistic-like condition who does not have severe or profound mental retardation (IQ <35) should, in our opinion, be given the WISC-R at some point in time during school age. In countries where the Wechsler Preschool and Wechsler Adult Intelligence Scales have been standardized they too can be used in the psychometric work-up of autism outside the school-age period. The typical WISC-R profile seen in autism—and often in high-functioning (or Asperger type) cases also—has been described in detail above.

Specific language tests tend to vary from one country to another. The best approach is to have a close collaboration with a speech therapist who will be able to accumulate experience in the field of speech–language evaluation in autism. The Peabody Picture Vocabulary Test (Dunn 1959) may be quite useful. My experience with the Illinois Test of Psycholinguistic Abilities (ITPA—Kirk *et al.* 1968), on the other hand, has been that it yields relatively little information about specific communication/language problems. In this connection it may be prudent to caution against the notion of autism as a speech–language disorder (or in some basic sense clearly associated with language disorders). Current concepts in autism stress the overall communicative deficits rather than specific language problems. Semantic–pragmatic problems and non-verbal communication deficits seem to be more typical of autism and autistic-like conditions than such 'autism-specific language peculiarities' as echolalia and pronoun reversal. We are much in need of a good battery for testing communicative skills in the field of speech and language and, in particular, in areas such as pragmatics, semantics, mime and gesture.

For those particularly interested in detailed analyses of autism spectrum problems, all sorts of other tests may be used. The Matching Familiar Figures Test and the Embedded Figures Test are but two examples of tests which have been scientifically validated in autism.

Summary and conclusions

Recent developments in autism have seen a formidable step forward for neuropsychology/cognitive psychology. Testable hypotheses suggesting that children with autism lack a 'theory of mind' and the strive for 'central coherence' have been forwarded and successfully put to the test. 'Old truths', such as IQ being the single best predictor of outcome, have again been highlighted. Autism is no longer conceptualized as a form of psychosis but as a developmental disorder. All these trends have led to a general consensus that all children with autism and autistic-like conditions need a proper psychometric evaluation. The WISC-R is clearly still the

173

best documented psychometric instrument in the field. The next few years will tell whether autism neuropsychology will become a firm branch of autism research or not. It seems clear already at this stage that some of the most interesting constructs in the whole field of autism have been generated by cognitive psychologists.

REFERENCES

Aurnhammer-Frith, U. (1969) 'Emphasis and meaning in recall in normal and autistic children.' *Language and Speech*, **12**, 29–38.
Baron-Cohen, S. (1988) 'Without a theory of mind one cannot participate in a conversation.' *Cognition*, **29**, 83–84.
—— (1989a) 'The autistic child's theory of mind: a case of specific developmental delay.' *Journal of Child Psychology and Psychiatry*, **30**, 285–297.
—— (1989b) 'Do autistic children have obsessions and compulsions?' *British Journal of Clinical Psychology*, **28**, 193–200.
—— (1990) 'Autism: a specific cognitive disorder of "mind-blindness".' *International Review of Psychiatry*, **2**, 81–90.
—— Leslie, A.M., Frith, U. (1985) 'Does the autistic child have a "theory of mind"?' *Cognition*, **21**, 37–46.
Bohman, M., Bohman, I.L., Björck, P.O., Sjöholm, E. (1983) 'Childhood psychosis in a northern Swedish county: some preliminary findings from an epidemiological survey.' *In:* Schmidt, M.H., Remschmidt, H. (Eds) *Epidemiological Approaches in Child Psychiatry, II.* Stuttgart: Thieme, pp. 164–173.
Clark, P., Rutter, M. (1979) 'Task difficulty and task performance in autistic children.' *Journal of Child Psychology and Psychiatry*, **20**, 271–285.
Dawson, G., Fernald, M. (1987) 'Perspective-taking ability and its relationship to the social behavior of autistic children.' *Journal of Autism and Developmental Disorders*, **17**, 487–498.
—— McKissick, F.C. (1984) 'Self-recognition in autistic children.' *Journal of Autism and Developmental Disorders*, **14**, 383–394.
Dunn, L. (1959) *Expanded Manual for the Peabody Picture Vocabulary Test.* Circle Pines, MN: American Guidance Services.
Freeman, B.J. (1976) 'Evaluating autistic children.' *Journal of Pediatric Psychology*, **1**, 18–21.
Frith, U. (1989a) *Autism: Explaining the Enigma.* Oxford: Basil Blackwell.
—— (1989b) 'Autism and "theory of mind".' *In:* Gillberg, C. (Ed.) *Diagnosis and Treatment of Autism.* New York: Plenum, pp. 33–52.
Gillberg, C. (1984) 'Infantile autism and other childhood psychoses in a Swedish urban region. Epidemiological aspects.' *Journal of Child Psychology and Psychiatry*, **25**, 35–43.
—— (1991) 'Outcome in autism and autistic-like conditions.' *Journal of the American Academy of Child and Adolescent Psychiatry*, **30**, 375–382.
—— Steffenburg, S. (1987) 'Outcome and prognostic factors in infantile autism and similar conditions: A population-based study of 46 cases followed through puberty.' *Journal of Autism and Developmental Disorders*, **17**, 273–287.
—— —— Jakobsson, G. (1987) 'Neurobiological findings in 20 relatively gifted children with Kanner-type autism or Asperger syndrome.' *Developmental Medicine and Child Neurology*, **29**, 641–649.
Gillberg, I.C., Gillberg, C. (1989) 'Asperger syndrome. Some epidemiological considerations: a research note.' *Journal of Child Psychology and Psychiatry*, **30**, 631–638.
Griffiths, R. (1970) *The Abilities of Young Children.* London: Children Research Centre.
Hermelin, B., O'Connor, N. (1970) *Psychological Experiments with Autistic Children.* Oxford: Pergamon.
Hobson, R.P. (1984) 'Early childhood autism and the question of egocentrism.' *Journal of Autism and Developmental Disorders*, **14**, 85–104.
—— (1986a) 'The autistic child's appraisal of expressions of emotion.' *Journal of Child Psychology and Psychiatry*, **27**, 321–342.
—— (1986b) 'The autistic child's appraisal of expressions of emotions: a further study.' *Journal of Child*

Psychology and Psychiatry, **27**, 671–680.

—— (1987) 'The autistic child's recognition of age- and sex-related characteristics of people.' *Journal of Autism and Developmental Disorders,* **17**, 63–79.

—— Ouston, J., Lee, A. (1988) 'Emotion recognition in autism: coordinating faces and voices.' *Psychological Medicine,* **18**, 911–23.

Hogrefe, G.J., Wimmer, H., Perner, J. (1986) 'Ignorance versus false belief: a developmental lag in attribution of epistemic states.' *Child Development,* **57**, 567–582.

Kirk, S., McCarthy, J., Kirk, W. (1968) *The Illinois Test of Psycholinguistic Abilities. Revised Edition.* Urbana, IL: University of Illinois Press.

Leslie, A.M. (1987) 'Pretence and representation: the origins of a "Theory of Mind".' *Psychological Review,* **94**, 412–426.

—— Frith, U. (1988) 'Autistic children's understanding of seeing, knowing and believing.' *British Journal of Psychiatry,* **4**, 315–324.

Lockyer, L., Rutter, M. (1970) 'A five to fifteen year follow-up study of infantile psychosis. IV: Patterns of cognitive ability.' *British Journal of Social and Clinical Psychology,* **9**, 152–163.

Lotter, V. (1967) *The Prevalence of the Autistic Syndrome in Children.* London: University of London Press.

O'Connor, N., Hermelin, B. (1988) 'Low intelligence and special abilities.' *Journal of Child Psychology and Psychiatry,* **29**, 391–396.

Ohta, M. (1987) 'Cognitive disorders of infantile autism: a study employing the WISC, spatial relationship conceptualization, and gesture imitations.' *Journal of Autism and Developmental Disorders,* **17**, 45–62.

Oshima-Takane, Y., Benaroya, S. (1989) 'An alterntive view of pronominal errors in autistic children.' *Journal of Autism and Developmental Disorders,* **19**, 73–85.

Premack, D., Woodruff, G. (1978) 'Does the chimpanzee have a "theory of mind?".' *Behavioral and Brain Sciences,* **4**, 515–526.

Prior, M., Dahlström, D., Squires, T.S. (1990) 'Autistic children's knowledge of thinking and feeling states in other people.' *Journal of Child Psychology and Psychiatry,* **31**, 587–601.

Raven, J. (1960) *Guide to the Standard Progressive Matrices.* London: H.K. Lewis.

Rumsey, J.M., Hamburger, S.D. (1988) 'Neuropsychological findings in high-functioning men with infantile autism, residual state.' *Journal of Clinical and Experimental Neuropsychology,* **10**, 201–221.

—— Creasey, H., Stepanek, J.S., Dorwart, R., Patronas, N., Hamburger, S.D., Duara, R. (1988) 'Hemispheric asymmetries, fourth ventricular size, and cerebellar morphology in autism.' *Journal of Autism and Developmental Disorders,* **18**, 127–137.

Rutter, M. (1983) 'Cognitive deficits in the pathogenesis of autism.' *Journal of Child Psychology and Psychiatry,* **24**, 513–531.

Shah, A., Frith, U. (1983) 'An islet of ability in autistic children: a research note.' *Journal of Child Psychology and Psychiatry,* **24**, 613–620.

—— Holmes, N. (1985) 'The use of the Leiter International Performance Scale with autistic children.' *Journal of Autism and Developmental Disorders,* **15**, 195–203.

Sigman, M., Ungerer, J.A. (1984) 'Attachment behaviors in autistic children.' *Journal of Autism and Developmental Disorders,* **14**, 231–244.

—— Mundy, P., Sherman, T., Ungerer, J. (1986) 'Social interactions of autistic, mentally retarded and normal children and their caregivers.' *Journal of Child Psychology and Psychiatry,* **27**, 647–656.

Treffert, D.A. (1989) *Extraordinary People.* New York: Harper & Row.

van Bourgondien, M.E., Mesibov, G. (1987) 'Humor in high-functioning autistic adults.' *Journal of Autism and Developmental Disorders,* **17**, 417–424.

Waterhouse, L., Fein, D. (1989) 'Social or cognitive or both?' *In:* Gillberg, C. (Ed.) *Diagnosis and Treatment of Autism.* New York: Plenum, pp. 53–62.

Whitehouse, D., Harris, J.C. (1984) 'Hyperlexia in infantile autism.' *Journal of Autism and Developmental Disorders,* **14**, 281–289.

Wing, L. (1980) *Early Childhood Autism. 2nd Edn.* Oxford: Pergamon.

—— (1981) 'Asperger's syndrome: a clinical account.' *Psychological Medicine,* **11**, 115–129.

—— Gould, J. (1979) 'Severe impairments of social interaction and associated abnormalities in children: epidemiology and classification.' *Journal of Autism and Developmental Disorders,* **9**, 11–29.

175

PART III

DISEASE ENTITIES THAT HAVE A SUBGROUP OF PATIENTS WITH AUTISTIC SYMPTOMS

16
CHROMOSOMAL ABERRATIONS

Introduction

Chromosomes are composed of deoxyribonucleic acid (DNA) embedded in a framework of various histones (Zellweger and Simpson 1977). The ability to test the chromosome complement of living humans developed late in the 1950s. This discovery was followed in the next decade by the cracking of the genetic code and the elucidation of the mechanisms of protein synthesis. These further discoveries led to the formulation of research projects interweaving the disciplines of paediatrics, genetics and developmental biology. Through cytogenetic techniques, the chromosomes could be visualized in individual patients. Through molecular biological methods, individual genes (DNA sequences) could now be identified. Particularly challenging was the possibility that molecular genetics might lead to understanding the CNS. Enthusiasm was so high that by the 1970s, lectures were being given and papers were being written entitled 'From gene to behavior' (Benzer 1971) and 'The genetics of behaviour' (Brenner 1973).

A generation later, it is now clear that the chromosomes and the genes that they carry are a most important but not solely determinative factor in cognition and behaviour. The study of the neurobiology of individuals with autism is an example of the complexities and limitations of a simple 'gene = behaviour' or 'chromosome aberration = misbehaviour' approach. In Chapter 8, the known patterns of genetic inheritance in autism were discussed; in this chapter, aberrations of the chromosomes noted in laboratory reports from patients with autism will be reviewed.

One of the first chromosome studies of children with infantile autism was stimulated in 1962 by the finding of a boy and a set of twin girls with severe behaviour disorders (called schizoid or schizophrenic at that time) and trisomy 22. This finding led to a further study of ten institutionalized children with the diagnosis of infantile autism or 'schizophrenia', but no further chromosomal abnormalities were detected (Biesele et al. 1962).

Almost 30 years later, it is interesting that the reports of chromosomal aberrations in patients with autistic symptoms show such a great variety of chromosomes as abnormal. In fact, with only four exceptions out of 23 pairs (chromosomes 7, 14, 19, 20), all the chromosomes have been reported to be aberrant in peripheral blood lymphocyte studies of one or more patients with an autistic syndrome. Although the relevance to brain dysfunction of these chromosomal aberration sightings remains to be determined in many cases the great range of these reports is of interest.

179

Autosomal aberrations

Chromosome 1. Aberrations of chromosome 1 are rare, probably because affected fetuses do not survive. Deletions of the short arm (1p) are very rare. A terminal deletion of 1p35 has been described in a boy who appeared to have a normal infancy (Wenger *et al.* 1988). However, by 2½ years of age, language delay, social difficulties and hyperactivity became apparent. He was placed in a special class for children with autism after unsuccessful placements in less restricted school environments and several psychiatric hospital admissions. At the age of 9, his weight increased from the 50th to the 90th centile in a year.

Chromosome 2. A deletion of the long arm of chromosome 2 (at 2q37) in combination with a partial trisomy (6p with duplications ranging from 6p21 to 6p25) has been reported in a child who met DSM-III-R criteria for infantile autism (see below). The authors (Burd *et al.* 1988) point out that this child differed from other individuals with partial trisomy 6p only by the presence of infantile autism and seizures, thus raising the possibility that the deletion of 2q37 may have been a factor in these particular symptoms.

Also, a case of non-homology between members of chromosome pair 2 (not further described) has been reported in a 5-year-old boy with autism (Ornitz *et al.* 1977). The authors described the chromosomal finding as incidental.

The folate-sensitive fragile site fra(2)(q13) has been reported in the literature in individuals with diagnoses of autism and Asperger syndrome (Jayakar *et al.* 1986, Saliba and Griffiths 1990). The clinical significance, if any, of autosomal fragile sites to autistic symptoms is unknown. Currently most investigators believe that they are coincidental findings. Many are commonly seen in the laboratory and can be induced in normal individuals.

Chromosome 3. A child has been described with a structual abnormality of chromosome 3—a replication, inversion and a deletion—together with an interstitial deletion on the short arm of chromosome 17 (Mariner *et al.* 1986). When examined at 17 years of age he had hypertelorism, prominent, low-set ears, scattered hypo- and hyperpigmented skin lesions, absence of eye contact, aloofness, echolalic speech, severe hyperactivity, catastrophic reaction to change, bizarre responses to aspects of his environment, scarring on his hand from self-biting, and a fascination for watches. He tested with an ABC-ASIEP* score of 139 (>68 suggestive of autism) and a CARS* score of 35.5, in the range of mild to moderate autism.

Chromosome 4. A *de novo* 4/10 balanced translocation has been observed in a high-functioning girl with autism (Pearl and Coleman 1992). Balanced translocations are found in normal individuals and their meaning is unclear. Recently it has been suggested that these inherited translocations may be associated with a higher

*ABC-ASIEP = Autism Screening Instrument for Educational Planning subtest of the Autistic Behavior Scale (Krug *et al.* 1979); CARS = Childhood Autism Rating Scale (Schopler *et al.* 1980).

incidence of developmental defects and mental retardation (Fryns *et al.* 1986).

Chromosome 5. Deletion of the short arm of chromosome 5, or the 5p– syndrome, is one of the most common deletion syndromes found in humans. The syndrome was named 'cri-du-chat' after the mewing cry of affected babies; this symptom is lost by about one third of the children by 2 years of age. The most common symptoms found in this patient group include microcephaly, hypertelorism, epicanthic folds, low-set ears and severe mental retardation. A study of 80 home-reared children with cri-du-chat syndrome examined many clinical factors but found only one that correlated with the size of the chromosomal deletion—there was a significant negative correlation between the individual's IQ and the size of the deletion (Wilkins *et al.* 1983). In describing development and behaviour in this patient group, Wilkins *et al.* reported that self-stimulatory behaviours such as head banging, hand waving and hand sucking, as well as mannerisms of withdrawal, were major problems in both the deletion and translocation subgroups of the children they were studying.

Regarding adults, two men with terminal deletions of 5p14 and 5p15 have been found in a cytogenetic survey of mentally retarded individuals with autistic behaviours in a state institution (Cantu *et al.* 1990). These individuals had not been previously diagnosed or identified as having physical signs of enough significance to warrant chromosomal testing; they were tested because they had autistic symptoms.

A balanced reciprocal translocation from the long arm of chromosome 5 to the long arm of chromosome 11 was identified in a female with an IQ of 33 who was tested as part of an epidemiological survey of autism (Ritvo *et al.* 1990). Her father also had this translocation.

Mariner *et al.* (1986) have described a patient with extra chromosomal material on the short arm of chromosome 5 (46,XY, 5p+) whose facial features were not dysmorphic. He had frequent, multiple self-stimulation, resistance to change, a unique attachment to objects and clothes and a CARS score of 33 (mild to moderate autism).

Chromosome 6. More than a dozen patients have been described with partial trisomy 6p; their break-points in the duplicated segment ranged from 6p21 to 6p25. The main features of the syndrome are rather non-specific: low birthweight, mental and growth retardation and failure to thrive. A boy with a breakpoint at 6p23 combined with a deletion of 2q37, who met DSM-III-R criteria for infantile autism, has been described by Burd *et al.* (1988) (Fig. 16.1). His mother had a balanced translocation. He had microcephaly, epicanthic folds with severe bilateral ptosis, low-set large ears with fleshy antitragus, bilateral frontal bossing and bow-shaped lips with a long philtrum. Many of these physical features are seen in the 6p partial trisomy syndrome; the clinical presentation of the deletion 2q is not described in the literature. Besides his autism, the boy also had seizures.

Three patients with autism and severe mental retardation associated with a

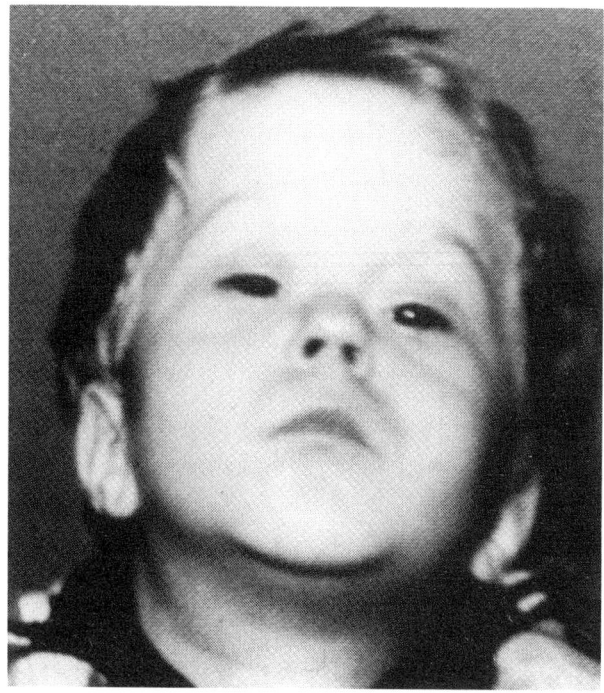

Fig. 16.1. 5-year-old boy with partial trisomy 6 syndrome and autism. He has a prominent forehead, low nasal bridge, pointed nose, bilateral ptosis, low-set ears and bow-shaped lips with long philtrum.

fragile site at 6q26 were reported by Gillberg and Wahlström (1985). Two of the three had epilepsy. The significance (if any) of the fragile site is unclear, considering that little is known about fragile sites of this kind and the presence of brain dysfunction.

Chromosome 8. Most individuals reported in the literature with a chromosomal error involving chromosome 8 have a 46/47 + 8 (normal/trisomy 8) mosaicism. Mild or severe mental impairment is usually described. A male with autism and an IQ of 36 has been described who had a partial trisomy of the distal tip of chromosome 8 and a probable partial deletion of the middle of the short arm of chromosome 8 (Ritvo *et al.* 1990). No evidence of mosaicism is mentioned.

Chromosome 9. The clinical presentation of the partial deletion of the short arm of chromosome 9 (the 9p– syndrome) has been fairly well delineated in the literature; the constant feature is moderate mental retardation. The patients are often described as content and happy (in contrast to the 9p+ [partial trisomy p] syndrome where antisocial behaviour is reported). A male with autism and an IQ of 60 has been reported to have the 9p– syndrome (Ritvo *et al.* 1990).

In a study in which children with autism were screened for the fragile X syndrome, a boy who was negative for that trait was incidentally found to have a balanced translocation t(9;17)(q12;q21), inherited from his father who was phenotypically normal (Ho and Kalousek 1989).

A finding of extra material in the heterochromatine region of chromosome 9 has been made in a patient with an autistic-like condition and severe mental retardation (C.G., personal case).

Chromosome 9 is also the site of the gene causing tuberous sclerosis in some families, a disease entity with a substantial number of patients with autistic symptoms (see Chapter 20).

Chromosome 10. A balanced 4/10 translocation has been described in a high-functioning girl with autism (Pearl and Coleman 1992).

Chromosome 11. A balanced reciprocal translocation from the long arm of chromosome 5 to the long arm of chromosome 11 has been described in a female with an IQ of 33 (Ritvo *et al.* 1990). Her father also had the translocation.

Like chromosome 9 (see above), chromosome 11 also appears to be the site of one of the genes causing tuberous sclerosis.

Chromosome 12. The long arm of chromosome 12 contains the human phenyl-alanine hydroxylase gene responsible for the metabolic disease phenylketonuria, which has a subgroup of untreated patients who in the past were mistakenly diagnosed as having Kanner autism (see Chapter 17).

Chromosome 13. Aberrations of the 13th chromosome—both trisomy 13 (Patau syndrome) and the 13 deletion syndrome—are well reported in the literature with many patients. Cases of trisomy 13 are often characterized by arhinencephaly or holoprosencephaly, a major developmental malformation of the brain, although the clinical picture varies from case to case. Often there are other malformations of the face, heart, gastrointestinal tract, genito-urinary tract and extremities. A boy with autism and severe mental retardation has been reported to have trisomy 13 (Steffenburg 1991).

The 13 deletion syndrome is usually caused by two cytogenetic variants. 13q– is a deletion of part of the long arm of chromosome 13; 13r, a ring chromosome, is produced by deletions in both arms and fusion of the two break-points. Both variants have a similar clinical picture including mild to profound mental retardation, usually with some degree of microcephaly, and holoprosencephaly in half the cases. Facial dysmorphic manifestations are common, as is retinoblastoma.

A 13 deletion syndrome was described in a patient with autism who had a retinoblastoma and reduced esterase D activity (Ritvo *et al.* 1988). In this patient, the deletion was on the long arm and involved band q13 and portions of bands q12 and q14. The patient had a second cousin who also had autism; however, the chromosome and esterase D studies in this individual were within the normal range. Another boy with autism and mental retardation has been reported with a deletion on the 13th chromosome but in this case it was a deletion of the short arm

(13p–) (Steffenburg 1991). His father was also mildly mentally retarded but had normal chromosomes.

Chromosome 15. This chromosome is reported to have deletions of the long arm in the q11 to q13 range presenting with markedly different clinical pictures. A well known example is the Prader–Willi syndrome, in which more than half of the cases have a cytogenetic finding of 15q11–13. In one study, in 21 of 24 patients the deletion derived from the father (Reik 1989). On the other hand, in individuals with Prader–Willi without any evidence of a deletion, it has been shown by DNA analysis that the patient received *both* chromosomes 15 from the mother (Nicholls *et al.* 1989). These findings suggest that the lack of a gene or genes in the paternally derived 15q11–13 region may cause the Prader–Willi phenotype.

This modification of gene expression by the parental origin of the gene is called *genomic imprinting*. Another example is the Angelman syndrome (formerly known as the 'happy puppet syndrome') which also involves the 15q11–13 region. The deleted chromosomal material from the long arm of chromosome 15 in these children has been shown by DNA analysis to be derived from the mother in all of nine cases studied (Pembrey *et al.* 1989, Reik 1989). It is possible that the lack of a gene or genes in the maternally-derived 15q11–13 region may cause the Angelman syndrome.

Thus, it appears that the Prader–Willi and Angelman syndromes share a common chromosome 15 deletion but differ in the parental origin of the deletion (Knoll *et al.* 1989). Why parental origin can be so important is not fully understood but one factor has been found from animal experiments. It appears that the passage of transgenes through the paternal germ line increases the frequency of undermethylation, and, conversely, transgenes that are maternally derived are more highly methylated (Surani *et al.* 1988). Although the deletions in both the Prader–Willi and Angelman syndromes appear to involve the same chromosomal bands, they involve extensive areas along the long arm of chromosome 15; current cytogenetic techniques have not distinguished small molecular differences between the deletions found in these two conditions.

Nevertheless, a patient has been described with a deletion in the q11–13 stretch of the long arm of chromosome 15 who did not have the symptoms of either the Prader–Willi or the Angelman syndrome. The evaluation of this patient recorded autistic symptomatology by 2 years of age and showed that she met the DSM-III-R criteria of an autistic disorder; she also had profound mental retardation and a bipolar disorder (manic–depressive illness) with a positive response to lithium (Kerbeshian *et al.* 1990). She had striking horizontal palpebral fissures with slight epicanthic folds, a low nasal bridge with a turned up and pointed nose, asymmetric nares and a flat philtrum (Fig. 16.2). She was observed to have numerous midline hand-wringing movements and to bite her hands. She suffered from insomnia, epilepsy and explosive behaviour. The authors of this report pointed out that the patient was very similar to another individual with autism

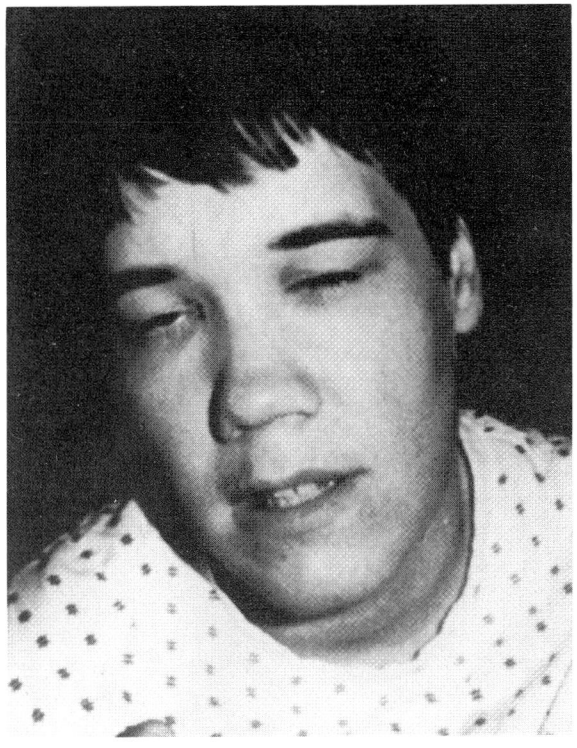

Fig. 16.2. 33-year-old woman with 15q12 deletion and autism. She has striking horizontal palpebral fissures and a low nasal bridge with pointed nose, asymmetrical nares and long philtrum.

recorded in the literature (Akuffo *et al.* 1986), in whom chromosomal findings were not recorded.

A recent study of six males with autism suggests that there may be a specific syndrome of autism, moderate to severe mental retardation, minor motor epilepsy, spinal deformities and minor physical anomalies associated with a marker chromosome (Gillberg *et al.* 1991). The extra chromosome appears to harbour genetically active material from chromosome 15. The typical phenotype is shown in Figure 16.3.

The q13 section of the long arm of chromosome 15 has been identified in marker chromosomes found in five patients with autism or autistic-like behaviour (Cantu *et al.* 1990, Schinzel 1990). Both males and females with 15q13 marker chromosomes have been reported, but the vast majority have been male.

Schreck *et al.* (1977) described a boy with severe infantile autism, moderate retardation, ptosis, exotropia, malocclusion and kyphosis, who had an extra chromosome which was thought to be derived from the short arm of chromosome 15.

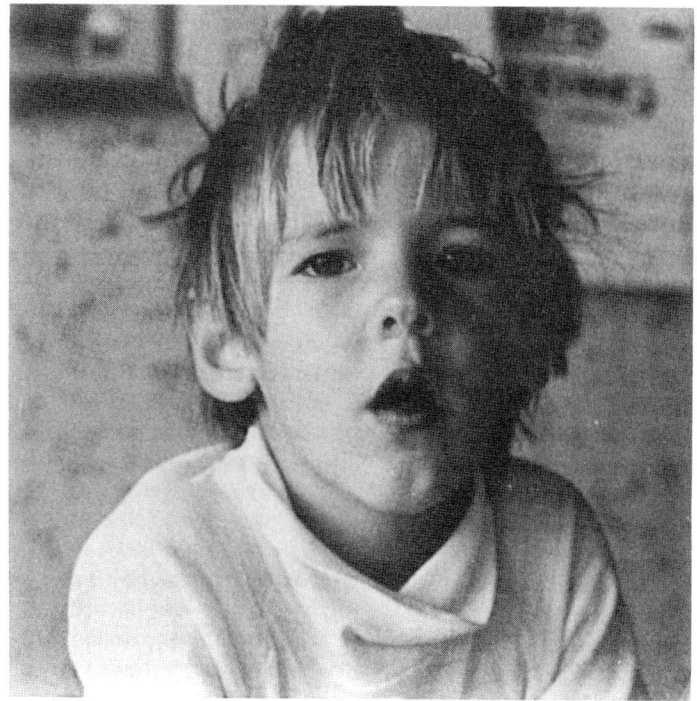

Fig. 16.3. Boy with marker chromosome 15 and autism.

Chromosome 16. A child has been reported with an inversion/duplication of chromosome 16 (Mariner *et al.* 1986). The girl, who would refer to herself only by her first name, had a history of echolalic and perseverative speech, an obesssion about ordering things in her environment, and unusual hand mannerisms (including holding her hand in front of her face like a microphone when she talked, hand wringing and hand flapping). Several psychiatrists diagnosed her as autistic; however her CARS score of 29 did not classify her as having full-blown autism.

Fragile sites on the long arm of chromosome 16 at the q23 level have been reported in 13 per cent of subjects in a chromosomal survey of children with infantile autism and other autistic-like conditions ('other childhood psychosis') (Gillberg and Wahlström 1985). Since this is one of the most common fragile sites seen in any population, the meaning is unclear. However, as the authors point out, the fact that two of the affected boys were first cousins implies that the finding cannot be summarily dismissed as unimportant. In some cases of autism, it could turn out to be a biological marker of brain dysfunction.

Chromosome 17. A child with an interstitial deletion on the short arm of chromosome 17 as well as structural abnormalities of chromosome 3 has been reported by Mariner *et al.* (1986) (see under Chromosome 3).

186

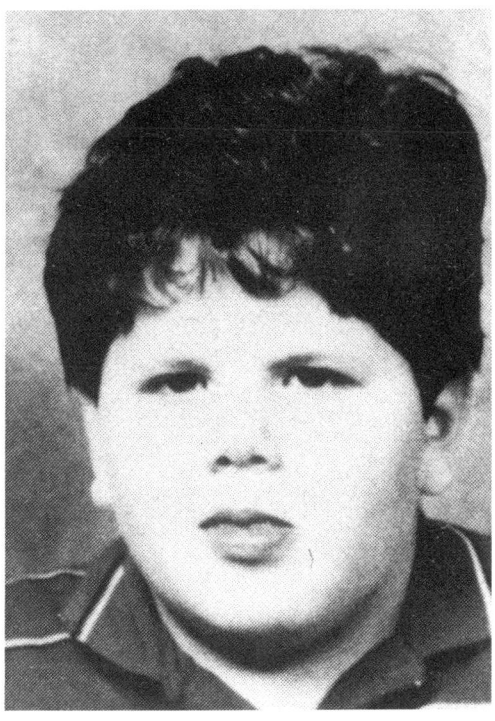

Fig. 16.4. 6-year-old boy with 18q12–21 deletion and 'autistic tendencies'. Onset of obesity was at 3 years. (Reproduced by permission from Wilson and Al Saadi 1989.)

In a chromosomal study of children with autism searching for the fragile X syndrome, a boy was incidentally found who had a balanced translocation t(9;17) (q12;q21) inherited from a father who was phenotypically normal (Ho and Kalousek 1989) (see above).

Deletion of chromosome 17 in a boy with severe mental retardation was also noted in a survey of children with autistic-like conditions (Steffenburg 1991).

Chromosome 18. Autistic tendencies have been described in a boy reported to have an interstitial deletion of chromosome 18 (q12.2q21.1) in his lymphocytes (Wilson and Al Saadi 1989). Developmental delay, perseveration, patterned movements and easy distractibility were described in the boy, who was obese (Fig. 16.4). Deletions on the long arm of chromosome 18 at an almost identical site have been described in patients who did not have autistic features (Wilson *et al.* 1979), so it is possible that detailed studies of this area on the long arm of chromosome 18 may reveal specific loci relevant to autistic symptoms.

Chromosome 21. There are a number of cases in the literature where Down syndrome (trisomy 21) and autism occur together (Knobloch and Pasamanick 1975, Campbell *et al.* 1978, Wakabayashi 1979, Wing and Gould 1979, Gillberg and

Wahlström 1985, Elia *et al.* 1990, Ritvo *et al.* 1990). Children with Down syndrome are more prone that other infants to the infantile spasms syndrome; in these cases, often the patient is left with subsequent autistic features. In Down syndrome as in other chromosomal disorders, the possibility that the chromosomally abnormal fetus might be more prone to perinatally acquired brain damage, which in turn might be related to autistic symptomatology, needs consideration.

Two children with both trisomy 21 and the fragile X syndrome are reported in the literature (Collacott *et al.* 1990).

Evaluating autistic features in a child with Down syndrome can sometimes be quite difficult (Rogers and Coleman 1992). For example, deciding about hearing and sensory processing can be misleading if the auditory problem is due to the recurrent otitis media from which so many children with Down syndrome suffer. Also, a child who is irritable, withdrawn and with poor eye contact may be developing an infection elsewhere, since this patient group is more prone in general to infections. Thus the diagnosis of autistic features should be made only if there is a consistent pattern well established over a period of time and other aetiologies of the symptoms have been ruled out.

There is an extensive literature stereotyping children with Down syndrome as being affectionate, easy in temperament and less likely to have psychiatric illness. However, using objective measures, some researchers find that many more children have been found to have serious behaviour disorders than had been identified by their parents, and the concept that these children are always 'easy' is clearly a myth (Gath and Gumley 1986). Nevertheless, teenagers with Down syndrome are less likely than other moderately to severely mentally retarded teenagers to have major psychiatric problems (Gillberg *et al.* 1986). It is likely, judging from the descriptions in the literature of patients who have a combination of trisomy 21 and autism, that—in at least some of the cases—additional brain dysfunction (such as regression of motor skills and minor signs of cerebral palsy) could be the true cause of the behaviour disorder, rather than the chromosomal abnormality as such.

Chromosome 22. Three cases of trisomy 22 associated with autism are described in the early chromosomal literature (Turner and Jennings 1961, Biesele *et al.* 1962). Also, there is a case history of a female with autism with a translocation between chromosome 22 and a chromosome characterized at that state of technology as 'in the D group' (13/14/15) (Hansen *et al.* 1977).

The sex chromosomes (gonosomes)
Fragile X syndrome
Lubs (1969) was possibly the first to describe this familial learning disorder syndrome associated with a specific chromosomal abnormality, a fragile site on the long arm of the X chromosome (later demonstrated to be at the location of q27.3). Several authors in the late 1970s and early '80s testified to the concurrence of a

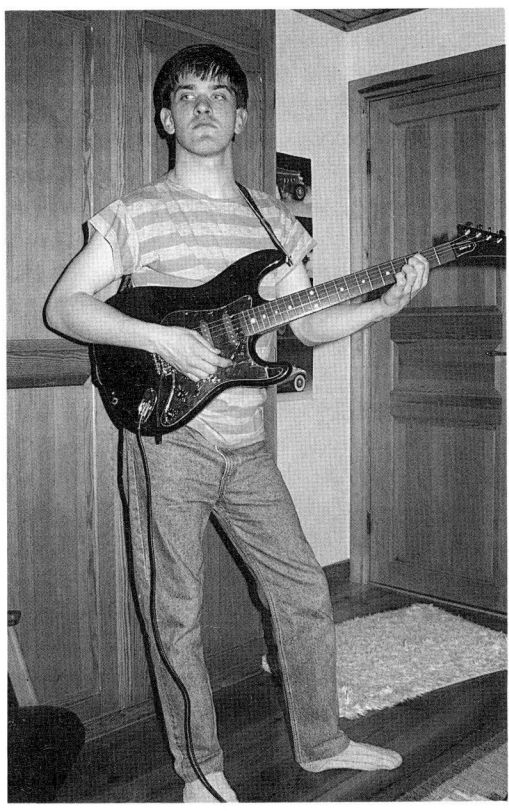

Fig. 16.5. Boy with fragile X syndrome, autism and mild mental retardation.

mental retardation syndrome in males associated with postpubertal hypertrophy of secondary sex characteristics, large ears and minor malformations of the hands and feet (see Hagerman 1989 for a review). The fragile Xq27.3 chromosome abnormality has since been shown to account for 5 to 7 per cent of all male cases of mental retardation (Blomquist *et al*. 1982, 1983) (Fig. 16.5). It has been estimated that the population prevalence is in the range of 0.7 to 0.9 per 1000. However, we are not aware of any population studies of fragile X prevalence, and the available estimates derive from a total screen of mentally retarded individuals in central England (Webb *et al*. 1986) and reviews of mental retardation and birth records (Herbst and Miller 1980).

In 1982, Brown *et al*. and Meryash *et al*. reported the concurrence of infantile autism and fragile X syndrome. Since then several hundred autism cases screened for fragile X have been reported in the literature. By the time of Hagerman's (1989) review, 693 male cases of autism subjected to adequate chromosomal analysis (in a folic acid depleted medium to facilitate detection of the fragile X chromosome

TABLE 16.1

Prevalence of fragile X in males with autism

Study	Cohort with autism N	Fra (X) N
In Opitz and Sutherland (1984)		
Leckman	25	0
Turner	70	1
Mikkelsen	20	1
Chudley	16	1
White	6	0
Jörgensen *et al.* (1984)	11	1
Venter *et al.* (1984)	40	0
Watson *et al.* (1984)	76	4
Blomquist *et al.* (1985)	43	5
Gillberg and Wahlström (1985)	40*	8
Goldfine *et al.* (1985)	34	0
Pueschel *et al.* (1985)	18	0
Brown *et al.* (1986)	183	24
Jayakar *et al.* (1986)	20	0
McGillivray *et al.* (1986)	40	3
Wright *et al.* (1986)	31	1
Gillberg *et al.* (1987)	15	3
Crowe *et al.* (1988)	20	2
Steffenburg *et al.* (1989)	20**	5
Steffenburg (1991)	26	2
Total	754	61 (8.1%)

*Population sample.
**Twins and triplets with autism (population sample).

abnormality) had been published and 51 (7.4 per cent) of these had the fragile X syndrome (those data, together with some more recently published, are listed in Table 16.1). Conversely, of 431 cases with the fragile X syndrome published before 1989, 61 (26 per cent) had autism or autistic-like conditions. In Steffenburg's (1991) population study, at least 6 per cent of all individuals with classical autism had the fragile X abnormality. In a previous population study from the same centre but relating to a different birth cohort, Gillberg and Wahlström (1985) found fragile Xq27.3 in 17 per cent of cases. The Swedish studies indicate that the concurrence of autism and the X chromosome abnormality is considerably higher than accounted for by the often concomitant mental retardation. Several authors have published non-retarded autism/Asperger syndrome cases with the fragile X abnormality (Gillberg *et al.* 1987, Hagerman 1987). This provides further evidence that autistic symptoms in the fragile X syndrome are not merely a consequence of mental retardation. Levitas *et al.* (1983) have suggested that a majority of male patients with the fragile X syndrome exhibit marked autistic features.

In the Nordic twin study of autism (Steffenburg *et al.* 1989), 21 per cent of all the (same-sex) twins and triplets in that study had a definite or probable fragile X chromosomal abnormality. This study included a set of identical triplets with fragile X (Gillberg 1983).

The bulk of the evidence suggested that the fragile X abnormality is reponsible for an important minority of male autism cases and that it is associated with autistic features in a majority of cases. However, as in other autism subgroups with a known aetiology, it may be possible to discern a particular behavioural phenotype (Gillberg 1992). This is described in more detail below.

The controversy as to just how large a proportion of the population with autism have the fragile X syndrome has been fuelled by problems in establishing a level of fragile X positivity (at the chromosomal level; most individuals with the fragile X syndrome show the abnormality only in a proportion of the examined cells, at least given our current methods of examination) which will not produce false positives or false negatives. At the moment, some authors seem to agree that 3 to 4 per cent of the examined cells should be fragile X positive for a diagnosis of the fragile X syndrome to be made (Bolton and Rutter 1990). However, there are many problems associated with accepting this approach. First of all, 3 per cent of 33 examined cells is equivalent to one cell. The risk that this might constitute a false positive case is probably greater than if three cells out of 300 examined turned out to be typical fragile Xq27.3 positive cells, but this would correspond to only 1 per cent of examined cells. Also, a number of studies have shown that unequivocal cases of the fragile X syndrome can occur with a frequency of less than 1 per cent of the examined cells being fragile X positive (*e.g.* Gillberg *et al.* 1991). There are also problems associated with the identification of the true fragile Xq27.3 chromosomal abnormality as such. There are a number of, possibly clinically unimportant, fragile sites occurring in the same region of the X chromosome that can easily be confused with the 'true' fragile X chromosomal anomaly. In conclusion, one can only say that (1) all cases of autism have to be screened for fragile X; (2) there is a need to be very critical when accepting low-count cases as fragile X positive, but extending the number of cells examined rather than accepting a percentage of an undefined number of cells will help in reducing the number of false positives; and (3) in families where there is a strong suspicion of fragile X a low count in one chromosomal culture should not lead to the conclusion that fragile X is not present.

In 1991 and 1992, progress in molecular biology resulted in the discovery of the genetic mechanism underlying the clinical presentation of fragile X syndrome. The pattern of inheritance had long been thought peculiar because, unlike the case with other X-linked disorders, the mothers of all affected children are considered to be obligate carriers and no new affected offsping arise as a direct result of a new mutation (Shapiro 1991). The responsible gene (FMR-1) has been cloned and it includes the DNA base pair sequence (CGG) that causes the fragile X mutation. It appears that the number of repeat CGGs is directly proportional to the increase in size of the unstable region of DNA and to the clinical presentaton. The research suggests that if a CGG segment is repeated six to 50 times, the individual is symptom-free, 52 to 200 repeats result in very mild retardation and risk of

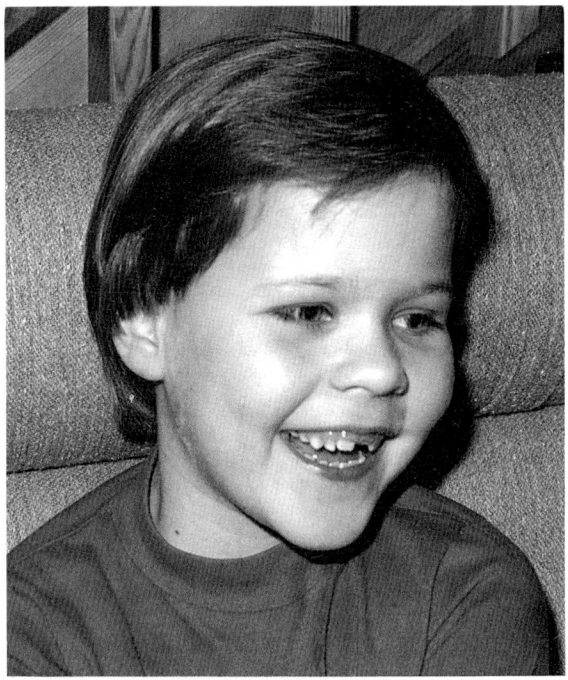

Fig. 16.6. 6-year-old girl with fragile X syndrome, autism and mild mental retardation (sister of boy in Fig. 16.5).

transmitting the severe form of the disease to offspring, and 230 to 1000 copies of the CGG region result in the severe form of the disease (Verkerk *et al.* 1991). Expanding DNA sequences, from generation to generation, might explain familial disease patterns where the clinical presentation worsens with each generation. The fragile X syndrome is not unique; other diseases, such as myotonic dystrophy and spinal bulbar atrophy, have also been found to have this new genetic pattern.

The fragile X abnormality in females was for several years considered not to predispose to autism. However, a number of studies from the late 1980s (Gillberg *et al.* 1988, LeCouteur *et al.* 1988; see also Hagerman 1989) indicate that autism may sometimes occur in fragile X positive females also (Fig.16.6). Some recent studies indicate that one of the main reasons for the failure to associate autism with the fragile X syndrome in females may have been the small number of female cases examined in previous studies. In the study by Cohen *et al.* (1989)—the largest to date in female autism/fragile X screening—four out of 31 females with autism were found to have the fragile X syndrome. The prevalence of the fragile X syndrome in females with autism is summarized in Table 16.2. According to the review, fragile X in autism may be only slightly less common in females than in males.

When autism coincides with the fragile X syndrome in males, it tends to be characterized by social avoidance, gaze avoidance, aversion of mutual gaze and a

192

TABLE 16.2
Prevalence of fragile X in females with autism

Study	Cohort with autism N	Fra (X) N
Jörgensen *et al.* (1984)	4	0
Venter *et al.* (1984)	17	0
Blomquist *et al.* (1985)	19	0
Goldfine *et al.* (1985)	3	0
McGillivray *et al.* (1986)	5	0
Wright *et al.* (1986)	9	0
Cohen *et al.* (1989)	33	4
Steffenburg *et al.* (1989)	14*	2
Steffenburg (1991)	5**	0
Total	109	6 (5.5%)

*Twins (population sample).
**Population sample.

greater sensitivity to parent's initiation of social gaze than other males with autism, turning away of the body on greeting, short echolalic bursts of speech, cluttering of speech, 'nervous' giggling, mounting anxiety after stimuli such as social inter-actions, occasional violent outbursts, hand-biting and other sterotypies (Levitas *et al.* 1983, Gillberg *et al.* 1986*b*, Bregman *et al.* 1988, Cohen *et al.* 1988, Wolff *et al.* 1989, Cohen *et al.* 1989, Hagerman 1989, Gillberg 1992). Much less is known about the behavioural phenotype in females. However, a few studies have suggested that females with the fragile X syndrome may have an increased rate of schizophrenia spectrum disorders and affective disorders. In particular there seems to be a case for a greater than chance concurrence of fragile X syndrome and schizoaffective disorders in females (Reiss *et al.* 1988, Reiss and Freund 1990, Steffenburg 1991).

There are both males and females with the fragile X syndrome who do not show autism or autistic behaviour. This group currently appears to be considerably larger among female cases, where autistic features and autism are likely to be present only in a minority. Nevertheless, there is growing evidence for unusual neuropsychological profiles in seemingly normal females with the fragile X syndrome (Hagerman 1989). Female heterozygotes without autism show social deficits—specifically shyness—even when IQ is normal. Such deficits have been suggested to be perhaps a mild form of the autistic spectrum.

The identification of a rather specific behavioural phenotype for autism cases with the fragile X syndrome illustrates how it is only after an aetiology has been found that the specificity of the behavioural syndrome can be established. Before the fragile X abnormality was disclosed, autism cases with the fragile X syndrome were considered 'classic' Kanner autism cases. Some authors have argued that autism is not associated with the fragile X syndrome (*e.g.* Einfeld *et al.* 1989). Conclusions to this effect usually rest on the basis of either few or no cases of the fragile X syndrome being diagnosed in (generally small) groups of patients with autism, or the comparison of individuals with so-called autism and individuals with so-called mental retardation with regard to prevalence of the fragile X chromosomal abnormality. A few authors have argued that just because autistic behaviour is no more common among fragile X positive individuals than among people with similar levels of mental retardation, there cannot be an association between autism and the fragile X syndrome (Einfeld *et al.* 1989). The conclusions are unwarranted in that (1) even though the fragile X syndrome may be the single most common associated disorder in autism, it is still relatively rare, and 30 or even 50 cases of autism without the chromosomal abnormality in a single non-population-based sample cannot be taken as evidence that the two are not associated; and (2) it is well known that moderate and severe mental retardation (the levels of intellectual functioning most often encountered in the fragile X syndrome) are often associated with autistic symptoms, and if you use an unselected mental retardation comparison group it will be likely to include autism cases caused by other disorders than the fragile X syndrome (as well as occasional cases with the fragile X syndrome, unless this abnormality has been screened out from the start). For instance, the report by Einfeld *et al.* of 45 fragile X positive individuals (with a mean age of almost 13 years, an age when many typical childhood autism cases no longer meet all the diagnostic criteria for autism) included as a comparison group patients with mental retardation associated with a number of conditions which have been proposed to be themselves associated with autism (cytomegalovirus infection, Williams syndrome, congenital hypothyroidism and 'epilepsy'). Furthermore, several of the comparison cases had not been screened for the occurrence of fragile X. Therefore, the findings that 9 per cent of individuals in each group met DSM-III-R criteria for autistic disorder and that similar percentages in both groups showed varying degrees of autistic behaviour may be taken to indicate that both groups are prone to autistic traits and autism.

Several small-scale folic acid, double-blind placebo-controlled crossover studies of fragile X syndrome have been performed in recent years (Levitas *et al.* 1983, Gillberg *et al.* 1986a, Hagerman 1989). Folic acid has usually been administered in doses of 0.5mg/kg/day. No obvious adverse effects have been noted. It is still too early to evaluate the importance of this possible pharmacological treatment in a subgroup of children with autism. A few studies have yielded results which could be taken to support starting treatment in early childhood, but the evidence is far from conclusive. There is some very limited evidence for a slight behaviourally positive effect of folic acid, whereas the findings so far are not in favour of a clear effect on cognition. Hagerman (1989) has speculated that, if there are positive effects of folic acid, these may not be specific to autistic features but rather be central stimulant effects which might enhance attention and so reduce meaningless, 'confused' activity.

Fragile sites other than Xq27.3
The significance, if any, of 'common' fragile sites (in autism mostly reported to be

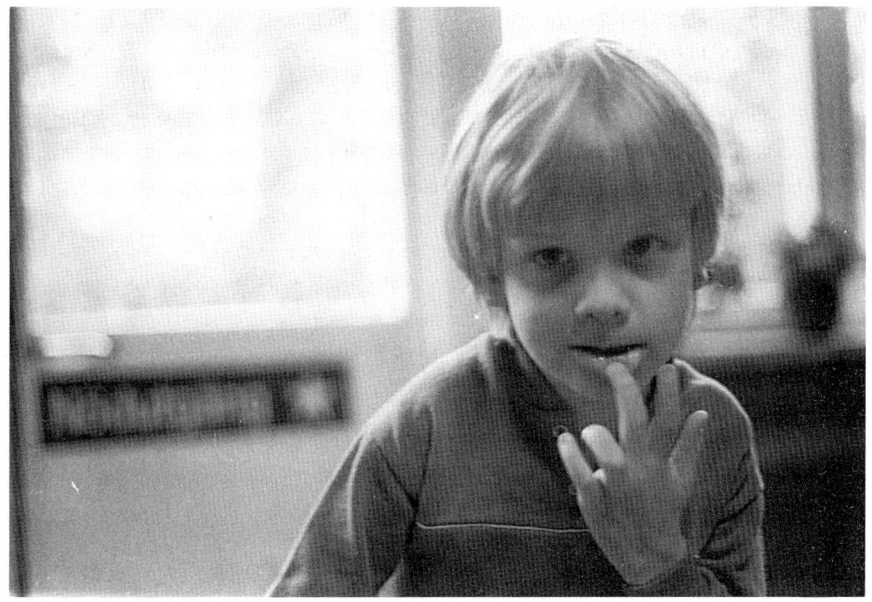

Fig. 16.7. Boy with XYY chromosomal abnormality and autism.

on chromosomes 2, 6 and 16) for the development of severe psychiatric or developmental disorders remains to be established. The status of fragile Xp22 is also unclear. It has been reported to be common in autism and Rett syndrome (Gillberg *et al.* 1984), but occurs in a percentage of normal people also.

Supernumerary sex chromosomes
The addition of an extra sex chromosome in the human karyotype is associated with a high rate of speech–language difficulties and learning disorders (Guichano *et al.* 1982, Bender *et al.* 1987). Crandall *et al.* (1973) evaluated 700 children referred to a child psychiatry clinic and found that 1.6 per cent had a sex chromosome abnormality and a behaviour problem. Sex chromosome abnormalities in the general population occur at a rate lower than 0.5 per cent. Autism has been occasionally reported in connection with supernumerary sex chromosomes. Of these, only the XYY abnormality has been reported in quite a number of cases, and by several different groups of researchers.

XYY SYNDROME
The XYY syndrome was long considered relatively harmless in respect to human psychiatric development. However, there is now good evidence that, apart from the fact that a small minority of persons with this karyotype develop into antisocial adults, speech–language and other learning disorders in childhood may be the rule

195

rather than the exception (Guichano *et al.* 1982; Bender *et al.* 1983, 1987).

Autism has been described in several individuals with the XYY syndrome (Abrams and Pergament 1971, Forsius *et al.* 1972, Mallin and Walker 1972, Nielsen *et al.* 1973, Gillberg *et al.* 1984), in such a way that pure coincidence is unlikely to be a plausible explanation. Furthermore, in the study by Nielsen *et al.*, poor social relatedness was reported in 13 of the 21 cases not given an autism diagnosis.

In the Swedish population study of chromosomes in autism and autistic-like conditions (Gillberg and Wahlström 1985), three out of 55 boys (5 per cent) showed either the complete XYY syndrome (one case—Fig. 16.7) or mosaicism involving a small number of cell populations containing an extra Y chromosome (two cases). Two of these boys had classic autism and the third was diagnosed as having Asperger syndrome (see Fig. 3.2, p. 48). The most probable explanation for the autism–sex chromosome abnormality link is a common speech language disorder, perhaps involving pragmatics. In combination with pre-, peri- or postnatal brain damage, the child already vulnerable to speech–language problems because of the XYY abnormality may develop autism. This seemed to be the case in at least one of the boys reported from the Swedish study (Gillberg *et al.* 1984).

XXX SYNDROME

One case of autism and the XXX syndrome has been reported in the literature so far (Wolraich *et al.* 1970). Fragile X has been reported in a 'normal' female with the XXX syndrome whose son has the fragile X syndrome (Fuster *et al.* 1988).

LONG Y VARIANTS

Judd and Mandell (1968) first reported a long Y variant in three of eight patients with autism. Hoshino *et al.* (1979) later reported that nine of 32 autism cases had 'long Y'. Several such cases were also reported by Gillberg and Wahlström (1985). However, even in the 'normal' population, 2 to 3 per cent of men show considerable variation of the length of the Y chromosome. Further, long Y chromosomes have been reported in other types of psychopathology than autism. Nevertheless, it appears that the rate of long Y chromosomes may be particularly high in autism.

ISODICENTRIC Y

A 3-year-old showing severe mental retardation and typical autism was demonstrated to have a normal X chromosome and an abnormal Y chromosome containing two centromeres. The abnormality was interpreted as an isochromosome Y composed of two copies of material from Ypter to Yq11.21. Thus this boy with autism had a male karyotype with an isodicentric Y chromosome. Both parents were healthy and had completely normal karyotypes.

The data implicating sex chromosome abnormalities in some cases of autism might, very speculatively, be linked with Lorna Wing's theory associating autism with normally occurring sex differences (Wing 1981). Autism might, in her view, be seen as perhaps the most extreme expression of normal male features. Most of the sex chromosome anomalies so far associated with autism indicate a relative decrease in the influence of normal 'female' chromosomes and hence a corresponding increase in the influence of the Y chromosomes.

Discussion

There has recently been a great deal of interest in what is described as the 'genetic influence' in autism (Smalley 1991) (see Chapter 8 for review). As can be seen from this list of patients with autism and chromosomal disorders, in some cases one of the parents carried a balanced translocation (thus not expressing the effect of the chromosomal deletion or duplication because of the balance). Hidden balanced translocations set the stage for one explanation of familial patterns in autism. However, familial patterns may be complex to diagnose even when the proband has a chromosomal error—an example is the case of a family in which one child with autism had a deletion on the long arm of chromosome 13 and a second cousin also with autism had a completely normal chromosome pattern (Ritvo *et al.* 1988).

Often patients with chromosomal errors are tested because of physical stigmata. This is an alerting sign to such a possibility in a patient with autism. However, as noted from this survey of the literature, the physical stigmata may be subtle, mild or non-evident. Even individuals with autism and a syndrome as distinctive as the cri-du-chat syndrome may be missed (Cantu *et al.* 1990). There is frequently considerable phenotypic variation from patient to patient with the same chromosomal syndrome, which may account for the inadequate diagnostic studies in some of these individuals.

In the autosomal aberrations, severe and profound retardation is usually found. One factor to consider in a severely retarded patient with autistic symptoms is the possibility of chromosomal karyotyping. However, it is necessary to keep in mind that high-functioning children with autism and individuals with Asperger syndrome have been found to have chromosomal abnormalities, particularly in the sex chromosomal syndromes.

The most striking thing about this review of the literature is the fact that abnormalities of so many different chromosomes have been found in studies of individuals with autism. In one of the largest epidemiological studies of autism ever done (233 patients with autism were located), 12 individuals (5 per cent) were found to have chromosomal anomalies (Ritvo *et al.* 1990). This is identical to the figure that Gillberg and Wahlström (1985) reported in 66 cases of autism and autistic-like conditions. In the Ritvo *et al.* study, half of the patients with autism and chromosomal abnormalities had Down syndrome (trisomy 21). A population-based study found that four of 35 individuals with autism had a definite chromosome disorder (Steffenburg 1991). These percentages compare favourably with the frequency of most of the other identified syndromes that present with autism. The exclusion of a chromosome disorder in a patient with autism is no longer a research procedure.

This survey of the chromosomal literature and autistic symptomatology reveals a paucity of trisomy syndromes and a greater frequency of deletion syndromes. Deletions are more difficult for laboratories to pinpoint in comparison to the immediately evident trisomy syndromes. Chromosomal testing in patients with autism needs to be done by high quality laboratories.

The following chapter will present diseases caused, not by duplication or deletion of entire chromosome areas, but by single genes that are carried on these chromosomes.

REFERENCES

Abrams, N., Pergament, E. (1971) 'Childhood psychosis combined with XYY abnormalities.' *Journal of Genetic Psychology*, **118**, 13–16.
Akuffo, E., MacSweeney, D.A., Gajwani, A.K. (1986) 'Multiple pathology in a mentally handicapped individual.' *British Journal of Psychiatry*, **149**, 377–378.
Bender, B.G., Linder, M.G., Robinson, A. (1987) 'Environment and developmental risk in children with sex chromosome abnormalities.' *Journal of the American Academy of Child and Adolescent Psychiatry*, **26**, 449–503.
Bender, L., Fry, E., Pennington, B., Puck, M., Salbenblatt, J., Robinson, A. (1983) 'Speech and language development in 41 children with sex chromosome abnormalities.' *Pediatrics*, **71**, 262–267.
Benzer, S. (1971) 'From gene to behavior.' *Journal of the American Medical Association*, **18**, 1015–1022.
Biesele, J.J., Schmid, W., Lawlis, M.G. (1962) 'Mentally retarded schizoid twin girls with 47 chromosomes.' *Lancet*, **2**, 403–405.
Blomquist, H.K., Gustavson, K.-H., Holmgren, G., Nordenson, I., Sweins, A. (1982) 'Fragile site X chromosomes and X-linked mental retardation in severely retarded boys in a northern Swedish county. A prevalence study.' *Clinical Genetics*, **21**, 209–214.
———————— Pålsson-Stråle, U. (1983) 'Fragile X syndrome in mildly mentally retarded children in a northern Swedish county. A prevalence study.' *Clinical Genetics*, **24**, 393–398.
—— Bohman, M., Edvinsson, S-O., Gillberg, C., Gustavson, K-H., Holmgren, G., Wahlström, J. (1985) 'Frequency of the fragile-X-syndrome in infantile autism. A Swedish multicenter study.' *Clinical Genetics*, **27**, 113–117.
Bolton, P., Rutter, M. (1990) 'Genetic influences in autism.' *International Review of Psychiatry*, **2**, 67–80.
Bregman, J.D., Leckman, J.F., Ort, S.I. (1988) 'Fragile X syndrome: genetic predisposition to psychopathology.' *Journal of Autism and Developmental Disorders*, **18**, 343–354.
Brenner, S. (1973) 'The genetics of behaviour.' *British Medical Bulletin*, **29**, 269–271.
Brown, W.T., Jenkins, E.C., Friedman, E., Brooks, J., Wisniewski, K., Raguthu, S., French, J.(1982) 'Autism is associated with the fragile X syndrome.' *Journal of Autism and Developmental Disorders*, **12**, 303–308.
———— Cohen, I.L., Fisch, G.S., Wolf-Schein, E.G., Gross, A., Waterhouse, L., Fein, D., Mason-Brothers, A., Ritvo, E., *et al.* (1986) 'Fragile X and autism: a multicenter survey.' *American Journal of Medical Genetics*, **23**, 341–352.
Burd, L., Martsolf, J.T., Kerbeshian, J., Jalal, S.M. (1988) 'Partial 6p trisomy associated with infantile autism.' *Clinical Genetics*, **33**, 356–359.
Campbell, M., Hardesty, A.S., Burdock, E.I. (1978) 'Demographic and perinatal profile of 105 autistic children: a preliminary report.' *Psychopharmacology Bulletin*, **14**, 36–39.
Cantu, E.S., Stone, J.W., Wing, A.A., Langee, H.R., Williams, C.A. (1990) 'Cytogenetic survey for autistic fragile X carriers in a mental retardation center.' *American Journal of Mental Retardation*, **94**, 442–447.
Chudley, A.E., Hagerman, R.J. (1987) 'Fragile X syndrome.' *Journal of Pediatrics*, **110**, 821–831.
Cohen, I.L., Fisch, G.S., Sudhalter, V., Wolf-Schein, E.G., Hanson, D., Hagerman, R., Jenkins, E.C., Brown, W.T. (1988) 'Social gaze, social avoidance, and repetitive behavior in fragile X males: a controlled study.' *American Journal of Mental Retardation*, **92**, 436–446.

—— Brown, W., Jenkins, E.C., Krawczun, M.S., French, J.H., Raguthu, S., Wolf-Schein, E.G., Sudhalter, V., Fisch, G., Wisniewski, K. (1989) 'Fragile X syndrome in females with autism.' *American Journal of Medical Genetics*, **34**, 302–303.

Collacott, R.A., Duckett, D.P., Mathews, D., Warrington, J.S., Young, I.D. (1990) 'Down's syndrome and the fragile X syndrome in a single patient.' *Journal of Mental Deficiency Research*, **34**, 81–86.

Crandall, B.F., Muller, M.M., Bass, H.N. (1973) 'Partial trisomy of chromosome number 15 identified by trypsin-giemsa banding.' *American Journal of Mental Deficiency Research*, **77**, 571–578.

Crowe, R.R., Tsai, L.Y., Murray, J.C., Patil, S.R., Quinn, J. (1988) 'A study of autism using X chromosome DNA probes.' *Biological Psychiatry*, **24**, 473–479.

Einfield, S., Molony, H., Hall, W. (1989) 'Autism is not associated with the fragile X syndrome.' *American Journal of Medical Genetics*, **34**, 187–193.

Elia, M., Bergonzi, P., Ferri, R., Musumeci, S.A., Paladino, A., Panerai, S., Ragusa, R.M. (1990) 'The etiology of autism in a group of mentally retarded subjects.' *Brain Dysfunction*, **3**, 228–240.

Forsius, H., Kaski, U., Schröder, J., de la Chapelle, A. (1972) 'Is there a common psychopathology of XYY boys? A clinical report on three cases of XYY and XY/XYY.' *Acta Paedopsychiatrica*, **39**, 28–41.

Fryns, J.P., Kleczkowska, A., Kubien, E., van den Berghe, H. (1986) 'Excess of mental retardation and/or congenital malformation in reciprocal translocations in man.' *Human Genetics*, **72**, 1–8.

Fuster, C., Templado, C., Miró, R., Barrios, L., Egozcue, J. (1988) 'Concurrence of the triple-X syndrome and expression of the fragile site Xq27.3.' *Human Genetics*, **78**, 293.

Gath, A., Gumley, D. (1986) 'Behavior problems in retarded children with special reference to Down's syndrome.' *British Journal of Psychiatry*, **149**, 156–161.

Gillberg, C. (1983) 'Identical triplets with infantile autism and the fragile-X syndrome.' *British Journal of Psychiatry*, **143**, 256–260.

—— (1992) 'Subgroups in autism. Are there behavioural phenotypes typical of underlying medical conditions?' *Journal of Intellectual Disability Research*, **36**, 201–214.

—— Wahlström, J. (1985) 'Chromosome abnormalities in infantile autism and other childhood psychoses: a population study of 66 cases.' *Developmental Medicine and Child Neurology*, **27**, 293–304.

—— Wahlström, J., Hagberg, B. (1984) 'Infantile autism and Rett's syndrome: common chromosomal denominator.' *Lancet*, **2**, 1094–1095. *(Letter.)*

—— Persson, E., Grufman, M., Themnér, U. (1986) 'Psychiatric disorders in mildly and severely mentally retarded urban children and adolescents: epidemiological aspects.' *British Journal of Psychiatry*, **149**, 68–74.

—— —— Wahlström, J. (1986) 'The autism–fragile-X syndrome (AFRAX). A population-based study of ten boys.' *Journal of Mental Deficiency Research*, **30**, 27–39.

—— Wahlström, J., Forsman, A., Hellgren, L., Gillberg, I.C. (1986) 'Teenage psychosis—epidemiology, classification and reduced optimality in the pre-, peri- and neonatal periods.' *Journal of Child Psychology and Psychiatry*, **27**, 87–98.

—— —— Jakobsson, G. (1987) 'Neurobiological findings in 20 relatively gifted children with Kanner-type autism or Asperger syndrome.' *Developmental Medicine and Child Neurology*, **29**, 641–649.

—— Ohlson, V-A., Wahlström, J., Steffenburg, S., Blix, K. (1988) 'Monozygotic female twins with autism and the fragile-X syndrome (AFRAX).' *Journal of Child Psychology and Psychiatry*, **29**, 447–451.

—— Steffenburg, S., Wahlström, J., Sjöstedt, A., Gillberg, I.C., Martinsson, T., Liedgren, S., Eeg-Olofsson, O. (1991) 'Autism associated with marker chromosome.' *Journal of the American Academy of Child and Adolescent Psychiatry*, **30**, 489–494.

Goldfine, P.E., McPherson, P.M., Heath, G.A., Hardesty, V.A., Beauregard, L.J. (1985) 'Association of fragile X syndrome with autism.' *American Journal of Psychiatry*, **142**, 108–110.

Guichano, M., Mattei, M.G., Mattei, J.F., Giraud, F. (1982) 'Genetic aspects of autosomal fragile X sites: a study of 40 cases.' *Journal de Génétique Humaine*, **30**, 183–197. *(In French.)*

Hagerman, R.J. (1987) 'Possible similarities between the fragile X and Asperger syndrome.' *American Journal of Diseases of Children*, **141**, 601–602. *(Letter.)*

—— (1989) 'Chromosomes, genes and autism.' *In:* Gillberg, C. (Ed.) *Diagnosis and Treatment of Autism.* New York: Plenum, pp. 105–132.

Hansen, A., Brask, B.H., Nielsen, J., Rasmussen, K., Sillesin, I. (1977) 'A case report of an autistic girl with an extra bisatellited marker chromosome.' *Journal of Autism and Childhood Schizophrenia*, **7**, 263–267.

Herbst, D.S., Miller, J.R. (1980) 'Nonspecific X-linked mental retardation. II: the frequency in British Columbia.' *American Journal of Medical Genetics*, **7**, 461–469.

Ho, H.H., Kalousek, D.K. (1989) 'Fragile X syndrome in autistic boys.' *Journal of Autism and Developmental Disorders*, **19**, 343–347.

Hoshino, Y., Yashima, Y., Tachibana, R., Kaneko, M., Watanabe, M., Kumashiro, H. (1979) 'Sex chromosome abnormality in autistic children—long Y-chromosome.' *Fukushima Journal of Medical Sciences*, **26**, 31–42.

Jayakar, R., Chudley, A.E., Ray, M., Evans, J.A., Perlov, J., Wand, R. (1986) 'Fra(2)(q13) and inv(9)(p11p12) in autism: causal relationship.' *American Journal of Medical Genetics*, **23**, 381–392.

Judd, L.L., Mandell, A.J. (1968) 'Chromosome studies in early infantile autism.' *Archives of General Psychiatry*, **18**, 450–457.

Jörgensen, O.S., Bröndum-Nielsen, K., Isager, T., Mouridsen, S.E. (1984) 'Fragile X chromosome among child psychiatric patients with disturbances of language and social relationships: a pilot study.' *Acta Psychiatrica Scandinavica*, **70**, 510–514.

Kerbeshian, J., Burd, L., Randall, T., Martsolf, J., Jalal, S. (1990) 'Autism, profound mental retardation and atypical bipolar disorder in a 33-year-old female with a deletion of 15q12.' *Journal of Mental Deficiency Research*, **34**, 205–210.

Knobloch, H., Pasamanick, B. (1975) 'Some etiologic and prognostic factors in early infantile autism and psychosis.' *Journal of Pediatrics*, **55**, 182–191.

Knoll, J.H.M., Nicholls, R.D., Magenis, R.E., Graham, J.M., Jalal, S. (1990) 'Angelman and Prader-Willi syndromes share a common chromosome 15 deletion but differ in parental origin of the deletion.' *American Journal of Medical Genetics*, **32**, 285–290.

Krug, D.A., Arick, J.R., Almond, P.J. (1979) 'Autism Screening Instrument for Educational Planning: background and development.' *In*: Gillam, J. (Ed.) *Autism: Diagnosis, Instruction, Management and Research*. Austin, TX: University of Texas Press.

Leckman, J.F., Cohen, D.J., Shaywitz, B.A., Caparulo, B.K., Heninger, G.R., Bowers, M.B. (1980) 'CSF monoamine metabolites in child and adult psychiatric patients.' *Archives of General Psychiatry*, **37**, 677–681.

LeCouteur, A., Rutter, M., Summers, D., Butler, L. (1988) 'Fragile X in female autistic twins.' *Journal of Autism and Development Disorders*, **18**, 458–460.

Levitas, A., Hagerman, R.J., Braden, M., Rimland, B., McBogg, P., Matus, I. (1983) 'Autism and the fragile X syndrome.' *Journal of Developmental and Behavioral Pediatrics*, **4**, 151–158.

Lubs, H.A. (1969) 'A marker X-chromosome.' *American Journal of Human Genetics*, **21**, 231–244.

Mallin, S.R., Walker, F.A. (1972) 'Effects of the XYY karyotype in one of 2 brothers with congenital adrenal hyperplasia.' *Clinical Genetics*, **3**, 490–494.

Mariner, R., Jackson, A.W., Levitas, A., Hagerman, R.J., Braden, M., McBogg, P.M., Smith, A.C., Berry, R. (1986) 'Autism, mental retardation, and chromosomal abnormalities.' *Journal of Autism and Developmental Disorders*, **16**, 425–440.

McGillivray, B.C., Herbst, D.S., Dill, F.J., Sandercock, J., Tischler, B. (1986) 'Infantile autism: an occasional manifestation of fragile X mental retardation.' *American Journal of Human Genetics*, **23**, 353–358.

Meryash, D.L., Szymanski, L.S., Gerald, P.S. (1982) 'Infantile autism associated with fragile X syndrome.' Journal of Autism and Developmental Disorders, **12**, 295–301.

Nicholls, R.D., Knoll, J.H.M., Butler, M.G., Karam, S., Lalande, M. (1989) 'Genetic imprinting suggested by maternal heterodisomy in non-deletion Prader-Willi syndrome.' *Nature*, **342**, 281–285.

Nielsen, J., Christensen, K.R., Friedrich, U., Zeuthen, E., Östergaard, O. (1973) 'Childhood of males with XYY syndrome.' *Journal of Autism and Childhood Schizophrenia*, **3**, 5–26.

Opitz, J.M., Sutherland, G.R. (1984) 'Conference report: international work-shop on the fragile X and X-linked mental retardation.' *American Journal of Medical Genetics*, **17**, 5–94.

Ornitz, E.M., Guthrie, D., Farley, A.J. (1977) 'The early development of autistic children.' *Journal of Autism and Childhood Schizophrenia*, **7**, 207–229.

Pembrey, M., Fennell, S.J., Van den Berghe, J., Fitchett, M., Summers, D., Butler, L., Clarke, C., Griffiths, S.M., Thompson, E., Super, M., *et al.* (1989) 'The association of Angelman's syndrome with deletions within 15q11-13.' *Journal of Medical Genetics*, **26**, 73–77.

Pueschel, S.M., Herman, R., Groden, G. (1985) 'Brief report: Screening children with autism for fragile-X syndrome and phenylketonuria.' *Journal of Autism and Developmental Disorders*, **15**, 335–338.

Reik, W. (1989) 'Genomic imprinting and genetic disorders in man.' *Trends in Genetics*, **5**, 331–336.

Reiss, A.L., Freund, L. (1990) 'Fragile X syndrome.' *Biological Psychiatry*, **27**, 223–240.

—— Hagerman, R.J., Vinogradov, S., Abrams, M., King, R.J. (1988) 'Psychiatric disability in female carriers of the fragile X chromosome.' *Archives of General Psychiatry*, **45**, 25–30.

Ritvo, E.R., Mason-Brothers, A., Freeman, B.J., Pingree, C., Jensen, W.R., McMahon, W.M., Petersen, P.B., Jorde, L.B., Mo, A., Ritvo, A. (1990) 'The UCLA–University of Utah epidemiologic survey of autism: the etiologic role of rare diseases.' *American Journal of Psychiatry*, **147**, 1614–1621.

—— —— Menkes, J.H., Sparkes, R.S. (1988) 'Association of autism, retinoblastoma, and reduced esterase D activity.' *Archives of General Psychiatry*, **45**, 600. *(Letter.)*

Rogers, P.T., Coleman, M. (1992) *Medical Care in Down Syndrome*. New York: Marcel Dekker.

Saliba, J.R., Griffiths, M. (1990) 'Brief report: Autism of the Asperger type associated with an autosomal fragile site.' *Journal of Autism and Developmental Disorders*, **20**, 569–575.

Schinzel, A. (1990) 'Autistic disorder and additional inv dup(15)(pter→q13) chromosome.' *American Journal of Medical Genetics*, **35**, 447. *(Letter.)*

Schopler, E., Reichler, R.J., DeVellis, R.F., Daly, K. (1980) 'Toward objective classification of childhood autism: Childhood Autism Rating Scale (CARS).' *Journal of Autism and Developmental Disorders*, **10**, 91–103.

Schreck, R.R., Breg, W.R., Erlanger, B.F., Miller, O.J. (1977) 'Preferential derivation of abnormal human G-group-like chromosomes from chromosome 15.' *Human Genetics*, **36**, 1–12.

Shapiro, L.R. (1991) 'The fragile X syndrome: a peculiar pattern of inheritance.' *New England Journal of Medicine*, **325**, 1736–1738.

Smalley, S.L. (1991) 'Genetic influences in autism.' *Psychiatric Clinics of North America*, **14**, 125–139.

Steffenburg, S. (1991) 'Neuropsychiatric assessment of children with autism: a population-based study.' *Developmental Medicine and Child Neurology*, **33**, 495–511.

—— Gillberg, C., Hellgren, L., Andersson, L., Gillberg, I.C., Jakobsson, G., Bohman, M. (1989) 'A twin study of autism in Denmark, Finland, Iceland, Norway and Sweden.' *Journal of Child Psychology and Psychiatry*, **30**, 405–416.

Surani, M.A., Reik, W., Allen, N.D. (1988) 'Transgenes as molecular probes for genomic imprinting.' *Trends in Genetics*, **4**, 59–62.

Turner, B., Jennings, A.N. (1961) 'Trisomy for chromosome 22.' *Lancet*, **2**, 49–50.

Venter, P.A., Op't Hof, J., Coetzee, D.J., Van der Walt, C.A., Retief, A.E. (1984) 'No marker (X) syndrome in autistic children.' *Human Genetics*, **67**, 107–111.

Verkerk, A.J.M.H., Pieretti, M., Sutcliffe, J.S., Fu, Y-H., Kuhl, D.P.A., Pizzuti, A., Reiner, O., Richards, S., Victoria, M.F., Zhang, F., *et al.* (1991) 'Identification of a gene (FMR-1) containing a CGG repeat coincident with a breakpoint cluster region exhibiting length variation in fragile X syndrome.' *Cell*, **65**, 905–914.

Volkmar, F.R., Cohen, D.J., Bregman, J.D., Hooks, M.Y., Stevenson, J.M. (1989) 'An examination of social typologies in autism.' *Journal of the American Academy of Child and Adolescent Pychiatry*, **28**, 82–86.

Wakabayashi, S. (1979) 'A case of infantile autism associated with Down's syndrome.' *Journal of Autism and Developmental Disorders*, **9**, 31–36.

Watson, M.S., Leckman, J.F., Annex, B., Breg, W.R., Boles, D., Volkmar, F.R., Cohen, D.J., Carter, C. (1984) 'Fragile X in a survey of 75 autistic males.' *New England Journal of Medicine*, **310**, 1462. *(Letter.)*

Webb, T.P., Bundey, S.E., Thake, A.I., Todd, J. (1986) 'Population incidence and segregation ratios in the Martin-Bell syndrome.' *American Journal of Medical Genetics*, **23**, 573–580.

Wenger, S.L., Steele, M.W., Becker, D.J. (1988) 'Clinical consequences of deletion 1p35.' *Journal of Medical Genetics*, **25**, 263.

Wilkins, L.E., Brown, J.A., Nance, W.E., Wolf, B. (1983) 'Clinical heterogeneity in 80 home-reared children with cri du chat syndrome.' *Journal of Pediatrics*, **102**, 528–533.

Wilson, G.N., Al Saadi, A.A. (1989) 'Obesity and abnormal behaviour associated with interstitial

201

deletion of chromosome 18 (q12.2q21.1).' *Journal of Medical Genetics*, **26**, 62–63.

Wilson, M.G., Towner, J.W., Forsman, I., Siris, E. (1979) 'Syndromes associated with deletion of the long arm of chromosome 18 [del(18q)].' *American Journal of Medical Genetics*, **3**, 155–174.

Wing, L. (1981) 'Sex ratios in early childhood autism and related conditions.' *Psychiatry Research*, **5**, 129–137.

—— Gould, J. (1979) 'Severe impairments of social interaction and associated abnormalities in children: epidemiology and classification.' *Journal of Autism and Developmental Disorders*, **9**, 11–29.

Wolff, P.H., Gardner, J., Paccia, J., Lappen, J. (1989) 'The greeting behavior of fragile X males.' *American Journal of Mental Retardation*, **93**, 406–411.

Wolraich, M., Bzostek, B., Neu, R.L., Gardner, L. (1970) Lack of chromosome aberrations in autism.' *New England Journal of Medicine*, **283**, 1231.

Wright, H.H., Young, S.R., Edwards, J.G., Abramson, R.K., Duncan, J. (1986) 'Fragile X syndrome in a population of autistic children.' *Journal of the American Academy of Child and Adolescent Psychiatry*, **25**, 641–644.

Zellweger, H., Simpson, J. (1977) *Chromosomes of Man. Clinics in Developmental Medicine No. 65/66.* London: Spastics International Medical Publications with Blackwell Scientific; Philadelphia: J.B. Lippincott.

17
METABOLIC DISORDERS

Inborn errors of metabolism underlie the autistic symptoms that are seen in some children. Unless these errors are sought for by laboratory testing, they are likely to be missed by the examiner.

These disease entities fall into two different patterns regarding the time of presentation. In one pattern, during gestation, the placenta of the mother often compensates or partially compensates for the fetus' inability to handle a particular metabolic pathway and the newborn appears quite asymptomatic. However, starting after birth and with the introduction of milk, the infant's metabolic system containing the inborn error is overwhelmed and there is a rapid build-up of minor metabolites which gradually cause brain dysfunction that soon becomes irreversible damage.

In the other pattern of presentation, the onset of the disease process is later than the newborn period. Although the child is at genetic risk for the disease, the enzyme involved may not decompensate immediately after birth, and the metabolic pathway may run normally at first. The failure of the genetically incorrectly programmed enzyme may occur later in the first year or even in the second year of life. Siblings with the same metabolic error tend to decompensate at about the same developmental stage; besides familial patterns, a serious illness or other major stress the infant experiences may decompensate the already barely functioning enzyme. In these cases, the age of presentation of symptoms can be any time up to 30 months of age.

Clinically, the exact age of presentation often tends to be hazy and has to be reconstructed after the fact. In the developing young brain, when progress is occurring daily, the mere plateauing of progress may signal the beginning of illness of the CNS. Although there is overlap with the mental retardation syndromes, the metabolic diseases which result in autistic symptoms have a slightly different work-up. This chapter discusses the known areas where inborn errors of metabolism have resulted in children with an autistic syndrome.

Diseases of amino acid metabolism
Phenylketonuria (PKU)
In 1960, Dr. C.E. Benda decided to try to convince psychiatrists that mental deficiency was a sector of child psychiatry. He took a group of psychiatrists to a ward to see several children with PKU and let them examine the children and make a diagnosis of childhood schizophrenia. Only afterwards did he tell them that the children were positive to PKU testing and had that metabolic disease (Benda 1960).

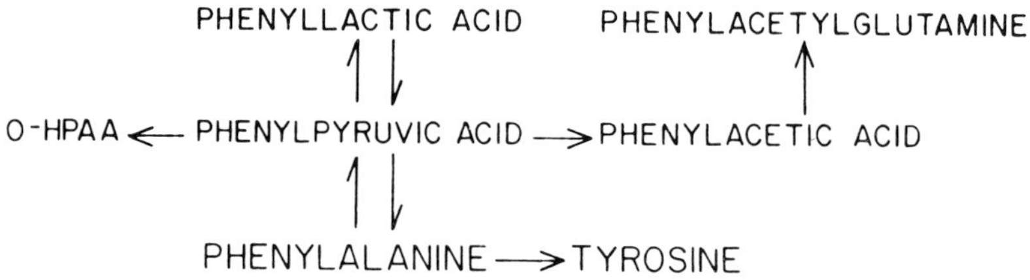

PHENYLLACTIC ACID   PHENYLACETYLGLUTAMINE
         ↑↓   ↑
O-HPAA ← PHENYLPYRUVIC ACID → PHENYLACETIC ACID
         ↑↓
    PHENYLALANINE → TYROSINE

Fig. 17.1. Minor metabolites build up to abnormal levels in the brain when the usual pathway from phenylalanine to tyrosine is blocked.

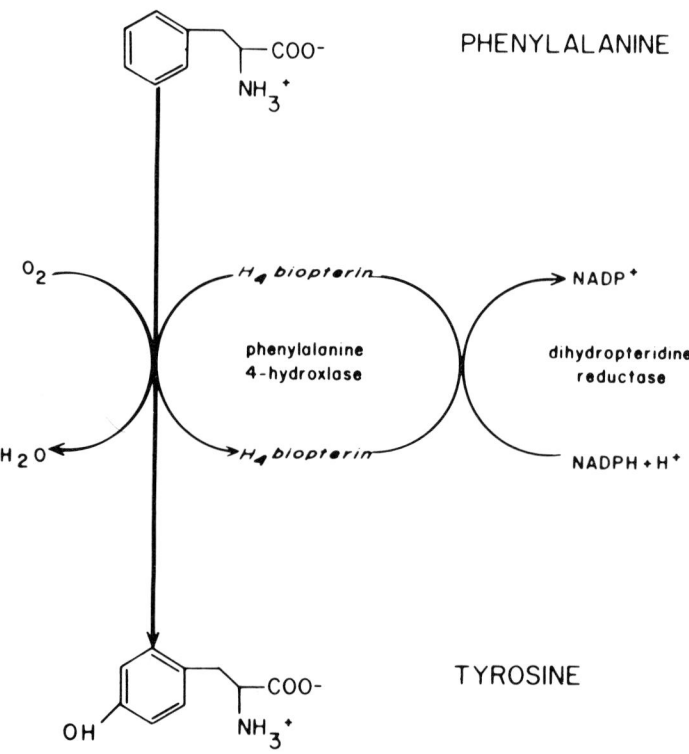

Fig. 17.2. The phenylalanine hydroxylase complex.

Nine years before Kanner described autism, Fölling (1934) had identified excessive phenylpyruvic acid in the urine of a group of retarded patients with a musty odour to their urine and thereby discovered PKU. By 1953, Jervis was able to demonstrate that the liver of these patients was deficient in the ability to convert phenylalanine to tyrosine. It is now understood that inadequate functioning of the enzyme phenylalanine hydroxylase (PAH, whose job it is to convert phenylalanine to tyrosine) results in a back-up of minor metabolites, such as phenylpyruvic acid and phenylacetic acid (the cause of the musty odour) spilling over into the urine (Fig. 17.1). Unfortunately, excessive levels of these metabolites also flood the CNS, gradually interfering with normal function.

After Fölling and Jervis found the biochemical basis for PKU, clinical descriptions of the patients began to appear in the literature. In a classic paper entitled 'The autistic syndrome and phenylketonuria', Friedman (1969) reviewed many of these papers. Referring to the behavioural descriptions of 11 out of 12 children with PKU in a paper by Kratter (1959), Friedman wrote 'What a complete description of an autistic child!' The clinical spectrum of PKU may be wider than originally thought—a patient with another psychiatric disease, anorexia nervosa, has also been found to have PKU (Clarke and Yapa 1991).

At first, it was thought that all patients with PKU had a single genetic error, which caused the enzyme to function so poorly. It is now clear that the phenylalanine hydroxylation reaction is the end result of a number of components: the enzyme itself, its essential cofactor (tetrahydrobiopterin), and a set of enzymes (and genes) for the production and maintenance of the cofactor (Fig. 17.2). The evidence now is that a genetic mutation could affect any one of the enzymes involved in this overall hydroxylation reaction and cofactor homeostasis. A physician diagnosing a patient with PKU needs to understand this because it directly affects the type of therapy chosen for the individual patient.

The human PAH gene resides on the long arm of chromosone 12, spans about 90,000 base pairs of DNA, has 13 exons and is decorated with a suite of highly informative DNA markers known as restriction fragment length polymorphisms (RFLPs). PAH haplotypes are derived from a set of eight RFLPs. More than 50 RFLP haplotypes have been documented at the human PAH locus (Woo 1988). Also, to date there have been 31 different PKU mutations and five instances of a PKU mutation occurring more than once in history (Scriver 1991).

Since PAH is an hepatic enzyme not present in serum or fibroblast cells, originally there was no available methodology for prenatal diagnosis of PKU; the cloning of the gene by Woo *et al.* in 1983 has now made this feasible. Not all mutations have yet been found, but even in families where the molecular defect (or defects) are not yet identified, the use of DNA linkage analysis can predict which siblings are carriers and the presence of absence of two abnormal genes in fetal tissue (Antonarakis 1989).

There is extensive polymorphism at the PAH locus, which varies in different areas of the world. European populations have at least 46 distinct RFLP haplotypes, while Asian families have at least 10 haplotypes. Four of the 46 haplotypes (1,2,3,4) account for more than 80 per cent of cases in European populations, while haplotype 4 alone accounts for approximately 80 per cent among the Chinese and Japanese (Levy 1989).

One of the debates in the field of autism has questioned whether child-rearing practices or biological factors in different parts of the world may account for different frequencies of autism among children in any particular geographical location. Although PKU is the aetiology of only a small fraction of the cases of autism, this kind of haplotype information can lead to a model of how biological factors may underlie different rates of a syndrome in different populations.

The successful treatment of PKU in a living infant depends upon early identification of the disease. Although they are reportedly normal at birth, there is some dispute in the literature as to whether affected children have a lower live-birth rate and a higher frequency of perinatal difficulties (Partington 1961, Rothman and Pueschel 1976). Sometimes neonatal nurses have noted a musty odour resulting from increased phenylacetic acid excretion. Increased frequency of vomiting occasionally results in surgery for suspected pyloric stenosis. Eczema also occurs soon after birth in a small percentage of patients. But often there is no evidence that alerts the medical staff to the presence of the serious disease about to engulf the infant.

Since the disease is almost always impossible to detect by clinical examination of the young infant and the successful treatment of PKU depends upon early identification of the abnormality, newborn screening laboratories exist around the world for the purpose of testing every baby for this inborn error of metabolism. In countries where newborn screening laboratories do not exist, children presenting with autism with underlying PKU are still being published in the medical literature. China is a country without newborn screening; Chen and Hsiao (1989) recently reported on a Chinese boy diagnosed as having infantile autism who was finally found to have PKU when 12 years old.

However, the fact that a country has newborn screening is not a guarantee that a patient with autism does not have PKU. The USA has newborn screening in all 50 states, yet Lowe et al. (1980) from the Yale University School of Medicine found three children with PKU while screening 65 children with autism and atypical childhood psychosis. A more recent study in the USA screened 38 boys with autism and found none with PKU (Pueschel et al. 1985). A recent Italian survey of mentally retarded persons with autism included one child with PKU (Elia et al. 1990).

How can the tragedy of a child developing autism due to PKU happen today? Alas, there are a number of possibilities. One set of problems are those related to logistics: the child can be born in a hospital without screenings (as in China); in hospitals which have screening, an infant can be accidentally missed during the screening process; an accident can happen to the specimen in the laboratory; the report can fail to reach the child's physician either by not being sent, getting lost *en*

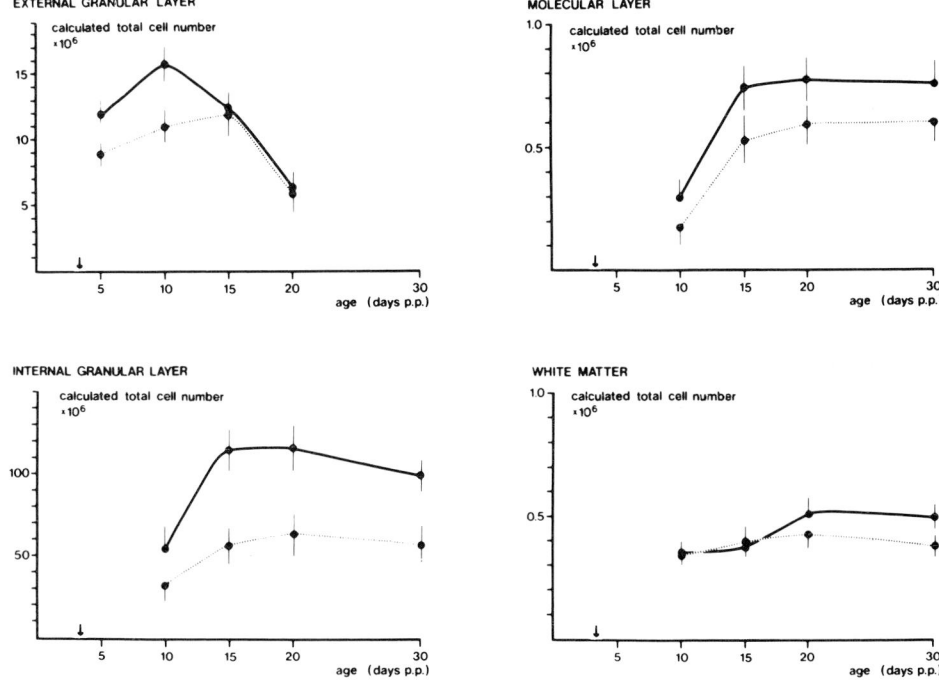

Fig. 17.3. Total cell numbers of individual cerebellar layers in suckling rats injected with phenylalanine and α-methylphenylalanine (dotted lines) compared to control rats injected with saline (solid lines). (Reproduced by permission from Huether *et al.* 1983.)

route or being misplaced in the doctor's office; or the physician can fail to act on the report when it comes.

Another set of problems is related to the age at which screening occurs. During gestation, the mother's liver effectively hydroxylyses the phenylalanine to tyrosine. In most cases, it is only after the baby is born and is handling the amino acids of milk on its own that the rise in the level of phenylalanine begins. As seen in Figure 17.3, total cell numbers in the cerebellum of suckling rats can be affected by excessive levels of phenylalanine. If infants are screened too early, they may not yet have developed an elevated level of phenylalanine and thus the screening test will miss them. Blood samples taken in the first 24 hours after birth may not yet be abnormal, yet many newborns leave the hospital at that age (McCabe *et al.* 1983).

But if a child is detected and appropriately diagnosed, this is a form of autism that should disappear because treatment is available. For most forms of PKU, a phenylalanine-restricted diet is effective if carefully monitored therapy is started under 3 months of age; the PKU Collaborative Study results indicate that the mean IQ can be in the normal range and behaviour can be normal (Dobson *et al.* 1977). Several types of phenylalanine-free products are available (Flannery *et al.* 1983).

However, some treated children still have learning disabilities (Berry *et al.* 1979) and some develop psychological and emotional difficulties in adolescence and early adulthood (Levy and Waisbren 1987). One area of debate concerns the possible need to continue the special diet well beyond childhood and perhaps indefinitely rather than reverting to a normal diet in middle childhood (Schuett and Brown 1984).

The first case of a special type of PKU or hyperphenylalaninaemia caused by the lack of a component of the phenylalanine hydroxylating system other than PAH was reported by Kaufman *et al.* (1975) who showed that a child, who did not respond to phenylalanine restriction, lacked dihydropteridine reductase (see Fig. 17.2) in biopsy samples of the liver and brain and in fibroblasts cultured from skin.

The therapy for this variant form of PKU involves more than restriction of phenylalanine intake and may include the administration of the precursors of the neurotransmitters catecholamines and serotonin. It must be geared to the individual patient (Butler *et al.* 1978). Besides genetic counselling and successful approaches to therapy, another reason to differentiate the subgroup of PKU patients who have dihydropteridine reductase deficiency is their sensitivity to a particular antibiotic, trimethoprim-sulphamethoxazole (Woody and Brewster 1990). A 4-year-old girl with this rare type of PKU developed parkinsonian symptoms when placed on the antibiotic; they rapidly disappeared when the antibiotic was discontinued.

Another variant form of PKU is the type in which both PAH and dihydropteridine reductase levels are normal but total biopterin levels in the liver, blood and urine are low (Bartholomé *et al.* 1977, Milstien *et al.* 1977) (see Fig. 17.2). These individuals have a block in the metabolic pathway for tetrahydrobiopterin (BH_4) and their therapy must compensate for that by the administration of BH_4 or synthetic analogues (Kaufman *et al.* 1983).

Regarding autistic symptoms in patients with PKU, three questions remain to be answered. The first one—What percentage of patients with PKU have autistic symptomatology?—may never be answered. This form of autism is disappearing thanks to newborn screening, and a series of untreated patients where such percentages can be calculated should never exist. If the question was not asked and answered in the past, it probably will remain unanswered. The closest we may get to an answer is the Friedman (1969) paper which does not offer final percentages but suggests that in some studies the percentage was disturbingly high.

The second question, a variation of the first, is—Since it is now possible to discover the molecular basis of the phenotypic heterogeneity in PKU (Okano *et al.* 1991), are there particular RFLP haplotypes of PKU likely to be associated with autistic symptomatology? This question may eventually be answered; early studies report the RFLP haplotypes are often closely correlated with phenylalanine levels (Guttler *et al.* 1987, Lyonnet *et al.* 1989).

The final question is related to therapy—Is there any value to starting therapy for PKU in an older infant or child past 3 months of age who has autistic symptoms?

Although the mental retardation cannot be prevented if therapy is started late, a few studies suggest that dietary treatment started at later ages can prevent further progress of the disability and might even have some behavioural benefit to the child (Lewis 1959, Gruter 1963, Lowe *et al.* 1980). Late onset therapy in PKU patients with autism remains an area of further evaluation. Some day somatic gene therapy might not only provide maximum benefit but might also eliminate the serious difficulties of maintaining the diet. However, this therapy cannot be developed until a great deal more is known about the PAH gene and its function (Levy 1989).

Our long-term goal is that this disease entity causing autistic symptoms will disappear from this type of textbook; it is theoretically possible with vigilant neonatal screening, prevention and early treatment.

Other amino acidopathies
PKU is the only inborn error of amino acid metabolism that is established as having produced a significant number of patients with autistic symptoms. In contrast to the studies on mental retardation syndromes which rapidly yielded quite a number of amino acidopathies when retarded children began to be tested, there is a scarcity of literature suggesting a correlation between the inborn errors of metabolism of amino acids and autism.

Histidinaemia has twice been reported in patients with the diagnosis of infantile autism (Rutter and Bartak 1971, Kotsopoulos and Kutty 1979). Originally, it was thought to be associated with mental retardation, but serious doubts have arisen. There is good evidence that, in many families, histidinaemia is a benign disorder as far as brain function is concerned (Levy *et al.* 1974). There remains the possibility that there is genetic heterogeneity in histidinaemia with two or more genetically distinct disorders: one that is clinically benign, another that results in mental retardation, and possibly one resulting in autistic symptoms. However, this seems unlikely based on present knowledge. It is more probable that this inborn error of metabolism was picked up incidentally because patients with mental retardation and autism often undergo extensive testing.

To date, however, most children with autism have not had a full medical work-up, and until this becomes standard practice the possibility of other amino acidopathies remains an open question.

Diseases of purines and pyrimidines
Purine autism
There now are a number of cases cited in the medical literature of patients who have autistic symptomatology and evidence of an error in purine metabolism. Perhaps this is not surprising, since the purine errors documented to date often have a behavioural or psychiatric component (Table 17.1). In some of the earlier patients described, autism was merely one feature of a much more complex syndrome such as spasticity or deafness, but more recently purine dysfunction has been found in patients with more classical infantile autism.

TABLE 17.1

Patients described in the literature with purine overproduction and CNS symptoms

Initial report	CNS signs					Aetiology
	Autistic symptoms	Deafness	Neurological symptoms	Other psychiatric symptoms	Mental retardation	
Lesch and Nyhan (1964)			Chorea, athetosis, spasticity	Severe self-mutilation, aggression	Moderate/severe	HPRT[1] level decreased
Sorensen and Benke (1967)			Chorea	Self-induced alopecia, antisocial behaviour		
Hooft et al. (1968)	Yes		Chorea, athetosis, spasticity	Mild self-mutilation	Severe	
Nyhan et al. (1969)	Yes	Yes			Moderate	PRPP[2] synthetase level increased
Rosenberg et al. (1970)		Yes	Ataxia, spasticity			
Coleman (1974)	'Childhood schizophrenia'			Psychosis	Moderate	
Coleman et al. (1974)			Seizures, ataxia	Social immaturity	Pseudo-retardation	CNS tumour excreting purines
Coleman (1976)	Yes (15 cases)		Adventitious movements, drooling, ataxia, tongue protrusion, abnormal EEG, toe-walking	Self-biting, irritability, 'less will'	Mild/moderate/severe	
Stoop et al. (1977)			Tetraparesis, tremor, ataxia			PNP[3] level decreased
Duran (1978)			Tetraparesis, cranial dysmorphism			Xanthine oxidase level decreased
Simmonds et al. (1982, 1985)		Yes	Hypotonia, infant 'head nods'		Mild	Nicotinamide adenine dinucleotide level decreased
Jaeken and van den Berghe (1984)	Yes (3 cases)		Hypotonia	Mild self-mutilation	Severe	Adenylosuccinase level decreased
Rosenberger-Debiesse and Coleman (1986)	Yes (6 cases)		Spasticity, febrile seizures, hypotonia	Self-mutilation, bruxism, irritability	Moderate/severe	

[1]HPRT = hypoxanthine phosphoribosyltransferase; [2]PRPP = phosphoribosylpyrophosphate; [3]PNP = purine nucleoside phosphorylase.

In 1968, Hooft *et al.* reported a child with an increased excretion of uric acid of 35 to 45mg/kg/day. The child had spasticity, choreoathetosis and self-mutilation and 'social contact was practically absent'. A low-purine diet was said to result in 'an undeniable improvement in the child's condition . . . whereas she had previously taken no interest in the outside world, she now even smiled at her parents.'

The following year Nyhan *et al.* (1989) described a 3-year-old boy with unusual autistic behaviour, failure to cry with tears, absence of speech, hypoplastic discoloured teeth and persistently pink urine. The description was of a boy 'very disturbed and autistic who seemed to be totally oblivious to the people around him.' Later studies also demonstrated deafness in this child. The research team documented an increased synthesis of purines *de novo* by the rate of conversion of glycine to uric acid which was seven times that of a control patient. In a later follow-up study on this patient, Becker *et al.* (1980) demonstrated that the excessive rate of uric acid synthesis in this child was probably explained by an increase in the purine enzyme phosphoribosylpyrophosphate synthetase in his fibroblasts.

Two siblings with autism whose grandparents were first cousins and another child with autism have been found to be deficient in another purine enzyme, adenylosuccinase (also called adenylsuccinate lyase) (Jaeken and van den Berghe 1984). The children had severe psychomotor retardation in addition to their autism. Four other patients with the syndrome have been reported in the literature (de Bree *et al.* 1986). It can be technically difficult to find succinylpurines in the urine and a simplified method has been proposed (Maddocks and Reed 1989). Detailed metabolic studies of cultured lymphoblasts from the two siblings with infantile autism suggested that structurally mutated adenylosuccinase was present in the mutant cells (Barshop *et al.* 1989).

Abnormal levels of inosinate dehydrogenase were reported in two patients with infantile autism (Gruber *et al.* 1985). It was not clear to the investigators whether the abnormality was primary or a secondary compensation for another, as yet unidentified, enzyme abnormality in these children.

In 1976, a United States research project involving 69 children with autistic symptoms (mean age 9 years) found that 15 (22 per cent) had elevated uric acid levels in the urine (hyperuricosuria), compared to 3 per cent of the age- and sex-matched controls (Coleman *et al.* 1976). None of the children had elevations of uric acid in the blood (hyperuricaemia). Ten years later, a similar survey in France examined 21 children with autism and found that six had hyperuricosuria and two of those also had hyperuricaemia (Rosenberger-Debiesse and Coleman 1986). More recently, a survey in Italy disclosed that 26 per cent of the Italian patients with autism had hyperuricosuria (Visconti, personal communication).

Lis *et al.* (1976), studying the urine of a small group of children with autism by chromatographic methods found low uric acid levels combined with high hypoxanthine levels in several patients.

Stubbs *et al.* (1982) investigated 18 unselected subjects with autism for the study of six purine enzymes: adenosine deaminase, nucleotide phosphorylase, hypoguanine phosphoribosyltransferase, adenine phosphoribosyltransferase, ecto-5-nucleotidase and adenosine kinase. The children were chosen at random—they were not selected by preliminary testing of blood or urinary uric acid levels—and were compared with normal children, mentally retarded children and children with cerebral palsy. There was much overlap of purine enzyme values between the experimental and control subjects; the authors interpreted this to mean that they were dealing with a heterogeneous population. Decreased levels of adenosine deaminase were found at a level of significance of $p<0.02$. This finding raised the question of problems of immune deficiency in autism, since hereditary absence of adenosine deaminase is known to cause severe combined immune deficiency disease (see Chapter 11).

Studies of purine metabolism in children are often based on 24-hour urine specimens instead of serum levels as is done in adults. Boss and Seegmiller (1982) noted that there is a chance of missing the diagnosis if one relies on a blood test rather than a 24-hour urine specimen in many of the purine syndromes seen in children. Puberty changes the equilibrium of the purine systems; after the onset of puberty, both blood and 24-hour urine studies are helpful in children with autism.

It is important to note that finding hyperuricosuria in a patient with autism does not establish that this is the relevant aetiology of the autistic symptoms in that child. As seen in the Coleman *et al.* (1976) study, a small percentage of children who are otherwise normal have hyperuricosuria. It is important in each patient to establish the mechanism that results in the hyperuricosuria. There are other disease entities, even including the presence of a debilitating illness, that can cause purine irregularities in children (for a differential diagnosis, see Coleman and Gillberg 1985). In evaluation of patients with hyperuricosuria, the initial finding is best confirmed by a uric acid clearance study which will establish if kidney function is intact and the abnormality is a metabolic rather than a renal one.

Since diagnosis of purine autism is in its infancy, treatment protocols are virtually non-existent. There are a couple of case studies which show possible response to a low-purine diet in children with autistic symptoms (Hooft *et al.* 1968, Coleman 1989). Rational therapy is based on specific enzymatic or DNA sequence findings in the individual patient, and these research challenges lie ahead.

Diseases of carbohydrate and lipid metabolism
Lactic acidosis
Lactic acidosis or hyperlactataemia without acidosis indicates some abnormality in the utilization of sugar, which increases the rate of lactate production relative to the rate of lactate utilization. Often the primary abnormality is in the rate of oxidation of glucose and the increase in lactate production appears to be caused by a decrease in the rate of lactate utilization in gluconeogenesis. Hyperlactataemia is not a specific biochemical abnormality in itself, but rather an indication that a particular patient may or may not have had an inborn error of metabolism in the family of

disorders of carbohydrate metabolism, including mitochondrial disorders. Sometimes the finding is merely related to the fact that a patient was struggling too hard when the blood was drawn, a characteristic of many children with autism.

Infantile spasms are a seizure syndrome of infancy that can be followed by an autistic clinical picture (see Chapter 6). In patients with infantile spasms and the acute onset of lactic acidosis without evidence of one of the more common aetiologies (*e.g.* sepsis, hypoxia), an inborn error of metabolism of a mitochondrial enzyme is possible (Robinson 1983). ACTH (adenocorticotrophic hormone) should be used with caution in such children (Rutledge *et al.* 1989).

Coleman and Blass (1985) described four patients who appeared to have the coexisting syndromes of autism and lactic acidosis. Three patients were male; one was female and was later diagnosed as having Rett syndrome (see Chapter 20). Research studies of one of the enzymes of the carbohydrate pathway, pyruvate dehydrogenase complex, are in progress with autism.

Mucopolysaccharidoses
Mucopolysaccharidoses are genetic metabolic errors that result from abnormalities of the biochemical constituents of connective tissue. The mucopolysaccharidoses that affect the CNS are associated with abnormal lysosomal degradation of polymers, with up to 100 sugar residues present in a chain. The clinical diseases result from dysfunction or virtual absence of an enzyme needed for catabolic degradation with subsequent accumulated storage within the lysosomes. In the early stages, these diseases are often hard to diagnose.

A number of patients have been mentioned in the literature with enzymatic diagnoses of mucopolysaccharidosis and autistic symptoms (Knobloch and Pasamanick 1975, Coleman 1976, Ritvo *et al.* 1990). One child with Hurler disease (α-L-iduronidase deficiency) detected by one of the present authors (M.C.) led to a screening test for mucopolysaccharidoses being added to the comprehensive research study at the Children's Brain Research Clinic (Coleman 1976); however no additional patients were found.

Two siblings with Sanfilippo syndrome (heparan-*N*-sulphatase deficiency) have been described in the UCLA–University of Utah epidemiologic survey of autism; they were both mentally retarded (Ritvo *et al.* 1990). Sanfilippo syndrome involves a mucopolysaccharidosis frequently associated with CNS pathology, often a severe seizure disorder.

Free fatty acids
Carbohydrate and lipid metabolism is a mostly untouched area in the evaluation of children with autism without a specific diagnosis. DeMyer *et al.* (1971) studied plasma free fatty acid metabolism in a mixed group of children with autism or schizophrenia and demonstrated greater variability than in controls. This suggested that the group was biochemically heterogeneous. No further studies are reported in the literature.

Conclusion

Very few investigators have evaluated groups of patients with autism looking for metabolic errors. Once such investigations become routine in evaluations, it is quite possible that other metabolic errors will be located. At this point, it appears that investigations into purines and pyrimidines may be a more fruitful area than amino acids.

REFERENCES

Antonarakis, S.E. (1989) 'Diagnosis of genetic disorders at the DNA level.' *New England Journal of Medicine*, **320**, 153–163.

Barshop, B.A., Alberts, A.S., Gruber, H.E. (1989) 'Kinetic studies of mutant human adenylosuccinase.' *Biochimica et Biophysica Acta*, **999**, 19–23.

Bartholomé, K., Byrd, D.J., Kaufman, S., Milstein, S. (1977) 'Atypical phenylketonuria with normal phenylalanine hydroxylase and dihydropteridine reductase activity in vitro.' *Pediatrics*, **59**, 757–761.

Becker, M.A., Raivio, K.O., Bakay, B., Adams, W.B., Nyhan, W.L. (1980) 'Variant human phosphoribosylpyrophosphate synthetase altered in regulatory and catalytic functions.' *Journal of Clinical Investigation*, **65**, 109–120.

Benda, C.E. (1960) 'Childhood schizophrenia, autism, and Heller's disease.' *In: Proceedings of the First International Metabolic Conference, Portland, ME.* New York: Grune & Stratton.

Berry, H.K., O'Grady, D.J., Perlmutter, L.J., Bofinger, M.K. (1979) 'Intellectual development and academic achievement of children treated early for phenylketonuria.' *Developmental Medicine and Child Neurology*, **21**, 311–320.

Boss, G.R., Seegmiller, J.E. (1982) 'Genetic defects in human purine and pyrimidine metabolism.' *Annual Review of Genetics*, **16**, 297–328.

Butler, I.J., Koslow, S.H., Krumholz, A., Holtzman, N.A., Kaufman, S. (1978) 'A disorder of biogenic amines in dihydropteridine reductase deficiency.' *Annals of Neurology*, **3**, 224–230.

Chen, C.H., Hsiao, K.J. (1989) 'A Chinese classic phenylketonuria manifested as autism.' *British Journal of Psychiatry*, **155**, 251–253.

Clarke, D.J., Yapa, P. (1991) 'Phenylketonuria and anorexia nervosa.' *Journal of Mental Deficiency Research*, **35**, 163–170.

Coleman, M. (1974) 'A crossover study of allopurinol administration to a schizophrenic child.' *Journal of Autism and Childhood Schizophrenia*, **4**, 231–240.

—— (1976) 'Introduction.' *In:* Coleman, M. (Ed.) *The Autistic Syndromes.* Amsterdam: North Holland; New York: Elsevier, pp. 1–10.

—— (1989) 'Autism: non-drug biological treatments.' *In:* Gillberg, C. (Ed.) *Diagnosis and Treatment of Autism.* New York: Plenum, pp. 219–235.

—— Blass, J.P. (1985) 'Autism and lactic acidosis.' *Journal of Autism and Developmental Disorders*, **15**, 1–8.

—— Gillberg, C. (1985) *The Biology of the Autistic Syndromes.* New York: Praeger.

—— Landgrebe, M.A., Landgrebe, A.R. (1974) 'Progressive seizures with hyperuricosuria reversed by allopurinol.' *Archives of Neurology*, **31**, 238–242.

—— —— —— (1976) 'Purine autism. Hyperuricosuria in autistic children: does this identify a subgroup of autism?' *In:* Coleman, M. (Ed.) *The Autistic Syndromes.* Amsterdam: North Holland; New York: Elsevier, pp. 183–195.

de Bree, P.K., Wadman, S.K., Duran, M., Fabery de Jonge, H. (1986) 'Diagnosis of inherited adenylosuccinase deficiency by thin-layer chromatography of urinary imidazoles and by automated cation exchange column chromatography of purines.' *Clinica Chimica Acta*, **156**, 279–288.

DeMyer, M.K., Schwier, H., Bryson, C.Q., Solow, E.B., Roeske, N. (1971) 'Free fatty acid response to insulin and glucose stimulation in schizophrenic, autistic and emotionally disturbed children.' *Journal of Autism and Childhood Schizophrenia*, **1**, 436–452.

Dobson, J.C., Williamson, M.L., Azen, C., Koch, R. (1977) 'Intellectual assessment of 111 four-year-old children with phenylketonuria.' *Pediatrics*, **60**, 822–827.

Duran, M., Beemer, F.A., Van de Heiden, C., Korteland, J., de Bree, P.K., Brink, M., Wadman, S.K. (1978) 'Combined deficiency of xanthine oxidase and sulfite oxidase. A defect of molybdenum metabolism or transport?' *Journal of Inherited Metabolic Disease*, **1**, 175–178.

Elia, M., Bergonzi, P., Ferri, R., Musumeci, A., Paladino, A., Panerai, S., Ragusa, R.M. (1990) 'The etiology of autism in a group of mentally retarded subjects.' *Brain Dysfunction*, **3**, 228–240.

Flannery, D.B., Hitchcock, E., Mamunes, P. (1983) 'Dietary management of phenylketonuria from birth using a phenylalanine-free product.' *Journal of Pediatrics*, **103**, 247–249.

Fölling, A. (1934) 'Phenylpyruvic acid as a metabolic anomaly in connection with imbecility.' *Zeitschrift für Physiologische Chemie*, **224**, 169–176.

Friedman, E. (1969) 'The "autistic syndrome" and phenylketonuria.' *Schizophrenia*, **1**, 249–261.

Gillberg, C., Steffenburg, S. (1987) 'Outcome and prognostic factors in infantile autism and similar conditions: a population-based study of 46 cases followed through puberty.' *Journal of Autism and Developmental Disorders*, **17**, 273–287.

Gruber, H.E., Jansen, I., Willis, R.C., Seegmiller, J.E. (1985) 'Alteration of the inosinate branchpoint enzymes in cultured human lymphoblasts.' *Biochemica et Biophysica Acta*, **846**, 135–144.

Gruter, W. (1963) *Angeborene Stoffwechselstorungen und Schwachsinn am Beispiel der Phenylketonurie*. Stuttgart: F. Enke.

Guttler, F., Ledley, F.D., Lidsky, A.S., DiLella, A.G., Sullivan, S.E., Woo, S.L.C. (1987) 'Correlation between polymorphic DNA haplotypes at phenylalanine hydroxylase locus and clinical phenotypes of phenylketonuria.' *Journal of Pediatrics*, **110**, 68–71.

Hooft, C., van Nevel, C., de Schaepdryver, A.F. (1968) 'Hyperuricosuric encephalopathy without hyperuricaemia.' *Archives of Disease in Childhood*, **43**, 734–737.

Huether, G., Neuhoff, V., Kaus, R. (1983) 'Brain development in experimental hyperphenylalaninaemia: disturbed proliferation and reduced cell numbers in the cerebellum.' *Neuropediatrics*, **14**, 12–19.

Jaeken, J., van den Berghe, G. (1984) 'An infantile autistic syndrome characterised by the presence of succinylpurines in body fluids.' *Lancet*, **2**, 1058–1061.

Jervis, G. (1953) 'Phenylpyruvic oligophrenia: deficiency of phenylalanine oxidizing system.' *Proceedings of the Society for Experimental Biology and Medicine*, **82**, 514–515.

Kaufman, S., Holtzman, N., Milstein, S., Butler, I.J., Krumholz, A. (1975) 'Phenylketonuria due to deficiency of dihydropteridine reductase.' *New England Journal of Medicine*, **293**, 785–790.

—— Kapatos, G., Rizzo, W.B., Schulman, J.D., Tamarkin, L., Van Loon, G.R. (1983) 'Tetrahydropterin therapy for hyperphenylalaninemia caused by defective synthesis of tetrahydrobiopterin.' *Annals of Neurology*, **14**, 308–315.

Knobloch, H., Pasamanick, B. (1975) 'Some etiologic and prognostic factors in early infantile autism and psychoses.' *Journal of Pediatrics*, **55**, 182–191.

Kotsopoulos, S., Kutty, K.M. (1979) 'Histidinemia and infantile autism.' *Journal of Autism and Developmental Disorders*, **9**, 55–60.

Kratter, F.E. (1959) 'The physiognomic, psychometric, behavioral and neurological aspects of phenylketonuria.' *Journal of Mental Science*, **105**, 421–427.

Lesch, M., Nyhan, W.L. (1964) 'A familial disorder of uric acid metabolism and central nervous system function.' *American Journal of Medicine*, **36**, 561–570.

Levy, H.L. (1989) 'Molecular genetics of phenylketonuria and its implications.' *American Journal of Human Genetics*, **45**, 667–670. (*Editorial.*)

—— Waisbren, S.E. (1987) 'The PKU paradigm: the mixed results from early dietary treatment.' *In:* Kaufman, S. (Ed.) *Amino Acids in Health and Disease: New Perspectives*. New York: Alan R. Liss, pp. 539–551.

—— Shih, V.E., Madigan, P.M. (1974) 'Routine newborn screening for histidinemia.' *New England Journal of Medicine*, **291**, 1214–1219.

Lewis, E. (1959) 'The development of concepts in a girl after dietary therapy for phenylketonuria.' *British Journal of Medical Psychology*, **32**, 282–287.

Lis, A.W., McLaughlin, D.I., McLaughlin, R.K., Lis, E.W., Stubbs, E.G. (1976) 'Profiles of ultra-absorbing components of urine from autistic children, as obtained by high-resolution ion-exchange chromatography.' *Clinical Chemistry*, **22**, 1528–1532.

Lowe, T.L., Tanaka, K., Seashore, M.R., Young, J.G., Cohen, D.J. (1980) 'Detection of phenylketonuria in autistic and psychotic children.' *Journal of the American Medical Association*,

215

243, 126–128.

Lyonnet, S., Caillaud, C., Rey, F., Berthelon, M., Frézal, J., Rey, J., Munnich, A. (1989) 'Molecular genetics of phenylketonuria in Mediterranean countries: a mutation associated with partial phenylalanine hydroxylase deficiency.' *American Journal of Human Genetics*, **44**, 511–517.

Maddocks, J., Reed, T. (1989) 'Urine test for adenylosuccinase deficiency in autistic children.' *Lancet*, **1**, 158–159.

McCabe, E.R., McCabe, B., Mosher, G.A., Allen, R.J., Berman, J.L. (1983) 'Newborn screening for phenylketonuria: predictive validity as a function of age.' *Pediatrics*, **72**, 390–398.

Milstien, S., Orloff, S., Spielberg, S., Berlow, S., Schulman, J., Kaufman, S. (1977) 'Hyperphenylalaninemia due to phenylalanine hydroxylase co-factor deficiency.' *Pediatric Research*, **11**, 460. *(Abstract.)*

Nyhan, W.L., James, J.A., Teberg, A.J., Sweetman, L., Nelson, L.G. (1969) 'A new disorder of purine metabolism with behavioral manifestations.' *Journal of Pediatrics*, **74**, 20–27.

Okano, Y., Eisen-Smith, R.C., Güttler, F., Lichter-Konecki, U., Konecki, D.S., Trefz, F.K., Dasovich, M., Wang, T., Henriksen, K., Lou, H., *et al.* (1991) 'Molecular basis of phenotypic heterogeneity in phenylketonuria.' *New England Journal of Medicine*, **324**, 1232–1238.

Partington, M. (1961) 'The early symptoms of phenylketonuria.' *Pediatrics*, **27**, 465–473.

Pueschel, S.M., Herman, R., Groden, G. (1985) 'Brief report: screening children with autism for fragile-X syndrome and phenylketonuria.' *Journal of Autism and Developmental Disorders*, **15**, 335–338.

Ritvo, E.R., Mason-Brothers, A., Freeman, B.J., Pingree, C., Jensen, W.R., McMahon, W.M., Petersen, C.B., Jorde, L.B., Mo, A., Ritvo, A. (1990) 'The UCLA–University of Utah epidemiologic survey of autism: the etiologic role of rare diseases.' *American Journal of Psychiatry*, **147**, 1614–1621.

Robinson, B.H. (1983) 'Inborn errors of pyruvate metabolism.' *Biochemical Society Transactions*, **11**, 623–628.

Rosenberg, A.L., Bergstrom, L., Troost, B.T., Bartholomew, B.A. (1970) 'Hyperuricemia and neurologic deficits: a family study.' *New England Journal of Medicine*, **282**, 992–997.

Rosenberger-Debiesse, J., Coleman, M. (1986) 'Brief report: Preliminary evidence for multiple etiologies in autism.' *Journal of Autism and Developmental Disorders*, **16**, 385–392.

Rothman, K., Pueschel, S. (1976) 'Birthweight of children with phenylketonuria.' *Pediatrics*, **58**, 842–844.

Rutledge, S.L., Snead, O.C., Kelly, D.R., Kerr, D.S., Swann, J.W., Spink, D.L., Martin, D.L. (1989) 'Pyruvate carboxylase deficiency: acute exacerbation after ACTH treatment of infantile spasms.' *Pediatric Neurology*, **5**, 249–252.

Rutter, M., Bartak, L. (1971) 'Causes of infantile autism: some considerations from recent research.' *Journal of Autism and Childhood Schizophrenia*, **1**, 20–32.

Schuett, V.E., Brown, E.S. (1984) 'Diet policies of PKU clinics in the United States.' *American Journal of Public Health*, **74**, 501–502.

Scriver, C.R. (1991) 'Phenylketonuria—genotypes and phenotypes.' *New England Journal of Medicine*, **324**, 1280–1281. *(Editorial.)*

Simmonds, H.A., Webster, D.R., Wilson, J., Lingam, S. (1982) 'An X-linked syndrome characterised by hyperuricaemia, deafness and neurodevelopmental abnormalities.' *Lancet*, **2**, 68–70.

—— —— Lingam, S., Wilson, J. (1985) 'An inborn error of purine metabolism, deafness and neurodevelopmental abnormality.' *Neuropediatrics*, **16**, 106–108.

Sorensen, L.B., Benke, P.J. (1967) 'Biochemical evidence for a distinct type of primary gout.' *Nature*, **213**, 1122–1123.

Stoop, J.W., Zegers, B.J.M., Hendricks, G.F.M., Siegenbeek van Heukelom, L.H., Staal, G.E.J., de Bree, P.K., Wadman, S.K., Ballieux, R.E. (1977) 'Purine nucleoside phosphorylase deficiency associated with selective cellular immunodeficiency.' *New England Journal of Medicine*, **296**, 651–655.

Stubbs, E.G., Litt, M., Lis, E., Jackson, R., Voth, W., Lindberg, A., Litt, R. (1982) 'Adenosine deaminase activity decreased in autism.' *Journal of the American Academy of Child Psychiatry*, **21**, 71–74.

Woo, S.L.C. (1988) 'Collation of RFLP haplotypes at the human phenylalanine hydroxylase (PAH) locus.' *American Journal of Human Genetics*, **43**, 781–783.

216

—— Lidsky, A.S., Guttler, F., Chandra, T., Robson, K.J.H. (1983) 'Cloned human phenylalanine hydroxylase gene allows prenatal diagnosis carrier detection of classical phenylketonuria.' *Nature*, **306**, 151–155.

Woody, R.C., Brewster, M.A. (1990) 'Adverse effects of trimethoprim-sulfamethoxazole in a child with dihydropteridine reductase deficiency.' *Developmental Medicine and Child Neurology*, **32**, 639–642.

18
INFECTIOUS DISEASES

In the mental retardation syndromes, both pre- and postnatal infections are known to be responsible for up to 10 per cent of the most severely damaging brain syndromes (Rostafinski 1964). Thus it seems possible that infectious aetiologies may be responsible for autism in some children, particularly those who present with symptoms in the neonatal period and those who develop concomitant severe mental retardation.

One piece of evidence in favour of this possibility is the finding that the incidence of births of children with autism is higher during the months of March and August (Bartlik 1981). The findings of this study, which was conducted in the warm/temperate climate of North Carolina, has since been confirmed by three additional studies in the colder climates of Canada (Konstantareas *et al.* 1986), North Dakota (Burd 1988) and Sweden (Gillberg 1990). The Canadian study showed March and early summer as peak times for births of children with autism, the North Dakota study reported March, July and August to have a higher birth rate for non-speaking children (not limited only to those with autism) and the Swedish study again found an excess of March births in a carefully diagnosed population matched with three sets of controls.

Seasonal variation in autism, if present, could indicate a number of possibilities. The underlying assumption is that some environmental pathogen is operating only during certain periods of the year. This is a pattern compatible with viral infections, which tend to occur in epidemics and often are worse in the winter season. Another possibility is related to nutrition, since maternal food intake can be seasonal and vitamin deficiencies are more likely in winter. (Winter would include part of the second trimester for March babies, the trimester believed to be implicated in many cases of autism.)

To study the possibility of an infectious aetiology in some cases of autism, Deykin and MacMahon (1979) did a retrospective epidemiological study of 163 individuals with autism and 355 unaffected siblings, using parent interviews and medical records. The number of cases for which an infectious aetiology could be established was small, indicating that the viruses studied were unlikely to have played a major role in any substantial proportion of the patients.

However, Deykin and MacMahon did note, in children whom they identifed as 'partially autistic', that there was a statistically significant difference between patients and sibling controls in prenatal maternal exposure to, or clinical illness with, rubella. In the 'fully autistic' children (although they were small in number) there were several findings. There was an increased frequency of combined (rubella

+ mumps) maternal illness/exposure for subjects in comparison to their sibling controls. They also noted that prenatal maternal influenza was four times as common among fully autistic children as among their siblings. In the postnatal period, exposure to mumps (either household exposure or the infant's clinical illness) was seen with increased frequency in fully autistic patients.

In an earlier study by Peterson and Torrey (1976), 78 subjects with autism and their matched controls had cultures collected for the presence of active cytomegalovirus and rubella virus infections. Most of the children were over 3 years of age; the study yielded negative results, which was not unexpected in view of the ages of the patients, since continued excretion of the virus is unusual in later childhood. Other negative results of that study were serum antibody titres for cytomegalovirus, rubella and rubeola viruses as well as serum immunoglobulins IgG, IgM and IgA. Young *et al.* (1977) studied immunoglobulins in the CSF of five children with autism and found no increase.

A further negative result of the Peterson and Torrey study related to the antibody titres for toxoplasmosis. Although six children with autism and two control children were positive, the mothers of all six children with autism were studied and found to be negative, ruling out the possibility of congenital toxoplasmosis infection.

In fact, the most positive finding of the Peterson and Torrey study was that two boys with autism, aged 4 and 8, tested positive for herpes simplex virus (HSV) type 2 antibodies. This type of HSV infection is usually transmitted by genital contact after puberty. In the case of these two patients, the mothers were screened and both were positive, making it possible, though not proven, that these children could have contracted clinical or subclinical HSV encephalitis either *in utero* or even during delivery. In the case of HSV type 1 infection (often responsible for oral lesions), antibodies were positive in 25 per cent of the children with autism compared to 13 per cent of the control children, a finding of unknown relevance.

These general surveys suggested the possibility of infectious aetiologies in a small number of patients but did not establish that brain infections were a major factor in autism. Since there appears to be growing evidence of immunological deficits in patients with autism (Warren *et al.* 1986, Yonk *et al.* 1990; see also Chapter 11), the exact role of CNS infections in this group of patients remains to be defined.

A review of the literature by aetiological agent follows; a summary is given in Table 18.1.

Prenatal infections
Prenatal infections are a difficult area to evaluate. Often the damage done to the fetus bears no relation to the severity of the disease in the mother. There is a most difficult dilemma if a mother becomes infected with a known fetal teratogen while pregnant. An effort to detect these types of damage during gestation has recently moved to a new level of testing. In addition to testing the sera of the mother, ultrasound techniques make it possible for antibodies to be detected in the fetus after the 22nd week of pregnancy when the fetus can make antibodies of its own. The presence of fetal antibodies would indicate that the fetus is infected.

Sometimes a pregnant woman who has no obvious infection at all may still give birth to a child severely damaged by an infection. Because of the immaturity of the brain and its protective systems, fetuses and infants up to 1 year of age are at especial risk for infectious, particularly viral, damage (Sells *et al.* 1975). Understanding of this phenomenon has led to a search for infectious causes of autism by a number of investigators.

Rubella
Rubella is a viral infection that occurs in epidemics. Since the introduction of rubella inoculation programmes (begun in the USA in 1968) these periodic epidemics have been virtually eliminated and the incidence of rubella pathology in children has decreased dramatically. Some countries do not yet have rubella

inoculation, and in such countries prenatal rubella remains in the differential diagnosis of a child with autism. Rimland (1964) was the first to call attention to the relationship of rubella to autism.

In the USA, one of the last documented epidemics occurred in 1964; it was estimated that at least 20,000 children were born damaged as a result of the epidemic. At New York University Medical Center, a rubella birth defect evaluation project was established in which 243 children were studied (Chess *et al.* 1971). 18 of these children were classified as having either full or partial autism. After this epidemic, other centres also reported cases of autism in children with congenital rubella (Desmond *et al.* 1967, Freedman *et al.* 1970, Ornitz *et al.* 1977, Deykin and MacMahon 1979).

Chess (1977) published a follow-up longitudinal study of the children with congenital rubella when they were all 7 years of age. Four *new* cases of autism were identified on follow-up; one child had full and the other three had partial autism. When they were 3 years of age, none of these children had behaved in a manner which fullfilled the criteria for either full or partial autism. Thus, in those rare cases when autistic symptoms develop after 30 months of age, the underlying presence of an infectious agent, such as rubella, needs to be considered in the differential diagnosis.

Most interestingly, Chess reported that of the original 18 cases, six patients had *recovered* and one other had improved regarding autistic symptoms. The children who did not recover or even became worse tended to be the more severely retarded ones. Five out of nine of the children with autism who also had severe or profound deafness were in the group who recovered from autism. In their original monograph, Chess *et al.* (1971) noted that 17 of the original 18 rubella patients with autism had some sensory impairment. However, many of the other children in the study had similar sensory impairments so their presence did not define the group with autism.

In more recent surveys of the aetiologies of autistic symptoms, in an institution for the mentally retarded in Italy (Elia *et al.* 1990) and in a population survey of autism in the state of Utah (Ritvo *et al.* 1990), rubella embryopathy continues to be suspected. It may be regarded as a triumph of modern vaccination programmes that in the Utah autism survey only one child was found with rubella embryopathy. This boy had microphthalmia and an antibody titre of 1:160; he also had three sisters with a diagnosis of autism.

Cytomegalovirus (CMV)
It is less clearly established that CMV infection is an aetiological agent in autism. Not only are there few reported cases in children with autism, but the high frequency of CMV in the population as a whole makes it more difficult to prove causality in any particular case. Between 0.5 and 1 per cent of newborns can be shown to have a congenital CMV infection (Starr *et al.* 1970).

Stubbs (1978) made the first report in the literature of congenital CMV infection in a child with autism and other disabilities. Subsequently at least seven more cases have been mentioned (Markowitz 1983, Ahlfors *et al.* 1984, Stubbs *et al.* 1984, Ivarsson *et al.* 1990, Ritvo *et al.* 1990). One of these cases was detected in a prospective study of congenital CMV infection in which 72 infants were followed for more than three years (Ahlfors *et al.* 1984). In another case there was documentation of the maternal infection which suggested a primary infection shortly before the 20th week of gestation (Ivarsson *et al.* 1990). There has been an attempt to treat one of these children with transfer factor immunotherapy (Stubbs *et al.* 1980). In most of these cases of congenital CMV infection/autism there were also concomitant neurological disorders such as seizures or spasticity.

Herpes simplex virus
Neonatal HSV infection is thought to be present in approximately one out of every 2000 live-born infants (Brown *et al.* 1991). Three boys reported to have congenital herpes (2 definite, 1 possible) were published in the population survey of autism recently performed for the state of Utah (Ritvo *et al.* 1990). One child had psychomotor seizures, another an abnormal EEG. The child with psychomotor seizures had a twin who died at 12 days of age of congenital herpes; he also had a severe hearing loss and scarring of the retina.

The possibility of prenatal infection with HSV type 2 in two children with autism (Torrey and Peterson 1976) has been discussed above.

Other prenatal infections recorded in the literature
There are no other prenatal infections with enough adequate documentation in the literature at this time to establish other infectious aetiologies for autistic syndromes. However, since relatively few patients with autism have received complete medical work-ups, it is premature to rule out any infectious agent at this stage of knowledge.

The cases reported so far include children with autism with evidence of infection by rubeola virus (Deykin and MacMahon 1979), *Treponema pallidum* (syphilis) (Rutter and Bartak 1971, Knobloch and Pasamanick 1975), *Toxoplasma gondii* (Rutter and Bartak 1971), varicella-zoster virus (Knobloch and Pasamanick 1975) and human immunodeficiency virus (Pizzo *et al.* 1991, Schmitt *et al.* 1991).

The term 'prenatal infection' refers to the presumed time of onset of the infection. It is relevant to note that in some cases the infection is known to continue into the postnatal period with the shedding of the viruses for months after birth.

Postnatal infections
Herpes simplex virus
Can an infection after birth cause an autistic syndrome? An important contribution to our understanding of this possibility was made by DeLong *et al.* (1981) in a paper entitled 'Acquired reversible autistic syndrome in acute encephalopathic illness in children.' The authors identified three cases with striking autistic features that had

developed in previously normal children in the course of an acute encephalopathic illness. The clinical presentation was compatible with the involvement of function ascribed to a temporal lobe location. In two of these cases the specific aetiology was not identified and the children eventually made a complete recovery. In the third child, HSV infection was suspected and extensive left temporal lobe necrosis was found on CT scans; a rise in serum titres for HSV was documented.

The interesting fact about these three cases is that a behavioural syndrome was acquired at a clearly definable time in the course of an acute encephalopathic illness in previously normal children and then was reversible. DeLong *et al.* pointed out that the postencephalitic syndrome in these children resembled the Kluver–Bucy syndrome of bilateral medial temporal lobe dysfunction after surgical ablation. They used the term 'autistic syndrome' to describe the behavioural manifestations that developed during this encephalitis even though these children did not meet the early age requirement of such a diagnosis.

Gillberg (1986) has also described a normal child who developed all the classical symptoms of autism at an older age (14 years) in the course of HSV encephalitis. A rise in serum titres for HSV was documented during the acute course of the illness. The autistic-like symptoms became apparent on day 10, and this patient never recovered. Eight years later, a CT scan revealed bilateral widespread destruction of brain parenchyma in the temporal lobes with some medial involvement of the lower portion of the parietal lobes.

These cases of HSV encephalitis are particularly interesting because they meet all the criteria except age for an autistic syndrome. Although the overwhelming number of patients with autism present at very early ages, apparently it is possible for a virtually identical syndrome to present in the course of HSV encephalitis throughout the age groups of childhood. This finding has theoretical implications in that it demonstrates that the early onset criterion does not delineate a syndrome with absolutely specific psychopathology.

Other postnatal infections recorded in the literature
With the exception of HSV, there are very few reports indeed where even the minimum criteria are met that could establish a postnatal infection as aetiological to autistic symptoms.

The only hint is regarding possible causes of the mild/moderate hydrocephalus syndrome seen in one subgroup of patients with autism and the subject of debate among the authors of imaging studies (see Chapter 13). Knobloch and Pasamanick (1975) have described a patient with autism whose hydrocephalus was secondary to bacterial meningitis. *Haemophilus influenzae* meningitis was recently reported in two children with autism (Ritvo *et al.* 1990), and epiglotitis with this agent was reported in an infant who developed autism in the month following infection (Gillberg *et al.* 1990). Deykin and MacMahon (1979), in their epidemiological study of children with autism, described eight who had a postnatal mumps virus infection. This may be of interest because of the literature on animal experimentation which suggests that mumps virus sometimes causes CSF blockage and mild hydrocephalus.

Summary

In summary, evidence in a few patients suggests that infectious agents in the prenatal or postnatal period may be a factor in the development of autism. The most common mechanism appears to be a direct toxic effect on brain cells from the infection (encephalitis). Another possible secondary mechanism may be related to altered pressure relationships within the brain, as are seen in types of hydrocephalus.

It is of interest that, in reports concerning both rubella and HSV infections, cases with late onset are found. An infectious aetiology is a strong contender in the differential diagnosis of autistic symptoms starting after 30 months of age.

REFERENCES

Ahlfors, K., Ivarsson, S.A., Harris, S., Svanberg, L., Holmqvist, R., Lernmark, B., Theander, G. (1984) 'Congenital cytomegalovirus infection and disease in Sweden and the relative importance of primary and secondary infections.' *Scandinavian Journal of Infectious Diseases*, **16**, 129–137.

Bartlik, B.D. (1981) 'Monthly variation in births of autistic children in North America.' *Journal of the American Medical Women's Association*, **36**, 363–368.

Brown, Z.A., Benedetti, J., Ashley, R., Burchett, S., Selke, S., Berry, S., Vontver, L.A., Corey, L. (1991) 'Neonatal herpes simplex infection in relation to asymptomatic maternal infection at the time of labor.' *New England Journal of Medicine*, **324**, 1247–1252.

Burd, L. (1988) 'Month of birth of non-speaking children.' *Developmental Medicine and Child Neurology*, **30**, 685–686. *(Letter.)*

Chess, S. (1977) 'Follow-up report on autism in congenital rubella.' *Journal of Autism and Childhood Schizophrenia*, **7**, 68–81.

—— Korn, S.J., Fernandez, P.B. (1971) *Psychiatric Disorders of Children with Congenital Rubella*. New York: Brunner/Mazel.

DeLong, G.R., Bean, S.C., Brown, F.R. (1981) 'Acquired reversible autistic syndrome in acute encephalopathic illness in children.' *Archives of Neurology*, **38**, 191–194.

Desmond, M.M., Wilson, G.S., Melnick, J.L., Singer, D.B., Zion, T.E., Rudolph, A.J., Pineda, R.G., Ziai, M.H., Blattney, R.J. (1967) 'Congenital rubella encephalitis.' *Journal of Pediatrics*, **71**, 311–331.

Deykin, E.Y., MacMahon, G. (1979) 'Viral exposure and autism.' *American Journal of Epidemiology*, **109**, 628–638.

Elia, M., Bergonzi, P., Ferri, R., Musumeci, S.A., Paladino, A., Panerai, S., Ragusa, R.M. (1990) 'The etiology of autism in a group of mentally retarded subjects.' *Brain Dysfunction*, **3**, 228–240.

Freedman, D.A., Fox-Kolenda, B.J., Brown, S.L. (1970) 'A multihandicapped rubella baby: the first 18 months.' *Journal of the American Academy of Child Psychiatry*, **9**, 298–317.

Gillberg, C. (1986) 'Brief report: onset at age 14 of a typical autistic syndrome. A case report of a girl with herpes simplex encephalitis.' *Journal of Autism and Developmental Disorders*, **16**, 369–375.

—— (1990) 'Do children with autism have March birthdays?' *Acta Psychiatrica Scandinavica*, **82**, 152–156.

—— Ehlers, S., Schaumann, H., Jakobsson, G., Dahlgren, S.O., Lindblom, R., Bågenholm, A., Tjuus, T., Blidner, E. (1990) 'Autism under age 3 years: a clinical study of 28 cases referred for autistic symptoms in infancy.' *Journal of Child Psychology and Psychiatry*, **31**, 921–934.

Gillberg, I.C. (1991) 'Autistic syndrome with onset at age 31 years. Herpes encephalitis as one possible model for childhood autism.' *Developmental Medicine and Child Neurology*, **33**, 920–924.

Ivarsson, S.A., Bjerre, I., Vegfors, P., Ahlfors, K. (1990) 'Autism as one of several disabilities in two children with congenital cytomegalovirus infection.' *Neuropediatrics*, **21**, 102–103.

Knobloch, H., Pasamanick, B. (1975) 'Some etiologic and prognostic factors in early infantile autism and psychosis.' *Journal of Pediatrics*, **55**, 182–191.

Konstantareas, M.W., Hauser, P., Lennox, C., Homatidis, S. (1986) 'Season of birth in infantile autism.' *Child Psychiatry and Human Development*, **17**, 53–65.

Markowitz, P.I. (1983) 'Autism in a child with congenital cytomegalovirus infection.' *Journal of Autism and Developmental Disorders*, **13**, 249–253.

Ornitz, E.M. Guthrie, D., Farley, A.H. (1977) 'The early development of autistic children.' *Journal of Autism and Childhood Schizophrenia*, **3**, 207–229.

Peterson, M.R., Torrey, E.F. (1976) 'Viruses and other infectious agents as behavioural teratogens.' *In:* Coleman, M. (Ed.) *The Autistic Syndromes*. Amsterdam: North-Holland; New York: Elsevier, pp. 23–42.

Pizzo, R.G., Albizzati, A., Cervini, R., Grioni, A., Musetti, L., Saccani, M., Rossetti, M., Guareschi, A., Cazzullo, A. (1991) 'Autistic symptoms in 5 sero-reverted HIV+ children.' *Brain Dysfunction.* *(In press.)*

Rimland, B. (1964) *Infantile Autism*. Englewood Cliffs, NJ: Prentice-Hall.

Ritvo, E.R., Mason-Brothers, A., Freeman, B.J., Pingree, C., Jenson, W.R., McMahon, W.M., Petersen, P.B., Jorde, L.B., Mo, A., Ritvo, A. (1990) 'The UCLA–University of Utah epidemiologic survey of autism: the etiologic role of rare diseases.' *American Journal of Psychiatry*, **147**, 1614–1621.

Rostafinski, M.J. (1964) 'The incidence of preventable forms of brain damage.' *Virginia Medical Monthly*, **91**, 22–26.

Rutter, M., Bartak, L. (1971) 'Causes of infantile autism: some considerations from recent research.' *Journal of Autism and Childhood Schizophrenia*, **1**, 20–32.

Schmitt, B., Seeger, J., Kreuz, W., Eneukel, S., Jacobi, G. (1991) 'Central nervous system involvement of children with HIV infection.' *Developmental Medicine and Child Neurology*, **33**, 535–540.

Sells, C.J., Levy, H.L., Mount, F.W. (1975) 'Sequelae of central nervous system enterovirus infections.' *New England Journal of Medicine*, **293**, 1–4.

Starr, J.G., Bart, R.D., Gold, E. (1970) 'Inapparent congenital cytomegalovirus infection: clinical and epidemiologic characteristics in early infancy.' *New England Journal of Medicine*, **282**, 1075–1078.

Stubbs, E.G. (1978) 'Autistic symptoms in a child with congenital cytomegalovirus infection.' *Journal of Autism and Childhood Schizophrenia*, **8**, 37–43.

—— Budden, S.S., Burger, D.R., Vanderbark, A.A. (1980) 'Transfer factor immunotherapy of an autistic child with congenital cytomegalovirus.' *Journal of Autism and Developmental Disorders*, **10**, 451–458.

—— Ash, E., Williams, C.P.S. (1984) 'Autism and congenital cytomegalovirus.' *Journal of Autism and Developmental Disorders*, **14**, 183–189.

Warren, R.P., Margaretten, N.C., Pace, N.C., Foster, A. (1986) 'Immune abnormalities in patients with autism.' *Journal of Autism and Developmental Disorders*, **16**, 189–197.

Yonk, L.J., Warren, R.P., Burger, R.A., Cole, P., Odell, J.D., Warren, W.L., White, E., Singh, V.K. (1990) 'CD4+ helper T cell depression in autism.' *Immunology Letters*, **25**, 341–346.

Young, J.G., Caparulo, B.K., Shaywitz, B.A., Johnson, W.T., Cohen, D.J. (1977) 'Childhood autism: cerebrospinal fluid examination and immunoglobulin levels.' *Journal of the American Academy of Child Psychiatry*, **16**, 174–179.

19
STRUCTURAL ENTITIES

As imaging technology improves, more and more evidence is developing regarding the source of the structural abnormalities in subgroups of patients with autism (see Chapter 13). Those found to date appear to be mostly congenital malformations of one type or another; the only exceptions to this observation are benign tumours and hydrocephalus secondary to postnatal cerebral infections.

Cortical malformations
Using CT imaging, a few obvious lesions have been reported in the CNS of patients with autism. A large left parietal/occipital porencephaly, a right frontal poren-cephaly connecting to the ventricular system, and a loss of substance in the area of the right lateral geniculate have been recorded in children with autism (Coleman and Gillberg 1985). Whether these lesions are secondary to perinatal trauma or developmental malformations is difficult to establish by the level of CT definition of the lesions.

Magnetic resonance imaging (MRI) may have an advantage over CT in that it appears to be more successful in detecting more subtle congenital malformations which result from a defect in the migration of neurons to cortical layers during the first six months of gestation, a period of major cell migration. (Technically, MRI can scan with precision at many more levels because there is no fear of excessive radiation; it has excellent multiplanar capability and high resolution.)

Regarding developmental cortical malformations, Ritvo et al. (1986) were the first to note polymicrogyria on autopsy of an individual with autism, a finding also recorded by Kemper (1988). Berthier et al. (1990) were studying Asperger syndrome with MRI techniques and were surprised to find polymicrogyria in two patients.

These findings led to a study of MRI scans rated for the presence or absence of cerebral cortical malformations in 13 high-functioning male subjects with autism compared to age-, sex- and IQ-matched controls (Piven et al. 1990). Seven of these individuals were found to have cortical malformations. Five had poly-microgyria, one had schizencephaly and macrogyria, and one had macrogyria. Perhaps because they were high-functioning individuals, at the time these results seemed astonishing.

In the mental retardation literature, neuronal migration abnormalities are usually associated with low-functioning individuals. However, there is great vari-ation in the clinical results of these neuronal migration defects, and the severity of the malformation as graded by the MRI may not be correlated with the severity of the clinical disease (Barkovitch *et al*. 1987). For example, severe lissencephaly is one of the most serious types of neuronal migration abnormality; it often can best be characterized as neuronal migration arrest, yet patients have been described who appear to be only mildly affected (Barkovitch *et al*. 1991).

These cortical abnormalities are not specific to autism and are reported in a number of other syndromes. Genetic diseases, infections during gestation and autoimmune disorders have been implicated in the origin of these defects (see Chapters 11, 16, 17 and 18).

The cortical malformations in the study by Piven *et al*. (1990) were not confined to any particular lobe and were detected at the same rate in both hemispheres. The failure of the lesions to coincide topographically suggests that it is unlikely that they have a direct role in the pathogenesis of autism, but rather that in the subgroup of individuals with autism with these findings, they are linked to the underlying aetiology and timing of the disorder.

The first MRI study of patients with autism (Gaffney and Tsai 1987) disclosed a left occipital heterotopia of grey matter, another neuronal migration type of defect, in a high-functioning individual. If these findings of cortical malformations are confirmed and enlarged with future MRI studies in patients with autism, there may be some reinterpretation of past findings. For example, what is temporal lobe atrophy to one observer (Jones and Kerwin 1990) may be a neuronal migration defect known as 'open operculum' to another (Piven *et al*. 1991).

Neuronal migration occurs before the 6th month of gestation. Identification of these abnormalities of neuronal migration can be useful regarding the timing of the insult to the CNS. These MRI studies give additional weight to the concept of autism as a second trimester syndrome, at least in some of the patients, as has been suggested by second trimester maternal bleeding and other clues (see Chapter 26).

Cysts

Only a few patients with autism have been described with cystic lesions in the CNS. Knobloch and Pasamanick (1975) reported a case of hydrocephalus secondary to a papilloma of the choroid plexus in a child with autism. Six cases have also been described of individuals with autisic symptoms and a middle fossa arachnoid cyst pressing on structures at the tip of the temporal lobe (Segawa *et al*. 1986). These patients all met DSM-III criteria for autism and all had abnormalities in the sleep–wakefulness cycle. In one case, clinical improvement was noted after a cyst–peritoneal shunt. One of the present authors (M.C.) also had a patient with a middle fossa arachnoid cyst which was detected by MRI after a CT scan failed to reveal any abnormalities.

Occult, mild and moderate hydrocephalus

One of the first cases of autism evaluated from a neurological point of view was in a child who was found to have arrested hydrocephalus (Schain and Yannet 1960). A number of other cases have since been added to the literature (Knobloch and

Pasamanick 1975, Damasio *et al.* 1980, Garreau *et al.* 1984, Coleman and Gillberg 1985). In some cases, the aetiology of the hydrocephalus is known—*e.g.*, secondary to meningitis or to the Dandy–Walker syndrome (Knobloch and Pasamanick 1975)—but often the mechanism leading to the increased intracranial pressure is not established. The only factor that occurs with any consistency is that the cases tend to be of the less severe type in the spectrum of hydrocephalus syndromes.

In summary, imaging techniques and autopsy studies are beginning to disclose that a number of patients with autism have structural abnormalities in the brain. This finding includes a number of high-functioning patients. Thus, it might be useful for any patient with autistic symptoms, of any level of intellectual functioning, to have an imaging study as part of the initial work-up.

REFERENCES

Barkovich, A.J., Chuang, S.H., Norman, D. (1987) 'MR of neuronal migration anomalies.' *American Journal of Roentgenology*, **150**, 179–187.
—— Koch, T.K., Carrol, C.L. (1991) 'The spectrum of lissencephaly: report of ten patients analyzed by magnetic resonance imaging.' *Annals of Neurology*, **30**, 139–146.
Berthier, M.L., Starkstein, S.E., Leiguarda, R. (1990) 'Developmental anomalies in Asperger's syndrome: neuroradiological findings in two patients.' *Journal of Neuropsychiatry*, **2**, 197–201.
Coleman, M., Gillberg, C. (1985) *The Biology of the Autistic Syndromes*. New York: Praeger.
Damasio, H., Maurer, R.G., Damasio, A.R., Chui, H.C. (1980) 'Computerized tomographic scan findings in patients with autistic behavior.' *Archives of Neurology*, **37**, 505–510.
Gaffney, G., Tsai, L. (1987) 'Brief report: Magnetic resonance imaging of high-level autism.' *Journal of Autism and Developmental Disorders*, **17**, 433–438.
Garreau, B., Barthélémy, C., Sauvage, D., Leddet, I., LeLord, G. (1984) 'A comparison of autistic syndromes with and without associated neurological problems.' *Journal of Autism and Developmental Disorders*, **14**, 105–111.
Jones, P.B., Kerwin, R.W. (1990) 'Left temporal lobe damage in Asperger's syndrome.' *British Journal of Psychiatry*, **156**, 570–572.
Kemper, T.L. (1988) 'Neuroanatomic studies of dyslexia and autism.' *In:* Swann, J.W., Messer, A. (Eds) *Disorders of the Developing Nervous System: Changing Views on their Origins, Diagnosis, and Treatments*. New York: Alan R. Liss.
Knobloch, H., Pasamanick, B. (1975) 'Some etiologic and prognostic factors in early infantile autism and psychosis.' *Journal of Pediatrics*, **55**, 182–191.
Piven, J., Berthier, M.L., Starkstein, S.E., Nehme, E., Pearlson, G., Folstein, S. (1990) 'Magnetic resonance imaging evidence for a defect of cerebral cortical development in autism.' *American Journal of Psychiatry*, **147**, 734–739.
—— Starkstein, S., Berthier, M.L. (1991) 'Temporal lobe atrophy versus open operculum in Asperger's syndrome.' *British Journal of Psychiatry*, 457–458. *(Letter.)*
Ritvo, E.R., Freeman, B.J., Scheibel, A.B., Duong, T., Robinson, H., Guthrie, D., Ritvo, A. (1986) 'Lower Purkinje cell counts in the cerebella of four autistic subjects: initial findings of the UCLA-NSAC Autopsy Research Report.' *American Journal of Psychiatry*, **143**, 862–866.
Schain, R., Yannet, H. (1960) 'Infantile autism: an analysis of 50 cases and a consideration of certain neuropsychological concepts.' *Journal of Pediatrics*, **57**, 560–567.
Segawa, M., Nomura, Y., Nagata, E., Hata, K., Saitoh, S. (1986) 'Autism with middle fossa arachnoid cyst.' *Journal of Child Neurology*, **1**, 276.

20

OTHER ESTABLISHED SYNDROMES REPORTED IN PATIENTS WITH AUTISM

Patients with autistic symptoms are reported from time to time who are found to have other established syndromes. In this chapter, syndromes are included if two criteria are met: (1) the syndrome is not otherwise described in this textbook under chapters describing, for instance, the chromosomal, metabolic or infectious connections to autism; (2) two or more patients with the syndrome have been diagnosed with either idiopathic (Kanner, infantile) autism or autistic-like symptoms.

Cornelia deLange syndrome

Knobloch and Pasamanick (1975) reported that a child with the deLange syndrome met the criteria for autism. One of the present authors (C.G.) also has a child with both autism and the deLange syndrome in his practice.

Fetal alcohol syndrome

Children with fetal alcohol syndrome have been included in the Hauser *et al.* (1975) report of pneumoencephalograms in a series of patients with autism and in a report by Elia *et al.* (1991) of institutionalized persons with autism. Unfortunately, the fetal alcohol syndrome is such a common syndrome that the description of a patient with a second syndrome, such as autism, could be due to chance occurrence.

Hypomelanosis of Ito

A considerable number of children with hypomelanosis of Ito (incontinentia pigmenti achromians) and autism or autistic-like features have been described in the literature. Two of these patients were originally referred to a specialist in autism with the tentative diagnosis of infantile autism by the local physician (Åkefeldt and Gillberg 1991). One child (just) fulfilled criteria for autistic disorder (DSM-III-R) at age 3 to 5 years, and the other clearly fitted the clinical picture described by Asperger (1944) and fulfilled the criteria for Asperger syndrome of Gillberg and Gillberg (1989). In these cases, detailed medical work-up by a specialist revealed the underlying syndrome of hypomelanosis of Ito. In two further children hypomelanosis of Ito had already been diagnosed at the time when autistic symptoms were evaluated—a girl with an 'autistic-like condition' with five of the six criteria for Asperger syndrome (Åkefeldt and Gillberg 1991), and a microcephalic girl with stereotypies of an 'autistic nature' (Griebel *et al.* 1989). Recently,

Zappella (1992) has identified hypomelanosis of Ito in more than 20 young patients with autistic behaviour in a child neuropsychiatry clinic in Siena, Italy.

Hypomelanosis of Ito can be suspected in a child with autism if there are hypomelanotic areas on the skin (see Fig. 25.1, p. 298). These skin changes consist of hypopigmented, sharply circumscribed spots or streaks, sometimes in whorl-like shapes or clustering in bizarre patterns anywhere on the body. The skin changes persist throughout childhood, but are said to be less clearly conspicuous in adults. The hypomelanotic areas are best seen under a Wood's lamp.

The CNS is involved in about half of the cases. Mental retardation and early-onset epilepsy seem to be fairly common features. There does not seem to be a correlation between the amount of affected skin and the severity of brain dysfunction (Ardinger and Bell 1986). Other parts of the body involved in hypomelanosis of Ito include the skeleton (in particular, scoliosis, unequal bone length and malformation of facial bones) and the eye (corneal opacities and choroidal atrophy).

The aetiology of hypomelanosis of Ito is not known. Chromosomal irregularities (mosaicisms in cultured fibroblasts and to a lesser extent leukocytes as well as translocations) have been reported. In the case of the patients with autistic symptoms, one girl had a mosaicism (45,X/46,XX) in 4 per cent of examined cells and a second child (a boy) had a mostly normal karyotype with a potpourri of single cells each with an unusual variant—an 8q– marker, loss of chromosome 8, loss of chromosome 18, loss of chromosome 19 and loss of the Y chromosome (Åkefeldt and Gillberg 1991). MRI studies of this boy also showed evidence of tissue damage above and adjacent to the lateral ventricles, a finding said to be common in hypomelanosis of Ito.

In the one study available, the prevalence of hypomelanosis of Ito cases in a population of individuals with autism was tentatively reported as 0.5 per cent (Åkefeldt and Gillberg 1991). The disorder is one of three neuroectodermal syndromes to date where some of the patients have been found to have autistic features (the others—neurobfibromatosis and tuberous sclerosis—are discussed later in this chapter), and it is therefore recommended that a meticulous examination of the epidermis, preferably by Wood's lamp, should become a standard part of the work-up of any patient presenting with autistic symptoms.

Joubert syndrome

The Joubert syndrome is an autosomal recessive disorder characterized by partial or complete agenesis of the cerebellar vermis and episodic tachypnoea alternating with prolonged apnoea (Joubert et al. 1969). Mental retardation, ataxia, abnormal eye movements, tongue protrusion and hypotonia are standard features. Two patients with Joubert syndrome have been described with autistic features (Holroyd et al. 1991), one of whom met DSM-III-R diagnostic criteria for autistic disorder.

It is interesting that both these individuals appeared to be functioning at a much better developmental level than almost all other patients with this syndrome, in which the mental retardation is usually characterized as severe or profound (Casaer *et al.* 1985). They had full scale IQs of 64 and 85, and much of the developmental delay in both children related to motor and expressive language rather than global cognitive disability.

This report is of particular interest because of the finding of cerebellar vermis abnormalities in some patients with idiopathic autism (see Chapter 13). Further study of individuals with Joubert syndrome is needed, with particular attention to associations between neuroanatomical and clinical behaviour patterns.

Lujan–Fryns syndrome
A type of X-linked mental retardation has been described by Lujan *et al.* (1984) and Fryns and Buttiens (1987) in males with a marfanoid habitus, craniofacial changes, hypernasal voice and hyperactive behaviour. Two individuals with this diagnosis have been described as autistic (Gurrieri and Neri 1991).

Moebius syndrome (congenital facial diplegia)
Congenital non-progressive bilateral facial diplegia, especially of cranial nerves VI and VII, combined with external ophthalmoplegia is a rare neurological syndrome described by Moebius as early as 1888. There are now a number of patients reported in the literature who have Moebius syndrome and autistic symptoms (Ornitz *et al.* 1977, Gillberg and Winnergard 1984). In a recent evaluation of 17 children and young adults with Moebius syndrome, Gillberg and Steffenburg (1989) discovered that seven showed all or many symptoms typical of an autistic syndrome. Both of the present authors have such a patient in their practice. Considering the rarity of this brain damage syndrome, it is possible that the concurrence with autism is more than coincidence.

Moebius syndrome is currently classified into four types based on clinical and autopsy results. Three of these types (interruption of the cranial nuclei *in utero*, aplastic or hypoplastic cranial nuclei, and destruction or necrosis of cranial nuclei) involve the brainstem directly—an area of the CNS also postulated to be affected in some cases of autism (see Chapter 24). The fourth type of Moebius syndrome (primary myopathic changes in the musculature of the face) should be considered in a separate category of disease (Sudershan and Goldie 1985). In patients who display both syndromes, it is tempting to suggest that the basic dysfunction of these children, both neurological and psychiatric, is associated with a common underlying defect at the brainstem level.

Neurofibromatosis
Neurofibromatosis is another disorder where some of the patients have been described with autistic symptoms (Fig. 20.1). Like tuberous sclerosis, this disease entity is classified as a phakomatosis—a group of disorders characterized by their dysplastic nature and proclivity to tumour formation in the CNS, skin and viscera.

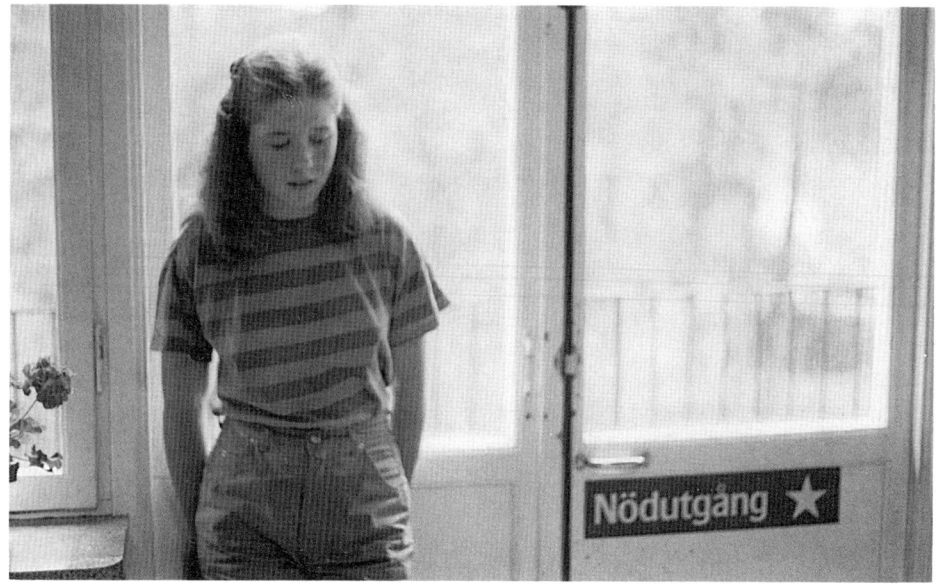

Fig. 20.1. 13-year-old girl with autism, mild to moderate mental retardation and extreme echolalia; at age 10 years, neurofibromatosis diagnosed and benign focal epilepsy begins.

The protean manifestations of neurofibromatosis make it a diagnostic challenge to clinicians; now symptoms of autism have been added to a long list of presenting problems in this patient group.

Cutaneous changes include café-au-lait spots, molluscum fibromas, hypo-pigmented spots (best seen with a Wood's lamp) or diffuse areas of pigmentation. Although hyperpigmented patches may be seen at birth, they usually appear later in the first decade and their number and degree of pigmentation is increased by adolescence. The characteristic lesion is the café-au-lait spot, an irregular hyperpigmented patch that varies in size from a few millimeters to many centimeters and tends to have a generalized distribution; any person with six or more café-au-lait spots measuring 1.5cm or more in diameter has a presumptive diagnosis of neurofibromatosis (Crowe *et al.* 1956). Neurofibromata and optic gliomas can be found. Another useful diagnostic aid is axillary or inguinal freckling. Mental retardation occurs in 10 to 20 per cent of cases. All neurofibromatosis patients with autistic symptoms in the literature or known to the authors of this book have been retarded. Lisch nodules (tiny melanocytic hamartomas projecting from the surface of the iris) appear to be of diagnostic value in differentiating the type 1 form of neurofibromatosis (Lubs *et al.* 1991).

Two major types of neurofibromatosis have now been distinguished by molecular cloning techniques (National Institutes of Health Consensus Development Conference 1988). The most common, neurofibromatosis type 1 (NF-1), can

232

be a genetic disorder due to autosomal dominant genetic mutations with 100 per cent penetrance; in one study there was complete penetrance documented by the age of 5 years in each patient (Huson *et al.* 1989). Chance mutations also account for many cases. The locus is on the long arm of chromosome 17 (the q11.2 area of the chromosome) and the gene is large, variously estimated at between 200 and 300kb in length encoding a protein of at least 2485 amino acids (Cawthon *et al.* 1990). Direct DNA diagnosis should become available in the near future, but because of the size of the gene many different mutations will probably be identified. A variety of types of mutational events can lead to expression of the NF-1 phenotype, including chromosome translocations, insertions, deletions and point mutations (Riccardi 1991). The population prevalence of NF-1 is around 1:3500 (Riccardi and Eichner 1986).

In the case of neurofibromatosis type 2 (NF-2), at present it is known that these patients do not carry the 17q11.2 mutation found in NF-1 but may have a gene for NF-2 on chromosome 22 (Rouleau *et al.* 1987). The cardinal feature of this condition is the development of bilateral acoustic neuromas in 96 per cent of cases. NF-2 patients also have fewer café-au-lait spots than are found in NF-1 (Huson and Thrush 1985). The exact incidence of NF-2 is unknown but is low, perhaps of the order of 0.2 per 100,000 (Clarke *et al.* 1990).

In reviewing series of patients with neurofibromatosis, children have been described who were 'exceedingly disturbed' (Crowe *et al.* 1956, Riccardi and Eichner 1986). The majority of children with neurofibromatosis display impulsivity and social imperception (Eliason 1988). However, neurofibromatosis was first specifically described in association with autism by the Swedish authors Gillberg and Forsell (1984) who published case reports of three children with autism or autistic-like conditions (two of whom were classic cases of Kanner autism) from a total population study of 51 cases. It is relevant to note that none of these children were diagnosed as having neurofibromatosis in infancy. The psychiatric symptoms had been present for many years before the underlying diagnosis of neurofibromatosis was made.

To date there are no other systematic studies corroborating the findings of the Swedish group, but in clinical studies the simultaneous appearance of the two disorders has been reported. Gaffney *et al.* (1988) reported on two patients selected for an MRI study of autism who were incidentally noted to have café-au-lait spots which led to later diagnosis of neurofibromatosis. A girl with autism and neurofibromatosis has been reported whose otherwise normal father also had neurofibromatosis (Steffenburg 1991). Clinical experience of one of the present authors (M.C.) also suggests that the concurrence of autism and neurofibromatosis is more common than would be expected by chance.

What is now needed are individual case studies to determine which of the types of neurofibromatosis (?or both) present with autistic symptoms. This will help hone the diagnostic skills of examiners of children with autism, since the two types have somewhat different clinical manifestations. In the meantime, meticulous examination of the skin of each patient presenting with autism, preferably with the help of a Wood's lamp, is warranted to rule out one of the neuroepidermal disorders in this patient group. In the case of neurofibromatosis, detailed ophthalmological examination is also a must.

Rett syndrome

Although autism is more common among boys, when autistic symptoms are seen in girls, Rett syndrome should be included in the differential diagnosis (Kerr and Stephenson 1985). Before Rett syndrome was well known, these girls were usually diagnosed as having 'early infantile autism' or 'disintegrative childhood psychosis'.

Working in Vienna, Andreas Rett (1966, 1968, 1977) published the first descriptions of a syndrome of cerebral atrophy in girls characterized by autistic behaviour and dementia, sterotypical use of the hands, apraxia of gait and loss of facial expression. Unaware of Rett's papers, investigators from other countries—Ishikawa *et al.* (1978) in Japan and Hagberg (1980) in Sweden—reported a similar clinical pattern found in girls. General awareness of the syndrome in the international medical community occurred after a combined report of 35 cases from several countries was published in an English-language journal (Hagberg *et al.* 1983). The incidence is estimated to be somewhere around 1:12,000 to 1:15,000 live female births (Kerr and Stephenson 1986, Witt-Engerström and Gillberg 1987). In 1990, the International Rett Syndrome Association, a parent/professional body, had registered 1420 cases worldwide.

Although autism is often the initial diagnosis in girls with Rett syndrome, there are a number of clinical details that help suggest the diagnosis of Rett syndrome (Olsson and Rett 1987, Gillberg 1989, Nomura and Segawa 1990). The ability to organize purposeful activities is lost (true apraxia) in girls with Rett syndrome, and hand wringing/washing/tapping and hand-to-mouth movements evolve with age as stereotypies that accompany the loss of purposeful hand function. Table 20.1 compares diagnostic criteria for Rett syndrome and infantile autism (Trevathan and Naidu 1988). It is confusing because many of the girls go through an autistic phase which can end as early as 4 years or persist into the 7 to 8 year age group (Olsson and Rett 1990). A further confusion is added by the appearance in the literature of a very occasional case of apparent Rett syndrome described in a boy (Coleman 1990, Topcu *et al.* 1991).

The Rett Syndrome Diagnostic Criteria Work Group (1988) has established a basis for the exact diagnosis of Rett syndrome using necessary, supportive and exclusion criteria (Table 20.2). The diagnosis is made by clinical symptoms alone, because to date no biological marker has been identified. Until the exact underlying aetiology of Rett syndrome is known and each patient can be tested for it, it will not be clear if this is a single syndrome or one that has a heterogeneous origin.

One of the most striking aspects of the syndrome is that grasping and other purposeful hand movements usually disappear by the age of 3 years and are replaced by characteristic stereotypic hand rubbing movements in front of the

234

TABLE 20.1

Comparison of Rett syndrome and infantile autism*

Rett syndrome	Infantile autism
1. Normal development to 6-18 months	1. Onset from early infancy
2. Progressive loss of speech and hand function	2. Loss of previously acquired skills does not occur
3. Profound mental retardation in all functional areas	3. More scatter of intellectual function. Visuospatial and manipulative skills often better than apparent verbal skills
4. Acquired microcephaly, growth retardation, decreased weight gain	4. Physical development normal in the majority
5. Stereotypic hand movements always present	5. Stereotypic behaviour is more varied in manifestation and is always more complex; midline manifestations rare
6. Progresive gait difficulties, with gait and truncal apraxia and ataxia; some may become non-ambulatory	6. Gait and other gross motor functions normal in first decade of life
7. Language always absent	7. Language sometimes absent; if present, peculiar speech patterns always present; markedly impaired non-verbal communication
8. Eye contact present, sometimes very intense	8. Eye contact with others typically avoided or inappropriate
9. Little interest in manipulating objects	9. Stereotypic ritualistic behaviour usually involves skilful but odd manipulation of objects or sensory self-stimulation
10. Seizures in at least 70% in early childhood (various seizure types)	10. Seizures (usually temporal–limbic complex partial) in 25% in late adolescence and adulthood
11. Bruxism, hyperventilation with air-swallowing and breath-holding common	11. Bruxism, hyperventilation and breath-holding not typical
12. Choreoathetoid movements and dystonia may be present	12. Dystonia and chorea not present†

*Reproduced by permission from Trevathan and Naidu (1988).
†Extrapyramidal signs may appear in some patients with autism after puberty.

mouth or chest. (These movements, however, are not exclusively seen in Rett syndrome patients, and the diagnosis must be made by full evaluation.)

The girls have apparently normal physical and mental development until sometime between the ages of 5 to 24 months. Although prodromal signs and symptoms are sometimes observed that indicate a process occurring already during the first months of life, there are no predictable manifestations of this disorder before deterioration sets in (Witt Engerström 1990). Some time during the first or second year of life, the girls enter Stage I of a four-stage progression; diagnostic characteristics of these stages wre developed by Hagberg and Witt Engerström (1986). Table 20.3 shows the clinical characteristics and differential diagnoses by these stages. Based on further experience, Witt Engerström (1990) suggested the creation of different pathways in the last two stages. Stage III is reserved for

TABLE 20.2
Diagnostic criteria for Rett syndrome*

Necessary criteria
1. Apparently normal prenatal and perinatal period
2. Apparently normal psychomotor development through first 6 months†
3. Normal head circumference at birth
4. Deceleration of head growth between ages 5 months and 4 years
5. Loss of acquired purposeful hand skills between ages 6 and 30 months, temporally associated with communication dysfunction and social withdrawal
6. Development of severely impaired expressive and receptive language, and presence of apparent severe psychomotor retardation
7. Stereotypic hand movements such as hand wringing/squeezing, clapping/tapping, mouthing, and 'washing'/rubbing automatisms appearing after purposeful hand skills are lost
8. Appearance of gait apraxia and truncal apraxia–ataxia between ages 1 and 4 years
9. Diagnosis tentative until 2 to 5 years of age

Supportive criteria
1. Breathing dysfunction
   a. Periodic apnoea during wakefulness
   b. Intermittent hyperventilation
   c. Breath-holding spells
   d. Forced expulsion of air or saliva
2. EEG abnormalities
   a. Slow waking background and intermittent rhythmic slowing (3–5Hz)
   b. Epileptiform discharges, with or without clinical seizures
3. Seizures
4. Spasticity often with associated development of muscle wasting and dystonia
5. Peripheral vasomotor disturbances
6. Scoliosis
7. Growth retardation
8. Hypotrophic small feet

Exclusion criteria
1. Evidence of intrauterine growth retardation
2. Organomegaly, or other signs of storage disease
3. Retinopathy or optic atrophy
4. Microcephaly at birth
5. Evidence of perinatally acquired brain damage
6. Existence of identifiable metabolic or other progressive neurological disorder
7. Acquired neurological disorders resulting from severe infections or head trauma

---

*Reproduced by permission from Trevathan and Naidu (1988).
†Development may appear normal until 18 months of age.

ambulatory girls who stay in the stage until they lose ambulation (Stage IV-A). Another path, called Stage III-IV, has been created for non-ambulatory girls, leading to Stage IV-B if they are not walking by 10 years of age (Fig. 20.2).

The disorder results in severe/profound levels of mental retardation (Perry *et al.* 1991). 68 per cent of patients eventually develop scoliosis, with a period of accelerated progression during the early teenage years, and eventually one-third lose ambulation skills (Coleman *et al.* 1988). In adults, there appears to be no further mental deterioration and less prominant seizures and breath holding.

Medical work-up of these girls is still in the research stage. Intermittent mild elevation of lactate, and to a greater extent pyruvate levels in blood and CSF, have been reported (Haas and Rice 1985, Budden *et al.* 1990). An MRI study on eight girls and eight age-matched controls revealed significant differences in the area and shape of the whole hemisphere (suggesting the hemispheres were dysplastic as the result of a diffuse process) and the caudate nuclei (Casanova *et al.* 1989). The left caudate in these children was distorted; this finding confirms the involvement of the striatum in this disease entity.

A number of apparently non-specific findings—also seen in other diseases of the CNS—have been reported. These include low CSF levels of the neurotransmitters dopamine, norepinephrine and serotonin, with elevated levels of tetrahydrobiopterin (Zoghbi *et al.* 1989). (Undernutrition—often seen in Rett syndrome—can be a factor in low levels of biogenic amines.) A selective loss of myelin-associated lipids and changes in gangliosides were demonstrated in the temporal white matter of five patients (Lekman *et al.* 1991).

PET studies of six patients showed that cerebral blood flow and oxygen metabolism were abnormal and that the cerebral metabolic rate of oxygen and oxygen extraction fraction were low (Yoshikawa *et al.* 1991). Impaired oxidative metabolism was suggested by this study. The mitochondria of the muscle (where the respiratory chain is located in a cell) have been found to be abnormally shaped with membrane changes and abnormal vacuoles suggesting mitochondrial energy dysfunction (Eeg-Olofsson *et al.* 1988, Ruch *et al.* 1989). Other researchers find that the mitochondria appear normal yet still contain mitochondrial enzyme deficiencies (Coker and Melnyk 1991). However, Federico *et al.* (1991), who also report the presence of swollen mitochondria and a decrease of activity of respiratory enzymes in isolated mitochondria, were unable to find any major deletions of mitochondrial DNA by southern blot analysis.

The genetics of the syndrome are yet to be fully worked out. Most cases appear to be sporadic: this is compatible with a mitochondrial disease. Another suggestion is that some families may have an X-linked dominant mutation lethal in males, but the gene responsible for the syndrome has yet to be identified (Ferlini *et al.* 1990). There is research underway evaluating the possibility of non-random X chromosome inactivation. Other hypotheses include an autosomal dominant pattern, a two-step mutation approach, and a search for uniparental disomy.

Less than 1 per cent of reported cases appear to be familial (Zoghbi *et al.* 1990). One woman with Rett syndrome has given birth after a 35-week gestation to a girl who appeared normal and well nourished at birth. After some possible prodromal signs in the first year, the child began a definite regression at 15 to 16 months of age (Witt Engerström, personal communication).

Neuropathological studies have shown that malnutrition is common before death and that diffuse brain atrophy is a non-specific finding; the degree of atrophy appears to be related to the duration of the disorder (Harding *et al.* 1985, Missliwetz and Depastas 1985, Jellinger and Seiteberger 1986, Brucke *et al.* 1988).

TABLE 20.3

Rett syndrome: clinical characteristics and differential diagnosis by stage*

Stage	Clinical characteristics	Differential diagnosis
Stage I Onset: 6–18mths Duration: mths	Developmental stagnation Deceleration of head/brain growth Lack of interest in play activity and environment Hypotonia EEG background: normal or minimal slowing of posterior rhythm	Benign cogenital hypotonia Prader–Willi syndrome Cerebral palsy
Stage II Onset: 1–3yrs Duration: wks to mths	Rapid developmental regression with irritability Loss of hand use Seizures Hand stereotypies: wringing, clapping, tapping, mouthing Autistic manifestations Loss of expressive language Insomnia Self-abusive behaviour (*e.g.* chewing fingers, slapping face) EEG: background slowing and gradual loss of normal sleep activity; focal or multifocal spike and wave	Autism Psychosis Hearing or visual disturbance Encephalitis Epileptic encephalopathy Neurocutaneous syndromes Neurodegenerative disorders Various disorders of organic acid and amino acid metabolism
Stage III Onset: 2–10yrs Duration: mths to yrs	Severe mental retardation/apparent dementia Amelioration of autistic features Seizures Typical hand sterotypies: wringing, tapping, mouthing Prominent ataxia and apraxia Hyperreflexia and progressive rigidity Hyperventilation, breath-holding, aerophagia during waking Weight loss with excellent appetite Early scoliosis Bruxism EEG: gradual disappearance of posterior rhythm, generalized slowing, absent vertex and spindle activity, epileptiform abnormalities activated during sleep	Spastic ataxic cerebral palsy Spinocerebellar degeneration Leukodystrophies or other storage disorders Neuroaxonal dystrophy Lennox–Gastaut syndrome Angelman syndrome

Continues ↓

Stage IV	Progressive scoliosis, muscle	Unknown degenerative disorder
Onset: 10+yrs	wasting and rigidity	
Duration: yrs	Decreasing mobility, wheelchair-dependent	
	Growth retardation	
	Improved eye contact	
	Virtual absence of expressive and receptive language	
	Trophic disturbance of feet	
	Reduced seizure frequency	
	EEG: poor background organization with marked slowing and mutilfocal spikes and slow spike and wave pattern activated by sleep	

*Reproduced by permission from Trevathan and Naidu (1988).

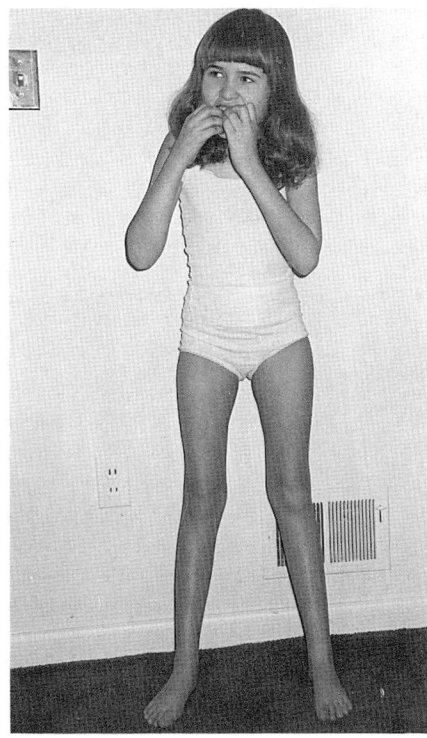 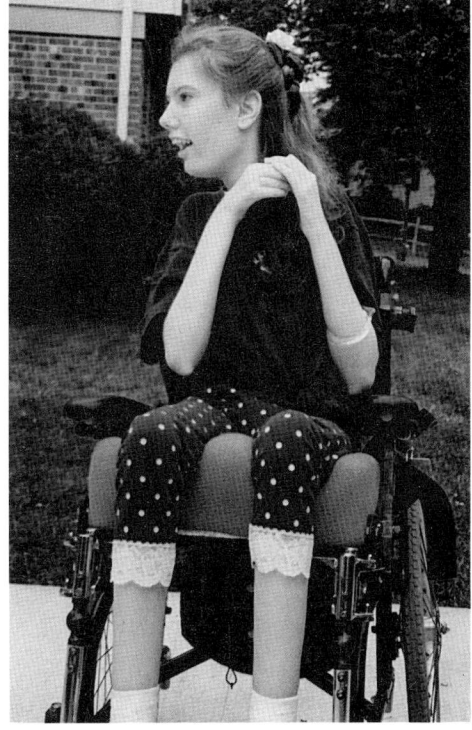

Fig. 20.2. Two teenage girls with Rett syndrome who followed different clinical courses. *Left:* Stage III (ambulatory). *Right:* Stage IV-B (non-ambulatory—see text for explanation of substaging).

No evidence of active degenerative disease has been reported.

No therapy is known that can cure Rett syndrome. Therapies are directed at maintaining or, if possible, improving function and preventing deformities. Seizure disorders need neurological treatment and monitoring. Treatments include physical therapies, occupational therapies, music therapy, hydrotherapy and appropriate orthopaedic treatment (Van Acker 1991).

Sotos syndrome (cerebral gigantism)

Cerebral gigantism is a non-progressive clinical syndrome originally described by Sotos *et al.* (1964). Affected children have macrocrania, hydrocephalus, excessive body size, accelerated growth, clumsiness, characteristic facies and a simulated appearance of acromegaly. A wide spectrum of intelligence has been reported from profound mental retardation to normal intelligence with specific deficits in language, visuomotor activities or mathematics. Precocious puberty has occurred in some patients.

Emotional and behavioural disturbances, including abnormalities of socialization, have been reported in this patient group (Livingwood and Borengasser 1981, Varley and Crnic 1984, Rutter and Cole 1991); however, the children described in these reports did not have all the characteristics of autism. Six male patients with the Sotos syndrome and the necessary criteria for a diagnosis of autism have been reported in the literature (Morrow *et al.* 1990, Zappella 1990). The 5-year-old reported by Morrow *et al.* had normal intelligence in spite of an early history of mild developmental delay (Fig. 20.3). All the 3- to 10-year-old patients described by Zappella had mental retardation as well as autism.

Gilles de la Tourette syndrome

The Tourette syndrome is a neurological disorder characterized by involuntary movements (motor tics) and vocalizations (phonic or vocal tics). In addition, patients may have obsessions, compulsions, the attentional deficit syndrome and other psychiatric symptoms. The disorder generally begins in childhood; the genetic mode of transmission is most compatible with autosomal dominant inheritance. The Tourette syndrome is thought to have a frequency of occurrence somewhat similar to that of autism (1:2500 vs. 1:2200).

The Tourette syndrome is related to autism in two ways. Several children have been described in the literature with original diagnoses of infantile autism followed by the development of Tourette symptoms often beginning around the time of puberty (Realmuto and Main 1982, Barabas and Mathews 1983, Burd *et al.* 1987, Ritvo *et al.* 1990). A study involving 12 children with autism who had also developed symptoms of the Tourette syndrome as they grew older reported that this particular subgroup scored higher on IQ tests and had better expressive language skills than children with autism in the same cohort who did not develop Tourette syndrome (Burd *et al.* 1987). The meaning of this observation, which has been confirmed by one of the present authors (M.C.), remains unknown, but it

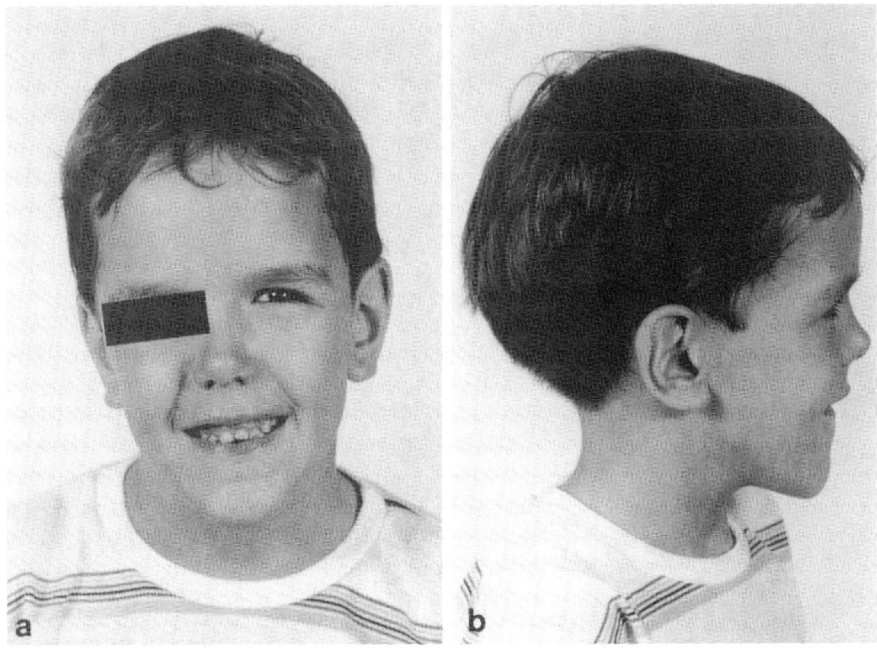

Fig. 20.3. 5-year-old boy with Sotos syndrome and autism. He has macrocephaly, dolichocephaly, triangular facies, downslanting palpebral fissures and a flat profile. (Reproduced by permission from Morrow *et al.* 1990.)

suggests that the children who later develop the Tourette syndrome in combination with autistic symptoms may be a distinct subgroup with a specific underlying pathology.

Tourette syndrome has also been reported in patients with autism who were receiving long-term neuroleptic medicine where the Tourette symptoms were thought to have been induced by the effect of the long-term therapy (Stahl 1980, Perry *et al.* 1989). Stahl coined the term 'tardive Tourette syndrome' to describe patients whose neuroleptic withdrawal takes the form of the Tourette syndrome. In such cases, it is hard to be sure exactly what is happening—the re-emergence of pre-existing stereotypies or the emergence of new ones, the appearance of the Tourette syndrome at this age or Tourette-like withdrawal dyskinesias. Careful review of past examinations and family history plus detailed monitoring of the future course can help distinguish between these various possibilities.

Tuberous sclerosis
Tuberous sclerosis, or the tuberous sclerosis complex as it is sometimes known, is a neurological disorder with behavioural manifestations including autism. It is a neurocutaneous disorder, one of three (along with neurofibromatosis and hypomelanosis of Ito—see above) that have been reported so far in connection with

241

autism and autistic-like conditions (including Asperger syndrome).

Severe tuberous sclerosis, which occurs in the general child population at a frequency of about 1:10,000, is an autosomal dominant disorder characterized by benign tumours (hamartomas, often called tubers—see Fig. 13.1, p.153) and malformations of one or more body systems including the CNS and skin. Skin manifestations include hypomelanotic macules and facial angiofibromas. Mental retardation is present in about half of the patients; 84 per cent have seizures (Gomez 1988). Linkage studies appear to show genetic heterogeneity, suggesting genes on several different chromosomes. Families with gene loci on chromosome 9 (q34) or 11 (q22–23) are known (Johnson and Gomez 1991), but there are other families with neither of these gene loci. Another possibility is a locus on chromosome 12 (Fafsold *et al.* 1991).

If the tuberous sclerosis literature is reviewed closely, it is seen that many children with autism or autistic-like symptoms have been reported. Dick and Ziegler (1967) were the first to report the association in the case of a 12-year-old boy with tuberous sclerosis and autistic-like features. Valente (1971) also described the association of autism with tuberous sclerosis. A few years, Lotter (1974) reported that indications of tuberous sclerosis might eventually develop in autism, even among children who had shown no major signs of the disorder in early childhood and did not have a family history. Since then, children and teenagers with tuberous sclerosis and autistic-like symptoms have been reported by a number of authors (Roth and Epstein 1971, Mansheim 1979, Gomez *et al.* 1982, Greenstein and Cassidy 1986, Fisher *et al.* 1987, Lawlor and Maurer 1987, Oliver 1987). There have also been descriptions of children and adults with tuberous sclerosis who are reported to meet the full criteria for autism (Taft and Cohen 1971, Curatolo and Cusmai 1987, Fisher *et al.* 1987, Jambaqué *et al.* 1991, Wakschlag *et al.* 1991).

A prevalence study of 'childhood pervasive developmental disorder' in the state of North Dakota (Fisher *et al.* 1986) identified three adults and one child who met the criteria for the disorder yet had the diagnosis of tuberous sclerosis. In fact, in this survey of a state with a small population, 25 per cent of patients with definitely diagnosed tuberous sclerosis met the criteria for classic or atypical autism. Hunt and Dennis (1987) also raised the possibility that tuberous sclerosis might be associated with autism much more often that hitherto believed.

In an excellent summary of the literature, Smalley *et al.* (1992) reveal that in published series of tuberous sclerosis patients in whom behavioural manifestations have been studied, autistic features have been described in from 17 to 58 per cent of subjects. The latter figure of 58 per cent was reported by Corbett and Hunt (1988) in a series of 88 children in England. In a recent study of 23 children with tuberous sclerosis (Jambaqué *et al.* 1991), six were described as autistic. These six, aged 8 to 11 years, were having frequent and intractable seizures. In this series, the persistence of active epileptic phenomena in both anterior and posterior areas of the brain (mostly related to tubers in these areas) seemed to play a major role in differentiating these children from the others with tuberous sclerosis who did not

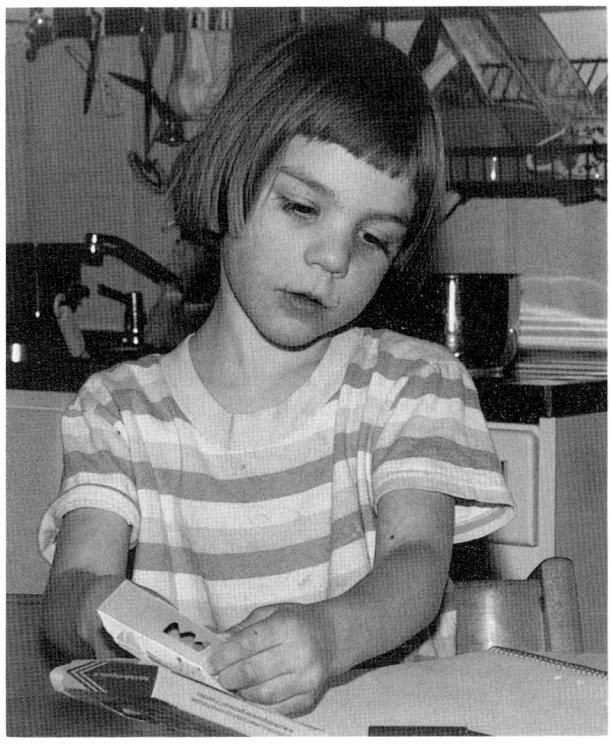

Fig. 20.4. 4-year-old girl with autism, epilepsy, near-normal intelligence and tuberous sclerosis.

show autistic features.

Looking at the problem from the other vantage point of patients presenting with autistic symptoms, most epidemiological studies of the autistic syndromes from Creak (1963) to the 1990 studies of Ritvo *et al.* and Elia *et al.* have included at least one case of tuberous sclerosis. These studies show a variation between 0.4 and 3 per cent in the frequency of tuberous sclerosis in a population of individuals with autism (Smalley *et al.* 1992). In the epidemiological study of autism by Wing and Gould (1979), 2 per cent of patients had autistic-like conditions, but none with classical autism had tuberous sclerosis. In the Gillberg and Steffenburg (1987) follow-up study of autism and autistic-like conditions, none of those with classical autism had tuberous sclerosis. In an ongoing study of autism in the Göteborg region, one of the present authors (C.G.) has encountered nine cases of tuberous sclerosis among 238 individuals with typical infantile autism, a rate of 4 per cent. Eight of these nine also had moderate or severe mental retardation and fits (infantile spasms, complex partial and generalized tonic–clonic seizures), whereas one had low-normal intelligence and occasional complex partial seizures (Fig. 20.4). In Steffenburg's (1991) population study of autism, the prevalence of tuberous sclerosis was 3 per cent.

243

However, if one limits the group under investigation to a subgroup of *individuals with autism and seizures*, in the two studies reported to date the frequency rises to 8 per cent (Riikonen and Simell 1990) or 14 per cent (Gillberg 1981). In a follow-up study of 214 children with infantile spasms, Riikonen and Amnell (1981) found that 25 per cent of children who had the combination of infantile spasms, infantile autism and normal levels of motor activity also had tuberous sclerosis.

The exact relationship between seizures, particularly early infantile spasms, in tuberous sclerosis patients, and the development of autistic symptoms is an important area of understanding. In most series of patients with tuberous sclerosis, individuals with autism have significantly more seizures and mental retardation than those without. However, there are always exceptions to the rule—Smalley *et al.* (1992) report a male with tuberous sclerosis and autism who has an estimated IQ of 116. Another finding of their study was that there were more male tuberous sclerosis patients with autism than females, despite the equal sex ratio in tuberous sclerosis itself.

Tuberous sclerosis patients with autism provide a striking illustration of the misconceptions of those who make a claim for a subdivision of autism into organic and non-organic cases. In many tuberous sclerosis–autism cases, there is no early indication of tuberous sclerosis at the time autism is diagnosed. In four of the cases seen by one of the present authors (C.G.), there were no signs of the physical genetic disorder before the age of 5 years, by which time they had all received their psychiatric diagnosis. One patient with autism and severe complex partial seizures had tuberous sclerosis revealed only after neurosurgery and removal of a diagnostic tumour.

Tuberous sclerosis patients with autism are often extremely difficult to care for. Not only do they show severe autistic behaviour disturbances, but they are often hyperkinetic and sometimes aggressive as well. Usually epileptic seizures are also present, yet parents and other caregivers often find the behaviour problems even more burdensome that the seizure disorder.

As further genetic information becomes available, it will be relevant to see if any particular genetic locus in tuberous sclerosis families is more associated with autistic features. One boy with tuberous sclerosis and autism is reported as belonging to a family with a probable error in chromosome 9 (Ritvo *et al.* 1990), but it is unclear whether this was verified in that individual patient.

Williams syndrome
Williams syndrome, also known as the elfin-face syndrome, presents in infancy with feeding difficulties, poor weight gain and irritability. It occurs in approximately 1:25,000 live births. The children have distinctive elfin-like facies, renal and cardiovascular abnormalities, and mental and growth retardation. Some but not all of the infants have raised levels of calcium in their blood (idiopathic infantile hypercalcaemia) but this corrects itself with time and usually does not persist

throughout childhood.

These patients often have high rates of behavioural and emotional disturbance compared with other mentally retarded children (Udwin *et al.* 1987). One problem seems to be the exact opposite of autism: over-friendliness. Yet this patient group does have several problems seen in autism, such as hyperacusis, social isolation and distractibility. Hypersensitivity to noise (vacuum cleaners, lawnmowers, electric shavers, thunder) results in the children putting their hands over their ears; as yet no auditory abnormalities have been found to explain this phenomenon. They also have a tendency to talk repetitively about topics which focus their attention. A recent study has shown that these unusual characteristics persist virtually unchanged into adult life (Udwin 1990).

Two children with both Williams syndrome and classical autistic features have been reported in the literature (Reiss *et al.* 1985). In contrast to the usual over-friendliness of patients with Williams syndrome, these two children exhibited social aloofness as well as ritualistic behaviours and deviant communication. Whole blood serotonin levels in these two patients were elevated. Two children with Williams syndrome and normal serotonin levels were recently described who did not exhibit autism (August and Realmuto 1989).

Single case reports
There are a number of single case reports in the medical literature regarding children with autistic symptoms and another established disease entity. In such cases, the role of coincidence in this association remains a likely hypothesis until proven otherwise.

• Achondroplasia and concurrent autistic symptoms have been observed by one of the present authors (C.G.).

• Classical autistic symptoms have been described in the Biedl–Bardet syndrome (Gillberg and Wahlström 1985). In one series, all the patients were described as having 'inappropriate mannerisms and shallow affect' (Green *et al.* 1989).

• A girl with the Coffin–Siris syndrome has been reported as having autistic behaviour (Hersh *et al.* 1982).

• A child with Duchenne muscular dystrophy was reported to have autistic symptoms (Komoto *et al.* 1984).

• The Lawrence–Moon–Biedl syndrome has been described in a patient who met DSM-III-R criteria for autism (Steffenburg 1991).

• An 11-year-old girl with congenital myotonic dystrophy and infantile autism has been reported (Yoshimura *et al.* 1989). Her mother also has myotonic dystrophy. Autistic behaviour appeared before 2 years of age and has persisted.

• A male with Noonan syndrome and autistic behaviour has been reported (Paul *et al.* 1983).

• In a series describing concomitant conditions in 74 children with autism, one 4-year-old-boy has been described as having oculocutaneous albinism (Ornitz *et al.* 1977).

Summary

The wide array of syndromes which have a subgroup of children with an autistic syndrome reinforces the concept that autism is a non-specific behavioural disorder. It is interesting to note that in several of the syndromes—hypomelanosis of Ito and the Joubert syndrome, for example—the patients described with autistic symptoms tend to be among the highest intellectually functioning children with that specific syndrome.

REFERENCES

Åkefeldt, A., Gillberg, C. (1991) 'Hypomelanosis of Ito in three cases with autism and autistic-like conditions.' *Developmental Medicine and Child Neurology*, **33**, 737–743.

Ardinger, H.H., Bell, W.E. (1986) 'Hypomelanosis of Ito. Wood's light and magnetic resonance imaging as diagnostic measures.' *Archives of Neurology*, **43**, 848–850.

Asperger, H. (1944) 'Die autistischen Psychopathen im Kindesalter.' *Archiv für Psychiatrie und Nervenkrankheiten*, **117**, 76–136.

August, G.J., Realmuto, G.M. (1989) 'Williams syndrome: serotonin's association with developmental disabilities.' *Journal of Autism and Developmental Disabilities*, **19**, 137–141.

Barabas, G., Mathews, W.S. (1983) 'Coincident infantile autism and Tourette syndrome: a case report.' *Journal of Developmental and Behavioral Pediatrics*, **4**, 280–281.

Brücke, T., Sofic, E., Killian, W., Rett, A., Reiderer, P. (1988) 'Reduced concentrations and increased metabolism of biogenic amines in a single case of Rett syndrome: a postmortem brain study.' *Journal of Neural Transmission*, **68**, 315–324.

Budden, S.J., Myer, E.C., Butler, I.J. (1990) 'Cerebrospinal fluid studies in the Rett syndrome: biogenic amines and β-endorphins.' *Brain and Development*, **12**, 81–84.

Burd, L., Fisher, W.W., Kerbeshian, J., Arnold, M.E. (1987) 'Is the development of Tourette disorder a marker for improvement in patients with autism and other pervasive developmental disorders?' *Journal of the American Academy of Child and Adolescent Psychiatry*, **26**, 162–165.

Casaer, P., Vles, J.S.H., Devlieger, H., Eggermont, E., Boel, M. (1985) 'Variability of outcome in Joubert syndrome.' *Neuropediatrics*, **16**, 43–45.

Casanova, M.F., Goldberg, T.E., Naidu, S., Khoromi, S., Kumar, A., Weinberger, D.R., Moser, H.W. (1989) 'Quantitative analysis of magnetic resonance imaging in Rett's syndrome.' *Biological Psychiatry*, **25**, 64A. *(Abstract.)*

Cawthon, R.M., Weiss, R., Xu, G., Viskochil, D., Culver, M., Stevens, J., Robertson, M., Dunn, D., Gesteland, R., O'Connell, P., *et al.* (1990) 'A major segment of the neurofibromatosis type 1 gene: cDNA sequence, genomic structure and point mutations.' *Cell*, **62**, 193–201. *(Erratum: **62**, following p. 608.)*

Clarke, A., Church, W., Gardner-Medwin, D., Sengupta, R. (1990) 'Intracranial calcification and seizures: a case of central neurofibromatosis.' *Developmental Medicine and Child Neurology*, **32**, 729–732.

Coker, S., Melnyk, A. (1991) 'Rett syndrome and mitochondrial enzyme deficiencies.' *Journal of Child Neurology*, **6**, 164–166.

Coleman, M. (1990) 'Is classical Rett syndrome ever present in males?' *Brain and Development*, **12**, 31–32.

—— Brubaker, J., Hunter, K., Smith, G. (1988) 'Rett syndrome: a survey of north American patients.' *Journal of Mental Deficiency Research*, **32**, 117–124.

Corbett, J., Hunt, A. (1988) 'Recent research on tuberous sclerosis.' *Journal of the Royal Society of Medicine*, **81**, 481–482.

Creak, E.M. (1963) 'Childhood psychosis: a review of 100 cases.' *British Journal of Psychiatry*, **109**, 84–89.

Crowe, F.W., Schull, W.J., Neil, J.W. (1956) *A Clinical, Pathological and Genetic Study of Multiple Neurofibromatosis.* Springfield, IL: C.C. Thomas.

Curatolo, P., Cusmai, R. (1987) 'Autism and infantile spasms in children with tuberous sclerosis.'

246

Developmental Medicine and Child Neurology, **29**, 550–551. *(Letter.)*

Dick, A.R., Ziegler, D.K. (1967) 'Tuberous sclerosis: a report of two cases.' *Journal of the Kansas Medical Society*, 102–116.

Eeg-Olofsson, O., al-Zuhair, A.G., Teebi, A.S., al-Essa, M.M. (1988) 'Abnormal mitochondria in the Rett syndrome.' *Brain and Development*, **10**, 260–262.

Elia, M., Bergonzi, P., Ferri, R., Musumeci, S.A., Paladino, A., Panerai, S., Ragusa, R.M. (1990) 'The etiology of autism in a group of mentally retarded subjects.' *Brain Dysfunction*, **3**, 228–240.

Eliason, M.J. (1988) 'Neurofibromatosis compared to developmental learning disorders.' *Neurofibromatosis*, **1**, 17–25.

Fahsold, R., Rott, H-D., Lorenz, P., Claussen, U., Schmalenberger, B. (1991) 'Evidence for a tuberous sclerosis locus on chromosome 12.' *Paper presented at the Fifth International Medical Symposium of the Tuberous Sclerosis Association of Great Britain, Sept. 1991.*

Federico, A., Dotti, M.T., Eusebi, M.P., Fabrizi, G., Malandrini, A., Manneschi, L. (1991) 'Mitochondrial changes in Rett syndrome.' *Brain Dysfunction. (In press.)*

Ferlini, A., Ansaloni, L., Nobile, C., Forabosco, A. (1990) 'Molecular analysis of the Rett syndrome using cDNA synapsin I as a probe.' *Brain and Development*, **12**, 136–139.

Fisher, W., Kolstoe, P., Kerbeshian, J., Burd, L. (1986) 'Tuberous sclerosis and autism.' *Developmental Medicine and Child Neurology*, **28**, 814–815. *(Letter.)*

—— Kerbeshian, J., Burd, L., Kolstoe, P. (1987) 'Tuberous sclerosis and autism.' *Journal of the American Academy of Child and Adolescent Psychiatry*, **26**, 700–703.

Fryns, J.P., Buttiens, M. (1987) 'X-linked mental retardation with marfanoid habitus.' *American Journal of Medical Genetics*, **28**, 267–274.

Gaffney, G.R., Kuperman, S., Tsai, L.Y., Minchin, S. (1988) 'Morphological evidence of brainstem involvement in infantile autism.' *Biological Psychiatry*, **24**, 578–586.

Gillberg, C. (1989) 'The borderland of autism and Rett syndrome: five case histories to highlight diagnostic difficulties.' *Journal of Autism and Developmental Disabilities*, **19**, 545–559.

—— (1991) 'The treatment of epilepsy in autism.' *Journal of Autism and Developmental Disorders*, **21**, 61–77.

—— Forsell, C. (1984) 'Childhood psychosis and neurofibromatosis—more than a coincidence?' *Journal of Autism and Developmental Disorders*, **14**, 1–8.

—— Steffenburg, S. (1987) 'Outcome and prognostic factors in infantile autism and similar conditions: a population-based study of 46 cases followed through puberty.' *Journal of Autism and Developmental Disorders*, **17**, 273–287.

—— —— (1989) 'Autistic behaviour in Moebius syndrome.' *Acta Paediatrica Scandinavica*, **78**, 314–316.

—— Wahlström, J. (1985) 'Chromosomal abnormalities in infantile autism and other childhood psychoses. A population study of 66 cases.' *Developmental Medicine and Child Neurology*, **27**, 293–304.

—— Winnergård, I. (1984) 'Childhood psychosis in a case of Moebius syndrome.' *Neuropediatrics*, **15**, 147–149.

Gillberg, I.C., Gillberg, C. (1989) 'Asperger syndrome—some epidemiological considerations: a research note.' *Journal of Child Psychology and Psychiatry*, **30**, 631–638.

Gomez, M. (1988) *Tuberous Sclerosis*. New York: Raven Press.

—— Kuntz, N.L., Westmoreland, B.R. (1982) 'Tuberous sclerosis, early onset of seizures and mental subnormality: study of discordant homozygous twins.' *Neurology*, **32**, 604–611.

Green, J.S., Parfrey, P.S., Harnett, J.D., Farid, N.R., Cramer, B.C., Johnson, G., Heath, O., McManamon, P.J., O'Leary, E., Pryse-Phillips, W. (1989) 'The cardinal manifestations of Bardet-Biedl syndrome, a form of Laurence-Moon-Biedl syndrome.' *New England Journal of Medicine*, **321**, 1002–1009.

Greenstein, M.A., Cassidy, S.B. (1986) 'Is tuberous sclerosis a cause of autism?' *New England Journal of Medicine*, **314**, 449. *(Letter.)*

Griebel, V., Krägeloh-Mann, I., Michaelis, R. (1989) 'Hypomelanosis of Ito: report of four cases and survey of the literature.' *Neuropediatrics*, **20**, 234–237.

Gurrieri, F., Neri, G. (1991) 'A girl with the Lujan-Fryns syndrome.' *American Journal of Medical Genetics*, **38**, 290–291. *(Letter.)*

Haas, R.H., Rice, M.A. (1985) 'Is Rett's syndrome a disorder of carbohydrate metabolism?

Hyperpyruvicacidemia and treatment by ketogenic diet.' *Annals of Neurology*, **18**, 418. *(Abstract.)*

Hagberg, B. (1980) 'Infantile autism, dementia and loss of hand use: a report of 16 Swedish girl patients.' *Paper presented at the Research Session of the European Federation of Child Neurology Societies, Manchester, England.*

—— Witt-Engerström, I. (1986) 'Rett syndrome: a suggested staging system for describing impairment profile with increasing age towards adolescence.' *American Journal of Medical Genetics*, **24**, 47–59.

—— Aicardi, J., Dias, K., Ramos, O. (1983) 'A progressive syndrome of autism, dementia, ataxia and loss of purposeful hand use in girls: Rett's syndrome: a report of 35 cases.' *Annals of Neurology*, **14**, 471–479.

Harding, B.N., Tudway, A.J., Wilson, J. (1985) 'Neuropathological studies in a child showing some features of the Rett syndrome.' *Brain and Development*, **7**, 342–344.

Hauser, S., DeLong, G., Rosman, N. (1975) 'Pneumographic findings in the infantile autism syndrome: a correlation with temporal lobe disease.' *Brain*, **98**, 667–688.

Hersh, J.H., Bloom, A.S., Weisskopf, B. (1982) 'Childhood autism in a female with Coffin-Siris syndrome.' *Journal of Developmental and Behavioral Pediatrics*, **3**, 249–251.

Holroyd, S., Reiss, A.L., Bryan, R.N. (1991) 'Autistic features in Joubert syndrome: a genetic disorder with agenesis of the cerebellar vermis.' *Biological Psychiatry*, **29**, 287–294.

Hunt, A., Dennis, J. (1987) 'Psychiatric disorder among children with tuberous sclerosis.' *Developmental Medicine and Child Neurology*, **29**, 190–198.

Huson, S.M., Thrush, D.C. (1985) 'Central neurofibromatosis.' *Quarterly Journal of Medicine, New Series*, **55**, 213–224.

—— Compston, A.S., Clark, P., Harper, P.S. (1989) 'A genetic study of von Recklinghausen neurofibromatosis in south-east Wales. I: Prevalence, fitness, mutation rate and effect of parental transmission on severity.' *Journal of Medical Genetics*, **26**, 704–711.

Ishikawa, A., Goto, T., Narasaki, M., Wokochi, K., Kitahara, H., Fukuyama, Y. (1978) 'A new syndrome (?) of progressive psychomotor deterioration with peculiar stereotyped movement and autistic tendency: a report of three cases.' *Brain and Development*, **3**, 258.

Jambaqué, I., Cusmai, R., Curatolo, P., Cortesi, F., Perrot, C., Dulac, O. (1991) 'Neuropsychological aspects of tuberous sclerosis in relation to epilepsy and MRI findings.' *Developmental Medicine and Child Neurology*, **33**, 698–705.

Jellinger, K., Seiteberger, F. (1986) 'Neuropathology of Rett syndrome.' *American Journal of Medical Genetics*, **24** (Suppl. 1), 259–288.

Johnson, W.G., Gomez, M.R. (Eds) (1991) *Tuberous Sclerosis and Allied Disorders. 2nd Edn.* New York: New York Academy of Sciences.

Joubert, M., Eisenring, J., Robb, J.P., Andermann, F. (1969) 'Familial agenesis of the cerebellar vermis.' *Neurology*, **19**, 813–825.

Kerr, A.M., Stephenson, J.B. (1985) 'Rett's syndrome in the west of Scotland.' *British Medical Journal*, **291**, 579–582.

—— —— (1986) 'A study of the natural history of Rett syndrome in 23 girls.' *American Journal of Medical Genetics*, **24** (Suppl. 1), 77–83.

Knobloch, H., Pasamanick, B. (1975) 'Some etiologic and prognostic factors in early infantile autism and psychosis.' *Journal of Pediatrics*, **55**, 182–191.

Komoto, J., Usui, S., Otsuki, S., Terao, A. (1984) 'Infantile autism and Duchenne muscular dystrophy.' *Journal of Autism and Developmental Disorders*, **14**, 191–195.

Lawlor, B.A., Maurer, R.G. (1987) 'Tuberous sclerosis and the autistic syndrome.' *British Journal of Psychiatry*, **150**, 396–397.

Lekman, A.Y., Hagberg, B.A., Svennerholm, L.T. (1991) 'Membrane cerebral lipids in Rett syndrome.' *Pediatric Neurology*, **7**, 186–190.

Livingwood, A.B., Borengasser, M.A. (1981) 'Cerebral gigantism in infancy: implications for psychological and social development.' *Child Psychiatry and Human Development*, **12**, 46–53.

Lotter, V. (1974) 'Factors related to outcome in autistic children.' *Journal of Autism and Childhood Schizophrenia*, **4**, 263–277.

Lubs, M-L.E., Bauer, M.S., Formas, M.E., Djokic, B. (1991) 'Lisch nodules in neurofibromatosis type 1.' *New England Journal of Medicine*, **324**, 1264–1266.

Lujan, J.E., Carlin, M.E., Lubs, H.A. (1984) 'A form of X-linked mental retardation with marfanoid habitus.' *American Journal of Medical Genetics*, **17**, 311–322.

Mansheim, P. (1979) 'Tuberous sclerosis and autistic behavior.' *Journal of Clinical Psychiatry*, **40**, 97–98.

Missliwetz, J., Depastas, G. (1985) 'Forensic problems in Rett syndrome.' *Brain and Development*, **7**, 326–328.

Moebius, P.J. (1888) 'Ueber angeborene doppelseitige Abducens-Facialis-Lähmung.' *Münchener Medizinische Wochenschrift*, **35**, 91–94.

Morrow, J.D., Whitman, B.Y., Accardo, P.J. (1990) 'Autistic disorder in Sotos syndrome: a case report.' *European Journal of Pediatrics*, **149**, 567–569.

National Institutes of Health Consensus Development Conference (1988) 'Neurofibromatosis: conference statement.' *Archives of Neurology*, **45**, 575–578.

Nomura, Y., Segawa, M. (1990) 'Clinical features of the early stage of the Rett syndrome.' *Brain and Development*, **12**, 16–19.

Oliver, B.E. (1987) 'Tuberous sclerosis and the autistic syndrome.' *British Journal of Psychiatry*, **151**, 560. *(Letter.)*

Olsson, B., Rett, A. (1987) 'Autism and Rett syndrome: behavioural investigations and differential diagnosis.' *Developmental Medicine and Child Neurology*, **29**, 429–441.

—— (1990) 'A review of the Rett syndrome with a theory of autism.' *Brain and Development*, **12**, 11–15.

Ornitz, E.M., Guthrie, D., Farley, A.H. (1977) 'The early development of autistic children.' *Journal of Autism and Childhood Schizophrenia*, **7**, 207–229.

Paul, R., Cohen, D.J., Volkmar, F.R. (1983) 'Autistic behaviors in a boy with Noonan syndrome.' *Journal of Autism and Developmental Disorders*, **13**, 433–434. *(Letter.)*

Perry, A., Sarlo-McGarvey, N., Haddad, C. (1991) 'Brief report: Cognitive and adaptive functioning in 28 girls with Rett syndrome.' *Journal of Autism and Developmental Disorders*, **21**, 551–556.

Perry, R., Nobler, M.S., Campbell, M. (1989) 'Tourette-like symptoms associated with neuroleptic therapy in an autistic child.' *Journal of the American Academy of Child and Adolescent Psychiatry*, **28**, 93–96.

Realmuto, G.M., Main, B. (1982) 'Coincidence of Tourette's disorder and infantile autism.' *Journal of Autism and Developmental Disorders*, **12**, 367–372.

Reiss, A.L., Feinstein, C., Rosenbaum, K.N., Borengasser-Caruso, M.A., Goldsmith, B.M. (1985) 'Autism associated with Williams syndrome.' *Journal of Pediatrics*, **106**, 247–249.

Rett, A. (1966) *Uber ein cerebral-atrophisches Syndrom bei Hyperammonämie*. Vienna: Hollinek.

—— (1968) 'Uber ein eigenartiges Hirnatrophisches Syndrom bei Hyperammonämie in Kindesalter.' *Weiner Medizinische Wochenschrift*, **116**, 723–738.

—— (1977) 'Cerebral atrophy associated with hyperammonemia.' *In:* Vinken, P.J., Bruyn, G.W. (Eds) *Handbook of Clinical Neurology, Vol. 29: Metabolic and Deficiency Diseases of the Nervous System Part 2*. Amsterdam: Elsevier/North-Holland, pp. 305–329.

Rett Syndrome Diagnostic Criteria Work Group (1988) 'Diagnostic criteria for Rett syndrome.' *Annals of Neurology*, **23**, 425–428.

Riccardi, V.M. (1991) 'Neurofibromatosis: past, present and future.' *New England Journal of Medicine*, **324**, 1283–1285.

—— Eichner, J.E. (1986) *Neurofibromatosis: Phenotype, Natural History and Pathogenesis*. Baltimore: Johns Hopkins University Press, pp. 29–36.

Riikonen, R., Amnell, G. (1981) 'Psychiatric disorders in children with earlier infantile spasms.' *Developmental Medicine and Child Neurology*, **23**, 747–760.

—— Simell, O. (1990) 'Tuberous sclerosis and infantile spasms.' *Developmental Medicine and Child Neurology*, **32**, 203–209.

Ritvo, E.R., Mason-Brothers, A., Freeman, B.J., Pingree, C., Jenson, W.R., McMahon, W.M., Petersen, C.B., Jorde, L.B., Mo, A., Ritvo, A. (1990) 'The UCLA–University of Utah Epidemiologic Survey of Autism: the etiologic role of rare diseases.' *American Journal of Psychiatry*, **147**, 1614–1621.

Roth, J.C., Epstein, C.J. (1971) 'Infantile spasms and hypopigmented macules: early manifestations of tuberous sclerosis.' *Archives of Neurology*, **25**, 547–551.

Rouleau, G.A., Wertelecki, W., Haines, J.L., Hobbs, W.J., Trofatter, J.A., Seizinger, B.R., Martuza, R.L., Superneau, D.W., Conneally, P.M., Gusella, J.F. (1987) 'Genetic linkage of bilateral acoustic neurofibromatosis to a DNA marker on chromosome 22.' *Nature*, **329**, 246–248.

Ruch, A., Kurczynski, T.W., Velasco, M.E. (1989) 'Mitochondrial alterations in Rett syndrome.' *Pediatric Neurology*, **5**, 320–323.

Rutter, S.C., Cole, T.R.P. (1991) 'Psychological characteristics of Sotos syndrome.' *Developmental Medicine and Child Neurology*, **33**, 898–902.

Smalley, S.L., Tanguay, P.E., Smith, M., Gutierrez, G. (1992) 'Autism and tuberous sclerosis.' *Journal of Autism and Developmental Disorders*, **22**, 339–355.

Sotos, J.F., Dodge, P.R., Muirhead, D., Crawford, J.D., Talbot, N.B. (1964) 'Cerebral gigantism in childhood: a syndrome of excessively rapid growth with acromegalic features and a non-progressive neurologic disorder.' *New England Journal of Medicine*, **271**, 109–117.

Stahl, S.M. (1980) 'Tardive Tourette syndrome in an autistic patient after long-term neuroleptic administration.' *American Journal of Psychiatry*, **137**, 1267–1269.

Steffenburg, S. (1991) 'Neuropsychiatric assessment of children with autism.' *Developmental Medicine and Child Neurology*, **33**, 495–511.

Sudarshan, A., Goldie, W.D. (1985) 'The spectrum of congenital facial diplegia (Moebius syndrome).' *Pediatric Neurology*, **1**, 180–184.

Taft, L.T., Cohen, H.J. (1971) 'Hypsarrhythmia and infantile autism: a clinical report.' *Journal of Autism and Childhood Schizophrenia*, **1**, 327–336.

Topcu, M., Topaloglu, H., Renda, Y., Berker, M., Turanli, G. (1991) 'The Rett syndrome in males.' *Brain and Development*, **13**, 62. *(Letter.)*

Trevathan, E., Naidu, S. (1988) 'The clinical recognition and differential diagnosis of Rett syndrome.' *Journal of Child Neurology*, **3** (Suppl.), S6–S16.

Udwin, O. (1990) 'A survey of adults with Williams syndrome and idiopathic infantile hypercalcaemia.' *Developmental Medicine and Child Neurology*, **32**, 129–141.

—— Yule, W., Martin, N. (1987) 'Cognitive abilities and behavioural characteristics of children with idiopathic infantile hypercalcaemia.' *Journal of Child Psychology and Psychiatry*, **28**, 297–309.

Valente, M. (1971) 'Autism: symptomatic and idiopathic—and mental retardation.' *Pediatrics*, **48**, 495–496. *(Letter.)*

Van Acker, R. (1991) 'Rett syndrome: a review of current knowledge.' *Journal of Autism and Developmental Disorders*, **21**, 381–406.

Varley, C., Crnic, K. (1984) 'Emotional, behavioral and cognitive status of children with cerebral gigantism.' *Journal of Developmental and Behavioral Pediatrics*, **5**, 132–134.

Wakschlag, L.S., Cook, E.H., Hammond, D.N., Leventhal, B.L., Hopkins, J. (1991) 'Autism and tuberous sclerosis.' *Journal of Autism and Developmental Disorders*, **21**, 95–97. *(Letter.)*

Wing, L., Gould, J. (1979) 'Severe impairments of social interaction and associated abnormalities in children: epidemiology and classification.' *Journal of Autism and Developmental Disorders*, **9**, 11–29.

Witt Engerström, I. (1990) 'Rett syndrome in Sweden: neurodevelopment—disability—pathophysiology.' *Acta Paediatrica Scandinavica*, Suppl. 396, 1–60.

—— Gillberg, C. (1987) 'Rett syndrome in Sweden.' *Journal of Autism and Developmental Disorders*, **17**, 149–150. *(Letter.)*

Yoshikawa, H., Fueki, N., Suzuki, H., Sakuragawa, N., Masaaki, I. (1991) 'Cerebral blood flow and oxygen metabolism in Rett syndrome.' *Journal of Child Neurology*, **6**, 237–242.

Yoshimura, I., Sasaki, A., Akimoto, H., Yoshimura, N. (1989) 'A case of congenital myotonic dystrophy with infantile autism.' *No To Hattatsu*, **21**, 379–384. *(Japanese.)*

Zappella, M. (1991) 'Autism and cerebral gigantism.' *Brain Dysfunction. (In press.)*

—— (1992) 'Hypomelanosis of Ito is frequently associated with autism.' *European Child and Adolescent Psychiatry*, **1**, 170–177.

Zoghbi, H.Y., Milstien, S., Butler, I.J., Smith, E.O., Kaufman, S., Glaze, D., Percy, A.K. (1989) 'Cerebrospinal fluid biogenic amines and biopterin in Rett syndrome.' *Annals of Neurology*, **25**, 56–60.

—— Percy, A.K., Schultz, R.J., Fill, C. (1990) 'Patterns of X chromosome inactivation in the Rett syndrome.' *Brain and Development*, **12**, 131–135.

21
AUDITORY AND VISUAL CONSIDERATIONS

In published series of children with autistic symptoms, blind and deaf children are frequently reported. In one typical study, among children with autism identified from inpatient and outpatient child psychiatry units in France, 7 per cent were blind and 5 per cent were deaf (Garreau *et al.* 1984). In addition to total blindness and deafness, other levels of auditory and visual impairment are common in populations of children with autism. In a population-based survey by Steffenburg (1990), 24 per cent of children with autism or autistic-like disorders (no difference between the two groups) had a hearing deficit of more than 25dB, while more than 50 per cent of those children whose vision could be properly evaluated had a refraction error (mostly hypermetropia, but myopia and astigmatism were diagnosed in many cases).

Looking at the problem from the opposite perspective, autistic symptoms have been described in many congenitally blind and deaf children (Valente 1971; see also Chapter 18 *in re* children born with congenital rubella). Fraiberg (1977) reported that approximately 25 per cent of the totally blind young children known to her had autism. Autistic symptoms have been described in children with several different aetiologies of severe visual impairment, including retrolental fibroplasia (Keeler 1958, Valente 1971, Chase 1972), Leber congenital amaurosis (Rogers and Newhart-Larson 1989) and morning glory syndrome (Nawratzki *et al.* 1985). Congenital deafness is also present (sometimes undetected) in some non-verbal children with autism and is associated with known aetiologies of autism, such as congenital rubella infection (Chess *et al.* 1971).

Most congenitally blind and deaf children are not autistic, and what distinguishes those with autistic symptoms from those without is not fully understood. A recent study looked at this question (Rogers and Newhart-Larson 1989): five visually impaired boys with Leber amaurosis were compared with five age- and sex-matched children who had total blindness from birth from causes other than Leber syndrome (retrolental fibroplasia, congenital glaucoma or corneal lens opacity). The boys with Leber amaurosis met the criteria for infantile autism and had remarkably similar developmental histories. Their general behaviour resembled that of sighted children with autism far more than it did blind children without autism. According to their teachers, the children with Leber amaurosis appeared to be more disabled by autism than by blindness; they described the problem as difficulties with 'relatedness'. In contrast, the comparison children did not have abnormal social relatedness, even if they exhibited stereotypic behaviours, and none met DSM-III-R criteria for infantile autism.

It is well understood that early blindness and deafness in any child may affect cognition, as pointed out in an excellent review by Rapin (1979). Rapin emphasized that the majority of such children do become competent adults if the severity of their disability is taken into consideration. It is theoretically interesting that manifestly non-autistic children who are congenitally blind may sometimes show autistic-like features such as personal pronoun difficulties, echolalia and impairments in symbolic play (Hobson 1991).

Evaluation of the visual system is most important in any child presenting with autism. Moderate visual acuity problems can be compensated for with corrective lenses, but first they must be identified. Many children have strabismus, which may need correction. In the Steffenburg study, after extensive evaluations, only one third of the children were considered to have normal visual acuity; one boy with the Lawrence–Moon–Biedl syndrome gradually became blind.

Fundus abnormalities have also been reported (Ritvo et al. 1990, Steffenburg 1990). In the series of Ritvo et al., one boy with autism had septo-optic dysplasia and optic nerve atrophy; another had optic nerve atrophy, hypoplastic optic nerves and lack of cone vision; and a third had retinitis pigmentosa and congenital herpes. The question has even been raised as to whether retinal pathology in children with autism is a biological marker for a subtype of autism (Ritvo et al. 1986). An electroretinogram study revealed that 13 of 27 patients with autism had subnormal b-wave amplitudes (Ritvo et al. 1988); this work needs replication.

Most hearing deficits in children with autism are thought to be of neurogenic origin. Some are genetic (Ritvo et al. 1990). Otitis media has been considered a contributory factor in some cases (Ritvo et al. 1990, Steffenburg 1991), and one study showed an increased incidence of middle-ear disease (Konstantareas and Homatidis 1987). The processing of auditory stimuli has been extensively studied by electrophysiological means in this patient group (see Chapter 12).

It appears that obtaining a specific diagnostic aetiology and comprehensive acuity testing can help sort out the type of disability of a sensory-impaired child with autism and lead to more individualized remedial work.

Education is particularly difficult in these multiply disabled children who have both a major sensory loss and autism. One of the main items separating deaf children with autism from other deaf children is the avoidance of eye contact (Meadow 1984). Teaching such a child challenges the ingenuity of the teacher. Similarly, a visually impaired child with autism who has problems tolerating sounds and at times appears 'deaf' is also very difficult to teach. One example of such ingenuity is the report by Konstantareas et al. (1982) of a successful programme of teaching sign language to a blind child with autism by relying primarily on tactile, kinaesthetic and auditory modalities.

The physician is an important part of the multiply disabled child's professional team. The doctor has a particular responsibility to perform a full medical examination of such a child (see Chapter 25). This is essential to ensure that everything possible has been done to obtain diagnostic information that might help indicate medical therapies for decreasing haptic defensiveness, lack of eye contact and poor attention span. Such assistance might be of value in altering the rate of learning and achieving success in the educational programming.

REFERENCES

Chase, J.B. (1972) *Retrolental Fibroplasia and Autistic Symptomatology.* New York: American Foundation for the Blind.
Chess, S., Korn, S.J., Fernandez, P.B. (1971) *Psychiatric Disorders of Children with Congential Rubella.* New York: Brunner/Mazel.
Fraiberg, S. (1977) *Insights from the Blind.* New York: Basic Books.
Garreau, B., Barthélémy, C., Sauvage, D., Leddet, I., LeLord, G. (1984) 'A comparison of autistic syndromes with and without associated neurological problems.' *Journal of Autism and Developmental Disorders,* **14**, 105–111.
Hobson, R.P. (1991) 'What is autism?' *Pediatric Clinics of North America,* **14**, 1–17.
Keeler, W.R. (1958) 'Autistic patterns and defective communication in blind children with retrolental fibroplasia.' *In:* Hoch, P.H., Zubin, J. (Eds) *Psychopathology of Communication.* New York: Grune & Stratton. pp. 64–83.
Konstantareas, M.M., Homatidis, S. (1987) 'Brief report: ear infections in autistic children.' *Journal of Autism and Developmental Disorders,* **17**, 585–594.
—— Hunter, D., Sloman, L. (1982) 'Training a blind autistic child to communicate through signs.' *Journal of Autism and Developmental Disorders,* **12**, 1–12.
Meadow, K. (1984) 'Social adjustment of preschool children: deaf and hearing, with and without other handicaps.' *In:* Fewell, R. (Ed.) *Topics in Early Childhood Special Education.* Austin, TX: Pro-Ed, pp. 27–40.
Nawratzki, I., Schwartzenberg, T., Zaubermann, H., Yanko, L. (1985) 'Bilateral morning glory syndrome with midline brain lesion in an autistic child.' *Metabolic, Pediatric and Systemic Ophthalmology,* **8**, 35–36.
Rapin, I. (1979) 'Effects of early blindness and deafness on cognition.' *In:* Katzman, R. (Ed.) *Congenital and Acquired Cognitive Disorders.* New York: Raven Press, pp. 189–245.
Ritvo, E.R., Freeman, B.J., Creel, D., Crandall, A.S., Pingree, C., Barr, R., Realmuto, G. (1986) 'Retinal pathology in autistic children—a possible biological marker for a subtype?' *Journal of the American Academy of Child Psychiatry,* **25**, 137. *(Letter.)*
—— Creel, D., Realmuto, G., Crandall, A.S., Freeman, B.J., Bateman, B., Barr, R., Pingree, C., Coleman, M., Purple, R. (1988) 'Electroretinograms in autism: a pilot study of b-wave amplitudes.' *American Journal of Psychiatry,* **145**, 229–232.
—— Mason-Brothers, A., Freeman, B.J., Pingree, C., Jenson, W.R., McMahon, W.M., Petersen, P.B., Jorde, J.B., Mo, A., Ritvo, A. (1990) 'The UCLA–University of Utah epidemiologic survey of autism: the etiologic role of rare diseases.' *American Journal of Psychiatry,* **147**, 1614–1621.
Rogers, S.J., Newhart-Larson, S. (1989) 'Characteristics of infantile autism in five children with Lebers' congenital amaurosis.' *Developmental Medicine and Child Neurology,* **31**, 598–608.
Steffenburg, S. (1990) *Neurobiological Correlates of Autism.* M.D. thesis, University of Göteborg.
—— (1991) 'Neuropsychiatric assessment of children with autism.' *Developmental Medicine and Child Neurology,* **33**, 495–511.
Valente, M. (1971) 'Autism: symptomatic and idiopathic—and mental retardation.' *Pediatrics,* **48**, 495–496. *(Letter.)*

PART IV

TREATMENTS CURRENTLY UNDER INVESTIGATION

22
PHARMACOLOGICAL THERAPIES

The pharmacology of autism is directed toward attempts either to treat the condition in general or to treat specific maladaptive behaviours such as hyperactivity, stereotypies, temper tantrums and aggressiveness directed toward the self or others. For the treatment of autism in general, there is wide agreement that pharmacotherapy should never be viewed as a sole treatment, but rather as part of a comprehensive therapy programme (Campbell 1989). In fact, for some clinicians, the principle use of pharmacotherapy is limited to behavioural problems which have failed to respond to behaviour modification or other psychosocial treatments (Campbell and Schopler 1987). A current consensus among many paediatric psychiatrists is that young patients with high IQs may not need drugs at all, but rather can be adequately treated with enriched environments and behavioural/educational help. Regarding treatment for specific clinical symptoms, it is clear that pharmacotherapy is of value to some patients. However, the ideal remains that drug therapies may someday be directed at the underlying disease entity which causes the autistic symptoms rather than the symptoms themselves.

Sometimes after a patient has completed the work-up and received a diagnosis, there is no specific or even research therapy available for that diagnosis. For example, such would be the case for a diagnosis of prenatal rubella causing autistic symptoms; medical approaches for such gestational lesions need to focus on prevention of the disease itself. Sometimes, even after a specific biochemical abnormality has been found, correction of the abnormality either makes no difference to clinical behaviour or makes the patient worse. Sometimes after the work-up is completed, there is still not even an underlying diagnosis. In these three situations, it may be necessary to move to one of the pharmacological therapies being developed for patients simply because they have autistic symptoms.

These drugs therapies will be reviewed in two sections. First, the trials of many different drugs that occurred prior to the 1980s will be reviewed, both for the historical perspective and because this information is still relevant for some patients. In more recent years, a better understanding of both the efficacies and side-effects of recommended drugs has developed. As the pharmacological mechanisms underlying the effective use of drugs are better understood, it is beginning to be possible to select a drug for any particular patient on a more rational basis. However, the development of drugs for autism is very much an ongoing process, as the search for new pharmacological agents, particularly those targeted toward selected symptoms, continues.

Early trials

For several decades researchers attempted, by trial and error, to find drugs that might alleviate some of the clinical symptoms seen in children with autism. However, the state of the art as it existed in the late 1970s was best summed up by Dr Magda Campbell, a major researcher in drug therapy in autism, as follows:

'Psychopharmacology of autistic and schizophrenic children and adolescents is still in a primitive state. Drug studies with large samples of diagnostically homogeneous populations, controlled for age, IQ, and other pertinent variables, are almost nonexistent. There is no evidence, based on well-controlled, double-blind studies in large samples of children, that pharmacotherapy is more effective than administration of placebo or any other treatment.' (Campbell 1978)

The story of drug experimentation in children with autism goes back to the early 1950s when it was discovered that chlorpromazine was very useful in the treatment of adult psychiatric patients. Because of the success in adult schizophrenia, investigators began exploring the use of the various psychoactive agents with children who also had psychiatric symptomatology, including in some studies subgroups of patients with autism.

In studying these patients with autism there were many difficulties based on contemporary methods of clinical testing of drugs. Perhaps the most serious problem was the diagnostic confusion that existed at that time between research groups in selecting patients who met criteria for autism. Thus, the populations of children usually were not homogeneous from a clinical point of view, many studies were done without adequate controls, many were done without blind or crossover techniques, and often there was no random assignment of subjects to treatment conditions. Also, the samples studied tended to include only small numbers of patients, making statistical analysis difficult.

Age ranges in some of these studies were excessively wide, combining pre- and post-pubescent children in the same research category—a procedure which is now known to be inappropriate in evaluating drugs in children, particularly those with autism. Some of the phenothiazines, for example, appear to be relatively ineffective in young children but to help with some of the symptoms seen in young adults with autism. On the other hand, the same general principle applies to drug therapy as to all forms of therapy in autism: the younger the child, the better the results. Therefore, until a drug has been tried on very young (2- and 3-year-old) children with autistic symptoms, it should probably not be ruled out with certainty as a possible therapy.

In these early studies, initially promising drugs in tests on a few patients often would turn out to be of little more than placebo value when studied on larger groups. However, in fairness, it needs to be pointed out that since these drugs did not have adequate and stringent trials by current standards, the failure of these drugs to become accepted does not mean that future development is totally ruled out.

TABLE 22.1

Pharmacotherapy in autism—early studies

Class	Drug	Sample reference studies
Phenothiazines	Chlorpromazine	Korein *et al.* (1971), Campbell *et al.* (1972*b*)
	Trifluoperazine	Fish *et al.* (1966), Wolpert *et al.* (1967)
	Fluphenazine	Faretra *et al.* (1970), Engelhardt *et al.* (1973)
Thioxanthenes	Thiothixene	Wolpert *et al.* (1967), Campbell *et al.* (1970), Waizer *et al.* (1972)
Tricyclics	Imipramine	Campbell *et al.* (1971)
	Loxapine	Pool *et al.* (1976)
Amphetamines	Dextroamphetamine	Campbell *et al.* (1972*a*)
	Levoamphetamine	Campbell *et al.* (1976)
Ergot alkaloids	Lysergic acid diethylamide	Bender *et al.* (1963)
	Methysergide	Fish *et al.* (1969)
Indole derivative	Molindone	Campbell *et al.* (1971)
Antihistamines	Diphenhydramine	Korein *et al.* (1971)

Trials of some of these drugs were not continued because of side-effects. The low-potency neuroleptics, including chlorpromazine, were found to be associated with sedation even at low doses in children with autism. Both chlorpromazine and imipramine are associated with a decrease of the seizure threshold, putting a child with autism at higher risk of seizures (Tarjan *et al.* 1957, Petti and Campbell 1975). Since many such children are seizure-prone (see Chapter 6), the research use of these drugs has to be quite judicious. Tardive dyskinesia as a possible long-term sequela of therapy with phenothiazines was described during this period (Paulson *et al.* 1975). Even the tardive Tourette syndrome was thought to have been caused in two patients with autism as a result of a gradual tapering off of long-term therapy with thioridazine (Stahl 1980) and haloperidol (Perry *et al.* 1989*b*). Thioridazine was also found in one report of hospitalized children to be a major cause of weight gain and possibly a factor in decelerating learning. Nevertheless, thioridazine still continues to be prescribed for moderately to profoundly retarded inpatients; a recent study found that some patients with a high level of stereotypies responded to large doses of the drug (Aman and White 1988).

Drugs tested in these early years which have never been successful in gaining a major place in the pharmacopoeia of autism are listed in Table 22.1. This table, where possible, has been limited to studies that used some type of research design, as opposed to completely open, non-blind studies.

In a group of patients who have a variable syndrome rather than a single disease entity, it is important to emphasize that the failure of any individual drug to be established in a large group study does not mean that the drug might not be of value for a small subgroup of patients within the syndrome who have a specific disease process not shared by other patients with the syndrome. For example, lithium was listed along with the other drugs without established efficacy in the first edition of this book (1985); since then it has been found to be of some value in one small patient group (see below) and has been removed from the updated Table 22.1.

A full discussion of the methodological problems of these early drug studies can be seen in the writings of Magda Campbell (1975, 1978).

Before leaving the subject of unestablished treatments for patients with autism we should mention the attempt at haemodialysis. Prior to 1980, there was some evidence to suggest that dialysis might have been helpful in some adults with chronic schizophrenia (Varley *et al.* 1979). However, a course of ten weekly haemodialyses on a young adult female with autism had no therapeutic effect (Varley *et al.* 1980).

More current views

As years of experience built up and increasingly sophisticated research trials of drugs were undertaken, the issue of drug therapy for children with autism began to clarify. Factors of efficacy and safety began to be sorted out by experience and published studies. More selective use of drug regimens—for specific age-groups or specific targeted symptoms—are in process of development.

In the last decade, as DSM-III (American Psychiatric Association 1980) became a standard diagnostic tool, different criteria of diagnosis in different studies were no longer a stumbling block. There was also a great deal of thought paid to research design of drug trials, attempting to get clearer answers at the end of each study (Campbell 1987). Assessment instruments, although no single one is consistently used in all studies, are also more comparable, and their strengths and weaknesses are better understood. As the efficacy of some drug therapies began to emerge from studies, it became possible to shift attention to the important issue of safety in children.

These pharmacological studies have become much more sophisticated and have begun to examine clinical subgroups of patients. Consideration is now given to the age of the child, the initial severity of the illness, the level of intellectual functioning, and, in many studies, to patterns of symptoms or target symptoms. Even the biochemistry of the patient may now have some relevance to the choice of a drug.

A list of investigators who have studied the main drugs administered to patients with autism in recent years is given in Table 22.2.

Haloperidol and pimozide

Haloperidol is a very potent neuroleptic and a virtually pure D2 dopamine receptor antagonist. In the late 1970s and early '80s it appeared to be a very promising drug

TABLE 22.2

Pharmacotherapy in autism—modern studies

Haloperidol	*Fenfluramine*
Campbell *et al.* (1978)	Geller *et al.* (1982)
Cohen *et al.* (1980)	Ritvo *et al.*(1983, 1984, 1986)
Naruse *et al.* (1982)	Gastaut (1984)
Anderson *et al.* (1984, 1989)	August *et al.* (1985)
Perry *et al.* (1985, 1989*a*,*b*)	Beisler *et al.* (1986)
Locascio *et al.* (1991)	Campbell *et al.* (1986*a*, 1987, 1988*b*)
Malone *et al.* (1991)	Ho *et al.* (1986)
	Piggott *et al.* (1986)
Lithium	Realmuto *et al.* (1986)
Campbell *et al.* (1972*a*)	Stubbs *et al.* (1986)
Gram and Rafaelson (1972)	Barthélémy *et al.* (1988)
Kerbeshian *et al.* (1987)	Aman and Kern (1989)
Steingard and Biederman (1987)	Bruneau *et al.* (1989)
	Ekman *et al.* (1989)
Naltrexone	Martineau *et al.* (1989)
Herman *et al.* (1986, 1987)	Sherman *et al.* (1989)
Campbell *et al.* (1986*b*, 1988*c*, 1989, 1990*a*)	Sloman (1991)
Leboyer *et al.* (1988, 1990)	
Walters *et al.* (1990)	*Pimozide*
Panksepp and Lensing (1991)	Naruse *et al.* (1982)
Scifo *et al.* (1991)	

for autism. Systematic studies of haloperidol under double-blind conditions demonstrated its superiority over placebo in decreasing hyperactivity, temper tantrums, irritability, stereotypies and withdrawal (see Table 22.2). These studies found it effective not only in controlling negative behaviours such as stereotypies, but also in improving discrimination learning (Anderson *et al.* 1984) and the positive effects of behaviour therapy (Campbell *et al.* 1978). A later short-term study by the same group who reported improvement in learning failed to confirm this finding but did replicate significant reduction of negative behaviours (Anderson *et al.* 1989).

However, these hopes were diminished when it was discovered that 25 to 30 per cent of children with autism treated with haloperidol developed early forms of tardive dyskinesia after they had been on the drug for two years (Perry *et al.* 1985). A literature developed studying tardive dyskinesia due to neuroleptics in children with autism and differentiating pretreatment stereotypies from tardive and withdrawal dyskinesias (Campbell *et al.* 1988*a*, 1990*b*; Meiselas *et al.* 1989). Some patients appeared more at risk for developing repeated episodes of dyskinesia following haloperidol withdrawal; in this group of children, each subsequent episode of dyskinesia tended to occur increasingly earlier and to last longer (Malone *et al.* 1991). The tardive dyskinesia has proved reversible in most reported cases. Also, there was a case of neuroleptic malignant syndrome in a 10-year-old girl with autism, caused by haloperidol and chlorpromazine, with altered consciousness persisting for months; it was finally reversed by amantadine (Horikawa *et al.*

1989). It was disappointing that these serious side-effects developed, because halo-peridol remained effective as long-term treatment for certain severe behavioural symptoms such as temper tantrums, aggressive and self-mutilating behaviours (Perry *et al.* 1989*a*).

Pimozide, another neuroleptic, was included in a study of 35 individuals with autism; there was a significant reduction of some forms of aggression in this study, both with pimozide and haloperidol (Naruse *et al.* 1982).

Because of the side-effects, particularly tardive dyskinesia, these neuroleptics are generally no longer recommended for people with autism (Gualtieri 1991). The use of haloperidol is now not considered unless the patient's medical work-up is unrevealing, more benign therapies have failed and the child's behavioural problems make management extremely difficult. In that limited situation, it should be used in combination with behaviour therapy and be time-limited.

Fenfluramine and buspirone
As it became more apparent that it was important to find a drug not associated with tardive dyskinesia, interest increased in fenfluramine. With only one exception—a dystonic reaction of the muscles of the neck, tongue and throat following a single dose (Sananman 1974)—fenfluramine did not induce tardive dyskinesia, although of course it had its own side-effects.

Fenfluramine entered the pool of drugs for autism with a splash. Three boys were reported in an open study to have improved cognitive and social functioning, including a child whose IQ was said to have doubled (Geller *et al.* 1982). This single uncontrolled report was then followed by a multicentre study involving 81 patients (Ritvo *et al.* 1986) and a series of additional studies (see Table 22.2). These studies used a fixed dose of fenfluramine of 1.5mg/kg/day and a crossover design, except for the study by Campbell *et al.* (1988*b*) which employed a parallel groups design, random assignment of patients to treatment conditions and a flexible dose schedule (1.25 to 2.068mg/kg/day), as well as multiple raters and multiple rating scales.

One main reason that interest in fenfluramine escalated so quickly when its effects were first reported was related to its effect on serotonin. Serotonin levels had been found to be elevated in the platelets of more than one quarter of many populations of children with autism (see Chapter 10). Originally introduced as a diet pill, an atypical stimulant with structural similarity to amphetamine, fenfluramine was also classified as a serotonin antagonist in rats (Costa *et al.* 1971). Many studies have shown decreasing levels of serotonin in rat brains with increasing doses of fenfluramine. Studies with patients with autism have further supported earlier literature; these studies showed that the level of serotonin bound in the platelets in the blood in children with autism dropped while the drug was taken, and rebounded, sometimes even higher than baseline, when it was discontinued. It seemed that a simple and rational drug therapy—based on the biochemistry of a patient with autism—had been located.

Or had it? The two assumptions underlying this concept are that (1) serotonin antagonists in experiments with rats have the same effect in humans, and (2) the level of serotonin in the human platelet is likely to be similar to the level in the human CNS. Regarding the first assumption, the actual mechanism of serotonin at the neurons (stimulating serotonin release and then inhibiting its uptake—Garrattini *et al.* 1975) is the pattern seen in drugs classified as agonists, not antagonists: if anything, the *functional* level of serotonin in the human CNS could be increased rather than decreased by fenfluramine, depending on dose level. Regarding the second assumption that levels in the platelets reflect levels in the brain, the only published autopsy data indicate just the opposite: many samplings of blood serotonin during the lifetime of a child showed consistently above-normal levels, while autopsy study disclosed below-normal levels in the CNS (Coleman *et al.* 1977). (For further review of this subject, see Chapter 10.)

Moreover, drugs are not pure targets for a single metabolic system; in the case of fenfluramine, additional effects on the catecholamine system may be observed at different dose levels. That this drug can lower serotonin levels in the platelets of patients is well demonstrated; that in the brain it may actually be causing the low levels of serotonin found in some patients with autism seems as likely a scenario as any. The effects of different neurotransmitters balance each other out; it is quite complex, depending on the systems involved and doses used. Thus the mechanism by which fenfluramine affects patients with autism is far from clear.

The results of the fenfluramine studies have been reviewed (Campbell 1988, Aman and Kern 1989, Sloman 1991). Some studies used electrophysiological measures to examine the effect of fenfluramine on children. Bruneau *et al.* (1989) reported that electrophysiological data were affected according to the clinical responsiveness to the drug; in the six (out of 13) children who were clinical responders, auditory evoked potentials increased and single-trial potential variability decreased, whereas in non-responders there was no electrophysiological modification. These six responders showed improvement in attention and a reduction of motility disorders, anxiety and mood disturbances (Martineau *et al.* 1989). (Such an approach to drug studies, if validated by other groups, offers an interesting, additional tool for evaluation of drug trials.)

Gastaut (1984) reported that fenfluramine prevented syncope self-induced by Valsalva manoeuvre in psychotic retarded children. A number of studies of fenfluramine in the USA have suggested improvements in a subgroup of the population with autism studied. These improvements were in the areas of social relatedness, reduced stereotypic behaviour, decreased hyperactivity and improved attention span; some studies even found improvement in cognitive levels. Often these findings were not substantiated by other studies (Sherman *et al.* 1989); for example, an increase rather than a decrease in stereotypic behaviours has been noted (Piggott *et al.* 1986). The study by Campbell *et al.* (1988*b*) even suggested that the drug may have a negative effect on cognition.

There have been many reports of side-effects to fenfluramine treatment. These include anorexia, transient weight loss, lethargy, irritability, sleep difficulties and gastrointestinal symptoms. More troubling is the experimentl literature which suggests that one of the effects of fenfluramine on serotonin terminals or cell bodies might be irreversible (Harvey *et al.* 1975, Schuster *et al.* 1986, Molliver and Molliver 1990). Of greatest concern are the changes in the hippocampal serotonin nerve terminals.

Sloman (1991) has summarized the present situation regarding fenfluramine as follows: 'Fenfluramine may cause improvement in social behavior, excessive motor behavior, and attention span in some autistic children, but these changes are of limited magnitude and, because of the unresolved issue about its safety, its use can be justified only under stringent research conditions.'

Another research drug that has appeared on the scene is buspirone, an antianxiety drug that has been tried on children with autism because of its antiserotonergic properties. It is a $5HT_{1A}$ receptor agonist with an α_2-adrenergic antagonist metabolite. It has been tried on only four children with autism to date in crossover comparison with fenfluramine and methylphenidate (Realmuto *et al.* 1989). Two of the four children showed some improvement; no side-effects were observed.

Naltrexone

Some of the symptoms of autism seem to mimic those seen in opiate addicts, such as labile affect, insensitivity to pain and withdrawal stereotypies. There is also some early evidence of abnormalities of peripheral and central endogenous opioids in patients with autism (see Chapter 10). This has led to trials of naltrexone, a potent and long-acting opioid antagonist, in small groups of patients. Early reports were encouraging, suggesting that withdrawal, fidgety behaviour, hyperactivity, uncooperative behaviour and stereotypies may be improved (see Table 22.2).

The optimum dose of naltrexone has yet to be determined; at this point, it appears that lower doses (0.5 to 1.0mg/kg) may be more effective than higher ones. In one double-blind study, no correlation was found between clinical status and plasma endorphin levels (Scifo *et al.* 1991). Based on studies to date, Campbell *et al.* (1988*c*, 1990*a*) find the drug not very powerful but also without many side-effects. It is interesting to note that serotonin modulates the opioid pathway in humans.

Self-injurious behaviour is one of the most difficult symptoms to treat in patients with autism. Whatever the long-term outcome of naltrexone as a treatment for other milder symptoms in autism, it may well play a part for occasional selected patients with severe self-injurious behaviour (Herman *et al.* 1987, Leboyer *et al.* 1988, Walters *et al.* 1990).

Lithium carbonate

Is a bipolar affective disorder (manic–depressive illness) coexistent with or part of the autistic syndrome in some patients? Trials of lithium in patients with autism started as early as 1972 and are still continuing intermittently as patients are selected for this therapy. The literature, reviewed in Table 22.2, is sparse but suggests that in patients who have symptoms of a bipolar disorder, there is a chance that aggression or manic symptoms may respond.

Other drugs

BETA BLOCKERS

The beta blockers—propranolol, nadolol, and atenolol—have been studied in individuals with autism and associated severe problems, such as rages, self-injurious behaviour or aggressiveness, that were resistant to more standard treatments. The trials were small open pilot studies, often with continuing use of other psychotropic agents such as neuroleptics necessary during the clinical trial. Ratey et al. (1987a,b) have reported good response, with rapid diminution of aggressiveness and even some speech improvements in eight consecutive adults with autism. Further studies are indicated under controlled conditions, since the beta blockers may be a tool for some of the most intractible symptoms seen in patients with autism.

BROMOCRIPTINE

Bromocriptine is a dopaminergic agonist. Despite the failure of trials of L-dopa in patients with autism (see Chapter 23), Simon-Soret and Borenstein (1987) tried bromocriptine. They reported improvement in patients with autism after an open trial of 7.5mg/day.

CLOMIPRAMINE

Some children with autism have symptoms similar to those seen in the obessive–compulsive disorders. Clomipramine, a serotonin re-uptake blocker, has been helpful to patients with obessions and compulsions, an effect which appears to be separate from its antidepressant properties. Thus it seemed like a reasonable drug to try with patients with autism who had those symptoms. Gordon et al. (1990) conducted a double-blind crossover trial on six children with autism with compulsive symptoms and found a good response. Further studies appear to be warranted.

METHYLPHENIDATE

Hyperactivity is often a problem in children with autism, and is treated in other paediatric groups with stimulant drugs. Although studies of the use of D- and L-amphetamine in children with autism (Campbell et al. 1972a, 1976) demonstrated decreased hyperactivity, the positive effects were outweighed by negative effects on irritability, stereotypies and cognition. Two trials of methylphenidate (Hoshino et al. 1977, Birmaher et al. 1988) both reported benefit to some children with autism. However, there has been some criticism of these studies related to shortcomings in research design, and further controlled trials are called for.

Seizure disorders

The surprisingly high incidence of epilepsy in the population of patients with autism was reviewed in Chapter 6. When a patient has a first seizure, an evaluation should be done to try to determine the aetiology of the seizure. The risk of recurrence of a single, unprovoked afebrile generalized tonic–clonic seizure in children is less than 50 per cent (Camfield *et al.* 1984). If therapy is needed, classification of the type of seizure may help choose the most effective drug. In choosing an anticonvulsant drug, considerations of effectiveness, effects on cognition, growth and development, incidence and severity of known side-effects, cost and frequency of monitoring all enter into the decision.

Barbiturate anticonvulsants, such as phenobarbitone, can cause or increase hyperactivity in children with autism, and should be avoided. Phenytoin, another common anticonvulsant, may also have behavioural toxicity and affect long-term learning. Usually the best anticonvulsants for children with autism are carbamazepine, valproic acid or acetazolamide. It is even possible that these anticonvulsants might be of value for some of the symptoms of autism, but this has not been established by adequate studies. No drug is without side-effects: anticonvulsants need to be closely monitored and given with care.

Conclusion

A recent review of the use of drugs in patients with autistic symptoms questions whether pharmacotherapy has any value at all (Sloman 1991). When discussing naltrexone, the author argues, 'Although a good rationale exists for trying naltrexone, there is an equally good rationale for arguing that autism cannot be effectively treated with any medication.'

A generation of hard-working investigators have failed to find a major drug to treat autism. Since it is a disorder with so many different aetiologies, this is perhaps unsurprising. However, the value of psychopharmacology in treating some deeply troubling symptoms is already known; a number of new drugs with target symptoms (*e.g.* rage, compulsions) may be on the horizon. In the end, as in all other disciplines of medicine, treatment must come out of specific and precise diagnosis of each patient.

REFERENCES

Aman, M.G., Kern, R.A. (1989) 'Review of fenfluramine in the treatment of the developmental disabilities.' *Journal of the American Academy of Child and Adolescent Psychiatry*, **28**, 549–565.
—— White, A.J. (1988) 'Thioridazine dose effects with reference to stereotypic behavior in mentally retarded residents.' *Journal of Autism and Developmental Disorders*, **18**, 355–366.
American Psychiatric Association (1980) *Diagnostic and Statistical Manual of Mental Disorders (DSM-III)*, *3rd Edn.* Washington, DC: APA.
Anderson, L.T., Campbell, M., Grega, D.M., Perry, R., Small, A.M., Green, W.H. (1984) 'Haloperidol in the treatment of infantile autism: effects on learning and behavioral symptoms.' *American Journal of Psychiatry*, **141**, 1195–1202.
—— —— Adams, P., Small, A.M., Perry, R., Shell, J. (1989) 'The effects of haloperidol on discrimination learning and behavioral symptoms in autistic children.' *Journal of Autism and*

Developmental Disorders, **19**, 227–239.

August, G.J., Raz, N., Baird, T.D. (1985) 'Brief report: Effects of fenfluramine on behavioral, cognitive and affective disturbances in autistic children.' *Journal of Autism and Developmental Disorders*, **15**, 97–107.

Barthélémy, C., Bruneau, N., Garreau, B., Lelord, G., Martineau, J., Roux, S. (1988) 'Auditory evoked potential modifications in autistic children under DL-fenfluramine treatment: relationships with behavioral and biochemical responsiveness.' *Journal of Physiology*, **406**, 183P. *(Abstract.)*

Beisler, J.M., Tsai, L.Y., Stiefel, B. (1986) 'Brief report: the effects of fenfluramine on communication skills in autistic children.' *Journal of Autism and Developmental Disorders*, **16**, 227–233.

Bender, L., Faretra, G., Cobrinik, L. (1963) 'LSD and UML treatment of hospitalized disturbed children.' *In:* Wortis, J. (Ed.) *Recent Advances in Biological Psychiatry, Vol. 5.* New York: Plenum, pp. 84–92.

Birmaher, B., Quintana, H., Greenhill, L.L. (1988) 'Methylphenidate treatment of hyperactive autistic children.' *Journal of the American Academy of Child and Adolescent Psychiatry*, **27**, 248–251.

Bruneau, N., Barthélémy, C., Roux, S., Jouve, J., Lelord, G. (1989) 'Auditory evoked potential modifications according to clinical and biochemical responsiveness to fenfluramine treatment in children with autistic behavior.' *Neuropsychobiology*, **21**, 48–52.

Camfield, P.R., Camfield, C.S., Dooley, J.M., Tibbles, A.R.T., Garner, B., Fung, T. (1984) 'Recurrence after a first unprovoked afebrile seizure in childhood.' *Annals of Neurology*, **16**, 379. *(Abstract.)*

Campbell, M. (1975) 'Pharmacotherapy in early infantile autism.' *Biological Psychiatry*, **10**, 399–423.

—— (1978) 'Pharmacotherapy.' *In:* Rutter, M., Schopler, E. (Eds) *Autism: a Reappraisal of Concepts and Treatment.* New York: Plenum, pp. 337–355.

—— (1987) 'Drug treatment of infantile autism: the past decade.' *In:* Meltzer, H.Y. (Ed.) *Psychopharmacology: the Third Generation of Progress.* New York: Raven Press, pp. 1225–1231.

—— (1988) 'Fenfluramine treatment of autism.' *Journal of Child Psychology and Psychiatry*, **29**, 1–10. *(Annotation.)*

—— (1989) 'Pharmacotherapy in autism: an overview.' *In:* Gillberg, C. (Ed.) *Diagnosis and Treatment of Autism.* New York: Plenum, pp. 203–217.

—— Schopler, E. (1987) 'Pervasive developmental disorders.' *In: Psychiatric Treatment Manual I (PTM-I), APA Task Force on Treatment of Psychiatric Disorders.* Washington, DC: American Psychiatric Association, p. 294.

—— Fish, B., Shapiro, T., Floyd, A. (1970) 'Thiothixene in young disturbed children: a pilot study.' *Archives of General Psychiatry*, **23**, 70–72.

—— —— —— —— (1971) 'Study of molindone in disturbed preschool children.' *Current Therapeutic Research*, **13**, 28–33.

—— David, R., Shapiro, T., Collins, P., Koh, C. (1972a) 'Response to triiodothyronine and dextroamphetamine: a study of preschool schizophrenic children.' *Journal of Autism and Childhood Schizophrenia*, **2**, 343–358.

—— Shapiro, T., Floyd, A. (1972b) 'Acute responses of schizophrenic children to a sedative and a "stimulating" neuroleptic: a pharmacologic yardstick.' *Current Therapeutic Research*, **14**, 759–766.

—— Small, A.M., Collins, P.J., Friedman, E., David, R., Genieser, N. (1976) 'Levodopa and levoamphetamine: a crossover study among young schizophrenic children.' *Current Therapeutic Research*, **19**, 70–86.

—— Anderson, L.T., Meier, M., Cohen, I.L., Small, A.M., Samit, C., Sachar, E.J. (1978) 'A comparison of haloperidol, behavior therapy and their interaction in autistic children.' *Journal of the American Academy of Child Psychiatry*, **17**, 640–655.

—— Perry, R., Polonsky, B.B., Deutsch, S.I., Palij, M., Lukashok, D. (1986a) 'Brief report: an open study of fenfluramine in hospitalized young autistic children.' *Journal of Autism and Developmental Disorders*, **16**, 495–506.

—— Sokol, M.S., Small, A.M., Palij, M., Perry, R., Nobler, M., Addrizzo, D. (1986b) 'Naltrexone in autistic children: an acute open dose study.' *In: Scientific Proceedings for the Annual Meeting of the American Academy of Child and Adolescent Psychiatry*, **2**, 34.

—— Small, A.M., Palij, M., Perry, R., Polonsky, B.B., Lukashok, D., Anderson, L.T. (1987) 'The efficacy and safety of fenfluramine in autistic children: preliminary analysis of a double-blind study.' *Psychopharmacology Bulletin*, **23**, 123–127.

267

—— Adams, P., Perry, R., Spencer, E.K., Overall, J.E. (1988a) 'Tardive and withdrawal dyskinesias in autistic children: a prospective study.' *Psychopharmacology Bulletin*, **24**, 251–255.

—— —— —— Curren, E.L., Overall, J.E., Anderson, L.T., Lynch, N., Perry, R. (1988b) 'Efficacy and safety of fenfluramine in autistic children.' *Journal of the American Academy of Child and Adolescent Psychiatry*, **27**, 434–439.

—— —— Small, A.M., Tesch, L.M., Curren, E.L. (1988c) 'Naltrexone in infantile autism.' *Psychopharmacology Bulletin*, **24**, 135–139.

—— Overall, J.E., Small, A.M., Sokol, M.S., Spencer, E.K., Adams, P., Foltz, R., Manti, K.M., Perry, R., Nobler, M., *et al.* (1989) 'Naltrexone in autistic children: an acute open dose range tolerance trial.' *Journal of the American Academy of Child and Adolescent Psychiatry*, **28**, 200–206.

—— Anderson, L.T., Small, A.S., Locascio, J.J., Lynch, N.S., Choroco, M.C. (1990a) 'Naltrexone in autistic children: a double-blind and placebo-controlled study.' *Psychopharmacology Bulletin*, **26**, 130–135.

—— Locascio, J.J., Choroco, M.C., Spencer, E.K., Malone, R.P., Kafantaris, V., Overall, J.E. (1990b) 'Stereotypies and tardive dyskinesia: abnormal movements in autistic children.' *Psychopharmacology Bulletin*, **26**, 260–266.

Cohen, I.L., Campbell, M., Posner, D., Small, A.M., Triebel, D., Anderson, L.T. (1980) 'Behavioral effects of haloperidol in young autistic children.' *Journal of the American Academy of Child Psychiatry*, **19**, 665–677.

Coleman, M., Hart, P.N., Randall, J., Lee, J., Hijada, D., Bratenahl, C.G. (1977) 'Serotonin levels in the blood and central nervous system of a patient with sudanophilic leukodystrophy.' *Neuropädiatrie*, **8**, 459–466.

Costa, E., Groppetti, A., Revuelta, A. (1971) 'Action of fenfluramine on monoamine stores of rat tissues.' *British Journal of Pharmacology*, **41**, 57–64.

Ekman, G., Miranda-Linne, F., Gillberg, C., Garle, M., Wetterberg, L. (1989) 'Fenfluramine treatment of twenty children with autism.' *Journal of Autism and Developmental Disorders*, **19**, 511–532.

Engelhardt, D.M., Polizos, P., Waizer, J., Hoffman, S.P. (1973) 'A double-blind comparison of fluphenazine and haloperidol in outpatient schizophrenic children.' *Journal of Autism and Childhood Schizophrenia*, **3**, 128–137.

Faretra, G., Dooher, L., Dowling, J. (1970) 'Comparison of haloperidol and fluphenazine in disturbed children.' *American Journal of Psychiatry*, **126**, 1670–1673.

Fish, B., Shapiro, T., Campbell, M. (1966) 'Long-term prognosis and the response of schizophrenic children to drug therapy: a controlled study of trifluoperazine.' *American Journal of Psychiatry*, **123**, 32–39.

—— Floyd, A. (1969) 'Schizophrenic children treated with methysergide (Sansert).' *Diseases of the Nervous System*, **30**, 534–540.

Garrattini, S., Jori, A., Buczko, W., Samanin, R. (1975) 'The mechanism of action of fenfluramine.' *Postgraduate Medical Journal*, **51** (Suppl. 1), 27–35.

Gastaut, H. (1984) 'Efficacité de la fenfluramine pour le traitement des troubles comportmentaux compulsifs des enfants psychotiques.' *Presse Medicale*, **13**, 2024–2025. *(Letter.)*

Geller, E., Ritvo, E.R., Freeman, B.J., Yuwiler, A. (1982) 'Preliminary observations on the effect of fenfluramine on blood serotonin and symptoms in three autistic boys.' *New England Journal of Medicine*, **307**, 165–169.

Gordon, C., Rapoport, J., Hamburger, M.S., Mannheim, G. (1990) *In: Proceedings of the Annual Meeting of the American Academy of Child and Adolescent Psychiatry.*

Gram, L.F., Rafaelsen, O.J., (1972) 'Lithium treatment of psychiatric children and adolescents: a controlled clinical trial.' *Acta Psychiatrica Scandinavica*, **48**, 253–260.

Gualtieri, C.T. (1991) 'The neuropsychiatric treatment of autistic people.' *In: Postgraduate Advances in Autism Disorder*. Berryville, VA: Forum Medicum, pp. 1–11.

Harvey, J.A., McMaster, S.F., Yunger, L.M. (1975) 'p-Chloroamphetamine: selective neurotoxic action in the brain.' *Science*, **187**, 841–843.

Herman, B.H., Hammock, M.K., Arthur-Smith, A., Egan, J., Chatoor, I., Zelnik, N., Appelgate, K., Beockx, R.L. (1986) 'Effects of naltrexone in autism: correlation with plasma opioid concentrations.' *Scientific Proceedings for the Annual Meeting of the American Academy of Child and Adolescent Psychiatry*, **2**, 11–12.

268

——— ——— ——— ——— Werner, A., Zelnik, N. (1987) 'Naltrexone decreases self-injurious behavior.' *Annals of Neurology*, **22**, 550–552.

Ho, H.H., Lockitch, G., Eaves, L., Jacobson, B. (1986) 'Blood serotonin concentrations and fenfluramine therapy in autistic children.' *Journal of Pediatrics*, **108**, 465–469.

Horikawa, M., Ninomiya, M., Nishi, M., Ando, H., Yamashita, Y., Terasawa, K., Katafuchi, Y. (1989) 'A ten-year-old autistic girl with neuroleptic malignant syndrome caused by neuroleptic agents.' *No To Hattatsu*, **21**, 486–490. *(In Japanese.)*

Hoshino, Y., Kumashiro, H., Keneko, M., Takahashi, Y. (1977) 'The effects of methylphenidate on early infantile autism and its relation to serum serotonin levels.' *Folia Psychiatrica Neurologica Japonica*, **31**, 605–614.

Kerbeshian, J., Burd, L., Fisher, W. (1987) 'Lithium carbonate in the treatment of two patients with infantile autism and atypical bipolar symptomatology.' *Journal of Clinical Psychopharmacology*, **7**, 401–405.

Korein, J., Fish, B., Shapiro, T., Gerner, E.W., Levidow, L. (1971) 'EEG and behavioral effects of drug therapy in children: chlorpromazine and diphenhydramine.' *Archives of General Psychiatry*, **24**, 552–563.

Leboyer, M., Bouvard, M.P., Dugas, M. (1988) 'Effects of naltrexone on infantile autism.' *Lancet*, **i**, 715. *(Letter.)*

——— ——— Lensing, P., Launay, J-M., Tabuteau, F., Arnaud, P., Waller, D., Plumet, M-H., Recasens, C., Kerdelhue, B., *et al.* (1990) 'The opioid excess hypothesis of autism: a double-blind study of naltrexone.' *Brain Dysfunction*, **3**, 285–298.

Locascio, J.J., Malone, R.P., Small, A.M., Kafantaris, V., Ernst, M., Lynch, N.S., Overall, J.E., Campbell, M. (1991) 'Factors related to haloperidol response and dyskinesias in autistic children.' *Psychopharmacology Bulletin*, **27**, 119–126.

Malone, R.P., Ernst, M., Godfrey, K.A., Locascio, J.J., Campbell, M. (1991) 'Repeated episodes of neuroleptic-related dyskinesias in autistic children.' *Psychopharmacology Bulletin*, **27**, 113–117.

Martineau, J., Barthélémy, C., Roux, S., Garreau, B., Lelord, G. (1989) 'Electrophysiological effects of fenfluramine or combined vitamin B_6 and magnesium on children with autistic behaviour.' *Developmental Medicine and Child Neurology*, **31**, 721–727.

Meiselas, K.D., Spencer, E.K., Oberfield, R., Peselow, E.D., Angrist, B., Campbell, M. (1989) 'Differentiation of stereotypies from neuroleptic-related dyskinesias in autistic children.' *Journal of Clinical Psychopharmacology*, **9**, 207–209.

Molliver, D.C., Molliver, M.E. (1990) 'Anatomical evidence for a neurotoxic effect of ($\pm$) fenfluramine upon serotonergic projections in the rat.' *Brain Research*, **511**, 165–168.

Naruse, H., Nagahata, M., Nakane, Y., Shirahashi, K., Takesada, M., Yamazaki, K. (1982) 'A multicenter double-blind trial of pimozide (Orap), haloperidol and placebo in children with behavioural disorders, using crossover design.' *Acta Paedopsychiatrica*, **48**, 173–184.

Panksepp, J., Lensing, P. (1991) 'Brief report: a synopsis of an open-trial of naltrexone treatment of autism in four children.' *Journal of Autism and Developmental Disorders*, **21**, 243–249.

Paulson, G.W., Rizvi, C.A., Crane, G.E. (1975) 'Tardive dyskinesia as a possible sequel of long-term therapy with phenothiazines.' *Clinical Pediatrics*, **14**, 953–955.

Perry, R., Campbell, M., Green, W.H., Small, A.M., Die Trill, M.L., Meiselas, K., Golden, R.R., Deutsch, S.I. (1985) 'Neuroleptic-related dyskinesias in autistic children: a prospective study.' *Psychopharmacology Bulletin*, **21**, 140–143.

——— ——— Adams, P., Lynch, N., Spencer, E.K., Curren, E.L., Overall, J.E. (1989*a*) 'Long-term efficacy of haloperidol in autistic children: continuous versus discontinuous drug administration.' *Journal of the American Academy of Child and Adolescent Psychiatry*, **28**, 87–92.

——— Nobler, M.S., Campbell, M. (1989*b*) 'Case report: Tourette-like symptoms associated with chronic neuroleptic therapy in an autistic child.' *Journal of the American Academy of Child and Adolescent Psychiatry*, **28**, 93–96.

Petti, T.A., Campbell, M. (1975) 'Imipramine and seizures.' *American Journal of Psychiatry*, **132**, 538–539.

Piggott, L.R., Gdowski, C.L., Villanueva, D., Fischhoff, J., Frohman, C.F. (1986) 'Side effects of fenfluramine in autistic children.' *Journal of the American Academy of Child and Adolescent Psychiatry*, **25**, 287–289.

Pool, D., Bloom, W., Mielke, D.H., Roniger, J.J., Gallant, D.M. (1976) 'A controlled evaluation of

269

Loxitane in 75 adolescent schizophrenic patients.' *Current Therapeutic Research*, **19**, 99–104.

Ratey, J.J., Bemporad, J., Sorgi, P., Bick, P., Polakoff, S., O'Driscoll, G., Mikkelsen, E. (1987*a*) 'Brief report: open trial effects of beta-blockers on speech and social behaviors in 8 autistic adults.' *Journal of Autism and Developmental Disorders*, **17**, 439–446.

—— Mikkelsen, E.J., Sorgi, P., Zuckerman, S., Polakoff, S., Bemporad, J., Bick, P., Kadish, W. (1987*b*) 'Autism: the treatment of aggressive behaviors.' *Journal of Clinical Psychopharmacology*, **7**, 35–41.

Realmuto, G.M., Jensen, J., Klykylo, W., Piggott, L., Stubbs, B., Yuwiler, A., Geller, E., Freeman, B.J., Ritvo, E. (1986) 'Untoward effects of fenfluramine in autistic children.' *Journal of Clinical Psychopharmacology*, **6**, 350–355.

—— August, G.J., Garfinkel, B.D. (1989) 'Clinical effect of buspirone in autistic children.' *Journal of Clinical Psychopharmacology*, **9**, 122–125.

Ritvo, E.R., Freeman, B.J., Geller, E., Yuwiler, A. (1983) 'Effects of fenfluramine on 14 outpatients with the syndrome of autism.' *Journal of the American Academy of Child Psychiatry*, **22**, 549–558.

—— —— Yuwiler, A., Geller, E., Yokota, A., Schroth, P., Novak, P. (1984) 'Study of fenfluramine in outpatients with the syndrome of autism.' *Journal of Pediatrics*, **105**, 823–829.

—— —— —— Schroth, P., Yokota, A., Mason-Brothers, A., August, G.J., Klykylo, W., Leventhal, B., *et al.* (1986) 'Fenfluramine treatment of autism: UCLA collaborative study of 81 patients at nine medical centers.' *Psychopharmacology Bulletin*, **22**, 133–140.

Sananman, M.L. (1974) 'Dyskinesia after fenfluramine.' *New England Journal of Medicine*, **291**, 422. *(Letter.)*

Schuster, C.R., Lewis, M., Seiden, L.S. (1986) 'Fenfluramine: neurotoxicity.' *Psychopharmacology Bulletin*, **22**, 148–151.

Scifo, R., Battecane, N., Quattropani, M.C., Spoto, G., Marchetti, B. (1991) 'A double blind trial with naltrexone.' *Brain Dysfunction. (In press.)*

Sherman, J., Factor, D.C., Swinson, R., Darjes, R.W. (1989) 'The effects of fenfluramine (hydrochloride) on the behavior of fifteen autistic children.' *Journal of Autism and Developmental Disorders*, **19**, 533–544.

Simon-Soret, C., Borenstein, P. (1987) 'Essai de la bromocriptine dans le traitement de l'autisme infantile.' *Presse Medicale*, **16**, 1286.

Sloman, L. (1991) 'Use of medication in pervasive developmental disorder.' *Pediatric Clinics of North America*, **14**, 165–182.

Stahl, S.M. (1980) 'Tardive Tourette syndrome in an autistic patient after long-term neuroleptic administration.' *American Journal of Psychiatry*, **137**, 1267–1269.

Steingard, R., Biederman, J. (1987) 'Lithium responsive manic-like symptoms in two individuals with autism and mental retardation: case report.' *Journal of the American Academy of Child and Adolescent Psychiatry*, **26**, 932–935.

Stubbs, E.G., Budden, S.S., Jackson, R.H., Terdal, L.G., Ritvo, E.R. (1986) 'Effects of fenfluramine on eight outpatients with the syndrome of autism.' *Developmental Medicine and Child Neurology*, **28**, 229–235.

Tarjan, C., Lowery, V.E., Wright, S.W. (1957) 'Use of chlorpromazine in two hundred seventy-eight mentally deficient patients.' *American Journal of Diseases of Children*, **94**, 294–300.

Varley, C., Kolff, C., Trupin, E., Reichler, R.J. (1979) 'Proposed study of hemodialysis as a treatment for early autism.' *Journal of Autism and Developmental Disorders*, **9**, 305–306.

—— —— —— —— (1980) 'Hemodialysis as a treatment for infantile autism.' *Journal of Autism and Developmental Disorders*, **10**, 399–404.

Waizer, J., Polizos, P., Hoffman, S.P., Engelhardt, D.M., Margolis, R.A. (1972) 'A single-blind evaluation of thiothixene with outpatient schizophrenic children.' *Journal of Autism and Childhood Schizophrenia*, **2**, 378–386.

Walters, A.S., Barrett, R.P., Feinstein, C., Mercurio, A., Hole, W.T. (1990) 'A case report of naltrexone treatment of self-injury and social withdrawal in autism.' *Journal of Autism and Developmental Disorders*, **20**, 169–176.

Wolpert, A., Hagamen, M.B., Merlis, S. (1967) 'A comprehensive study of thiothixene and trifluoperazine in childhood schizophrenia.' *Current Therapeutic Research*, **9**, 482–485.

270

23
OTHER MEDICAL THERAPIES

Besides drugs (discussed in Chapter 22), other medical therapies have been used to treat patients with autism. More often, these therapies are directed at a particular disease entity which causes autism or at a particular biochemical finding in a patient with autism. If a treatment is effective be it a drug or some other medical therapy, it must have pharmacological activity, so this division into two chapters is made for reasons of custom rather than actual pharmacology. Diets, amino acids, vitamins and minerals may have pharmacological efficacy in appropriate situations; they also, like drugs, may have side-effects and paradoxical effects. The choice of a medical therapy must be based on as rational as possible an approach to the overall clinical and laboratory information available on a patient.

Diets
Diet therapy for phenylketonuria
The metabolic disease phenylketonuria (PKU; see Chapter 17) was one of the first forms of mental retardation for which a successful therapy was developed. In these patients, functional levels of enyzme in the liver are inadequate to convert the first amino acid (phenylalanine) to the second (tyrosine) in the important pathway that produces catecholamines in the brain (see Fig. 10.2, p. 121). The resultant shunting off of phenylalanine to minor pathways results in the accumulation of otherwise rare metabolites; at such abnormal levels, these minor metabolites appear to be quite toxic to the brain, although the exact mechanism causing brain damage in children with untreated PKU is still not clearly defined. Treatment consists of reducing phenylalanine in the diet to the point where the intake is minute (Koch *et al.* 1970).

To be successful, the diet must be started in the first few weeks of life. If infants with PKU are identified by neonatal screening and the diet is instituted early, the patients are spared a lifetime of mental retardation (Hsia *et al.* 1958) and, in some cases, autism. To the clinician who makes the diagnosis of PKU in an older child, the question arises, is there any value in starting treatment? There is not adequate experience in starting dietary treatment at later ages. However, what literature does exist suggests that it can prevent further progression of the disability and may even have some behavioural benefit to the child (Lewis 1959, Grüter 1963, Lowe *et al.* 1980). Major reversal seems out of the question. Variations on the diet, such as low-protein diets or new, more palatable phenylalanine-free dietary supplements, are alternative therapies currently under investigation for older patients. For example, with Product 196, subjective behavioural improvement was noted in six of ten older PKU subjects; no significant changes in intelligence were noted (Crowley *et al.* 1990).

This form of autism should be a disease entity of the past wherever adequate neonatal screening exists. Yet, some countries do not yet have such screening programmes, and unfortunately, even where they do exist, they can miss PKU in up to 20 per cent of liveborn infants (Sepe *et al.* 1979). The problem of treatment of older children with PKU and autistic symptoms is still with us.

Research diet therapies

A few patients with autism have been described with lactic acidosis (see Chapter 17). A case history of a boy with autism and lactic acidosis who responded to the ketogenic diet has been published (Coleman 1989). Research currently underway appears to have found an intermittent deficiency in the pyruvate dehydrogenase complex in this child. A single case is a preliminary finding; the value and type of dietary treatment in this subgroup of patients with autism still needs to be established.

In several countries a large subgroup of children with autism have been found to have hyperuricosuria (see Chapter 17). A research therapy, the administration of the purine compound adenosine, is being tried in one subgroup of these children with a demonstated adenylosuccinate lyase metabolic error. For the great majority of children who have hyperuricosuria yet do not have this metabolic error, the only available therapy at this time is a trial of a low purine diet, a diet which is reported to have been helpful in at least one child with autism; however, it has no effect on most patients (Coleman 1989). Exact treatment will depend, in the future, upon the determination in each patient of the specific aetiology of the hyperuricosuria.

Is there a subgroup of patients with autism whose autistic symptoms are related to malabsorption and/or food allergies? Do some such patients need to be on diets that avoid wheat or other foods? Some children with autism have been diagnosed by their paediatricians as having coeliac disease, malabsorption or food allergies. Although it is clear that patients occasionally have steatorrhoea (Goodwin *et al.* 1971) and that these same patients may have hypocalcinuria (Coleman *et al.* 1976), the only specific study of gluten sensitivity in autism was negative. After being loaded with gluten for weeks, jejunal biopsy of children with autism whose parents gave a history of wheat sensitivity showed no evidence of coeliac disease (McCarthy and Coleman 1979). Food allergies are an area of controversy in the field of gastroenterology. A case study of a 9-year-old retarded boy with autistic behaviours failed to show that suspected dietary substances had any effect on his behaviour (Bird *et al.* 1977). A double-blind, crossover study has shown benefit to some hyperactive children of food withdrawal diets (Egger *et al.* 1985) but there has been no comparable study in autism.

Experimental administration of amino acids

Several studies have been conducted on the results of the administration of L-dopa in autism, given to enhance dopamine levels (see Fig. 10.2, p. 121). The first one studied the effect of L-dopa over a six-month period; no changes were observed in the clinical course, measures of endocrine function or the percentage of REM sleep (Ritvo *et al.* 1971). The next studies also included administration of the dopamine agonists D-amphetamine and L-amphetamine (Campbell *et al.* 1972, 1976). Again, no clinical improvements were found; in fact, there was worsening and development of new sterotypies. A more recent trial of L-dopa therapy was not promising (Segawa *et al.* 1987). (On the other hand, dopamine antagonists, such as haloperidol, appear to be of value to some patients—see Chapter 22.)

The precursor of serotonin, 5-hydroxytryptophan (see Fig. 10.1, p. 116) has also been administered to patients with autistic symptoms (Sverd *et al.* 1978, Segawa *et al.* 1987). In the first of these trials, Sverd *et al.* administered up to 500mg of 5-hydroxytryptophan, combined with a decarboxylase inhibitor designed to facilitate entrance to the brain, to three children for 20 weeks; they found no clinical improvement. Much smaller daily doses of 25 to 30mg were given by Segawa *et al.*, who reported improvement in about half the patients. These were open, uncontrolled studies.

Vitamins

Vitamin B₆

There are six biologically active forms of vitamin B_6: pyridoxine, pyridoxal, pyridoxamine, and their respective phosphates; these six forms are interconvertable. Humans cannot synthesize the vitamin *de novo*. Vitamin B_6 is the co-enzyme of one enzyme in the serotonin pathway: L-aromatic amino acid decarboxylase (L-AAAD); and of two enzymes in the catecholamine pathway: L-AAAD and dopamine-β-hydroxylase (DBH). It also effects all non-oxidative enzymatic transformations of the other amino acid pathways, catalysing such reactions as decarboxylation, transamination, racemization, beta-elimination and gamma-elimination. Vitamin B_6 is also involved in the biosynthesis of lipids, protein, carbohydrates, nucleic acids and sphingosine bases; the effect of the vitamin is ubiquitous. It has been called the brain vitamin since it affects so many different aspects of CNS metabolism.

Large doses of pyridoxine are used as established therapy in several disease entities which affect the CNS: schizophrenia and/or mental retardation due to the cystathionine synthase deficiency form of homocystinuria (Braunwald *et al.* 1987); hereditary pyridoxine-dependent seizures which can even occur *in utero* (Swaiman and Milstein 1970); and mental retardation due to hereditary pyridoxine-dependent xanthurenic aciduria (Tada *et al.* 1968).

Research trials of large doses of vitamin B_6 have also been conducted in many other disease entities: autism, mental retardation in general, schizophrenia in general, Down syndrome, hyperactivity, on healthy adults and elderly people regarding memorization, dementia and psychological functioning, and on normal children regarding intelligence. According to Kleijnen and Knipschild (1991) who

273

reviewed the extensive literature on these research studies, most of which were controlled blind studies, encouraging results have been reported only in autism.

The trials of pyridoxine on children with autism grew out of clinical observations; there is no laboratory evidence of a deficiency—a study of levels of pyridoxine and other vitamins in 125 children admitted to a psychiatric unit showed no apparent decrease of vitamin levels in that patient group (Sankar 1979). In 1965, Heeley and Roberts were studying the tryptophan pathway in children with autism; when they administered one of the co-enymes of the tryptophan pathway, vitamin B_6 (see Fig. 10.1), they noted improvement in the tryptophan loading test (Heeley and Roberts 1966). This led to an open trial of pyridoxine by Bönisch (1968) which noted some marked improvements in the patients. Next, Rimland (1973, 1974) reported on the treatment with an experimental multi-vitamin regimen of 200 children with autistic symptoms. He noted that a subgroup of the patients appeared to respond to the pyridoxine, relapsed on withdrawal, and improved when the vitamin was reinstituted. Callaway (1977) also noted this finding. He and Rimland (together with Dreyfus) undertook a double-blind crossover evaluation of the effectiveness of pharmacological doses of vitamin B_6 on this previously identified subgroup (Rimland *et al.* 1978). In this study, they were able to correctly identify 11 out of 15 periods when the children with autism were on either placebo or vitamin B_6, using only the behavioural data.

In the ensuing studies by the Lelord group in France, it was confirmed that a group of patients with autism responded to vitamin B_6 in a double-blind crossover protocol (Lelord *et al.* 1978, 1981, 1982). These reseachers had added magnesium to their protocol because in a separate study by their group (Barthélémy *et al.* 1981) a trial of B_6 alone and of magnesium alone was found ineffective compared to the combination of pyridoxine and magnesium together. In addition to adding magnesium, the Lelord group also examined the effect of pyridoxine on averaged evoked potentials in the patients and reported an increase in amplitude of middle latency evoked potentials in the children receiving vitamin B_6 (Lelord *et al.* 1979; Martineau *et al.* 1981, 1982). Other studies also confirmed positive results in a subgroup of patients with autism (Ellman *et al.* 1983; Jonas *et al.* 1984; Martineau *et al.* 1985, 1986). Pyridoxine was also reported to improve elevated levels of homovanillic acid (HVA) in patients with autism (Barthélémy *et al.* 1983, Martineau *et al.* 1988).

One interesting recent study looked at the deficit in children with autism of the ability to form cross-modal associations. Evoked potential conditioning was used to compare two therapies: vitamin B_6 + magnesium vs. fenfluramine (Martineau *et al.* 1989). For the B_6–magnesium-sensitive children, there was an apparition of a conditioning phenomenon and a demonstrated ability to form cross-modal associations. For the fenfluramine-sensitive children, an enhancement of C_z evoked response amplitudes and frequencies was found, but no change was observed on the conditioning phenomenon. Such interesting work needs further replication.

The current consensus is that there is a subgroup of patients with autism who have some improvement of symptoms when they receive pharmacological doses of pyridoxine. No-one is claiming that pyridoxine therapy totally reverses autism. It seems clear that the clinical effects are sustained longer if magnesium is administered with the vitamin. Irritability, sound sensitivity and enuresis are less of a problem if magnesium is given simultaneously (Rimland *et al.* 1978).

Both major and minor side-effects may accompany pyridoxine therapy. Based on what we know so far, these are more likely to occur in adults than in children. The major side-effect is a sensory peripheral neuropathy (Schaumburg *et al.* 1983); the minor ones include blistering of those parts of the skin exposed to the sun (seen mostly in southern climates), stomach upset and irritability. Rarely, sound sensitivity and enuresis may occur. In a study in another patient group (children with Down syndrome), 0.5 per cent of the children developed the peripheral neuropathy, which appeared to be directly correlated with a developing niacin deficiency, probably secondary to the chronic administration of pyridoxine (Coleman *et al.* 1985).

A great deal remains to be learned about this therapy. Which clinical symptoms in patients with autism are likely to suggest a good outcome with a trial of pyridoxine? The role of magnesium needs further clarification, since it may be having a separate effect (see Chapter 10). One possible way of identifying the subgroup that might respond to this therapy while simultaneously selecting a dosage for such patients is to find children with autism who have two laboratory abnormalities—elevation of urinary HVA and depression of whole blood serotonin. The dose of pyridoxine would be that which brings these two abnormalities in the individual patient into the normal range for age. However, this is a temporary strategy to be used until the mechanism of this treatment is better understood. In children with autism who are responders, the identification of the specific biochemical pathway being corrected by this therapy remains a major research goal.

Folic acid
The level of folic acid, another of the water-soluble vitamins, has been shown to be within the normal range in children with psychiatric diagnoses (Sankar 1979, Lowe *et al.* 1981). However, trials of large doses of folic acid have been undertaken in children with fragile X syndrome, after it was shown that the fragile X abnormality would disappear in the chromosomal culture if oral folate supplements were given to the patients (see Chapter 16).

A number of studies of patients with fragile X syndrome have been completed, and although the answer is far from clear at this point, it appears that there may be a very slim hope of benefit to younger children but no such hope for therapy started after puberty (Lowe *et al.* 1981, Brown *et al.* 1986, Froster-Iskenius *et al.* 1986, Gillberg *et al.* 1986, Hagerman *et al.* 1986, Barthélémy *et al.* 1988). Doses ranged from 10 to 2500mg/day.

Ions

Magnesium

Magnesium levels have been found to be depressed in the serum and erthyrocytes in studies of groups of children with autism (see Chapter 10). The only studies which have detailed therapy for magnesium were part of the development of pyridoxine therapy (see above). This is an area where further work is needed. Is there a metabolic pathway using up the magnesium in the subgroup of children with autism who are deficient? Is their intake or absorption inadequate? Do they need supplements? There are no firm answers at this time.

Calcium

Some children with autistic symptoms have been found to have hypocalcinuria (see Chapter 10). The aetiology of this biochemical finding has so far resisted all attempts to define it. All forms of vitamin D, calcitonin, parathormone and so on are within the normal range in the most severely hypocalcinuric children with autism. Monitoring of the serum is not of value, since blood levels are almost always within the normal range no matter how severe the hypocalcinuria.

Improvement of this hypocalcinuria is possible with the use of calcium supplements, often combined with a special diet. Correction is difficult to achieve in this patient group, and massive supplements are sometimes necessary to bring the level of calcium in the urine up into the normal range. In one open series, the motor use of language was accelerated in conjunction with correction of the hypocalcinuria in 8 per cent of patients (Coleman 1989). A recent paper by Coleman (1992) indicates that when ocular self-injury occurs in conjunction with hypocalcinuria in patients with autism, correction of the calcium abnormality may give symptomatic relief of the self-injurious tendencies.

Conclusion

Many biological treatments other than drugs have been suggested as trials in autism. Since autism have multiple aetiologies, the best medical therapy will be the one designed to meet the underlying cause in each individual patient. Such approaches are in their infancy. Except for pyridoxine, which is a symptomatic rather than a curative therapy, no therapies so far suggested have been established.

REFERENCES

Barthélémy, C., Garreau, B., Leddet, I., Ernouf, D., Muh, J.P., Lelord, G. (1981) 'Behavioral and biological effects of oral magnesium, vitamin B_6 and combined magnesium-vitamin B_6 administration in autistic children.' *Magnesium Bulletin*, **3**, 150–153.
—— —— —— Sauvage, D., Muh, J.P., Lelord, G., Callaway, E. (1983) 'Intérêt des échelles de comportement et des dosages de l'acide homovanilique urinaire pour le contrôle des effets d'un traitement associant vitamine B_6 et magnésium chez des enfants ayant un comportement autistique.' *Neuropsychiatrie de l'Enfance et de l'Adolescence*, **31**, 289–301.
—— —— Buneau, N., Martineau, J., Jouve, J., Roux, S., Lelord, G. (1988) 'Biological and behavioral effects of magnesium and vitamin B_6, folates and fenfluramine in autistic children.' *In:* Wing, L.

(Ed.) *Aspects of Autism: Biological Research*. London: Royal College of Psychiatrists, pp. 59–73.

Bird, B.L., Russo, D.C., Cataldo, M.F. (1977) 'Considerations in the analysis and treatment of dietary effects on behavior: a case study.' *Journal of Autism and Childhood Schizophrenia*, 7, 373–382.

Bönisch, E. (1968) 'Erfahrungen met Pyrithioxin bei hirgeschädigten Kindern mit autistischen Syndrom.' *Praxis de Kinderpsychologie*, 8, 308–310.

Braunwald, E., Isselbacher, K.J., Petersdorf, R.G., Wilson, J.D., Martin, J.B., Fauci, A.S. (Eds) (1987) *Harrison's Principles of Internal Medicine*. New York: McGraw-Hill.

Brown, W.T., Cohen, I., Fisch, G., Wolf-Schein, E.G., Jenkins, V.A., Malik, M.N., Jenkins, E.C. (1986) 'High dose folic acid treatment of fragile X males.' *American Journal of Medical Genetics*, 23, 263–271.

Callaway, E. (1977) 'Response of infantile autism to large doses of B$_6$.' *Psychological Bulletin*, 13, 57–58.

Campbell, M., Fish, B., David, R., Shapiro, T., Collins, P., Koh, C. (1972) 'Response to triiodothyronine and dextroamphetamine: a study of preschool schizophrenic children.' *Journal of Autism and Childhood Schizophrenia*, 2, 343–358.

—— Small, A.M., Collins, P.J., Friedman, E., David, R., Genieser, N. (1976) 'Levodopa and levoamphetamine: a crossover study in young schizophrenic children.' *Current Therapeutic Research*, 19, 70–86.

Coleman, M. (1989) 'Autism: non-drug biological treatments.' *In:* Gillberg, C. (Ed.) *Diagnosis and Treatment of Autism*. New York: Plenum, pp. 219–236.

—— (1991) 'Ocular self-mutilation in autistic children: its relationship to hypocalcinuria.' *Brain Dysfunction. (In press.)*

—— Landgrebe, M.A., Landgrebe, A.R. (1976) 'Celiac autism: calcium studies and their relationship to celiac disease in autistic patients.' *In:* Coleman, M. (Ed.) *The Autistic Syndromes*. Amsterdam: North Holland; New York: Elsevier, pp. 197–208.

—— Sobel, S., Bhagavan, H.N., Coursin, D.B., Marquardt, A., Guay, M., Hunt, C. (1985) 'A double blind study of vitamin B$_6$ in Down's syndrome infants. Part I—Clinical and biochemical results.' *Journal of Mental Deficiency Research*, 29, 233–240.

Crowley, C., Koch, R., Fishler, K., Wenz, E., Ireland, J. (1990) 'Clinical trial of "off diet" older phenylketonurics with a new phenylalanine-free product.' *Journal of Mental Deficiency Research*, 34, 361–369.

Egger, J., Carter, C.M., Graham, P.J., Gumley, D., Soothill, J.F. (1985) 'Controlled trial of oligoantigenic treatment in the hyperkinetic syndrome.' *Lancet*, i, 540–545.

Ellman, G., Mendel, B., Silverstein, C.I., Callaway, E. (1983) 'Vitamin B$_6$ and autism.' *Paper presented at the meeting of the American Association on Mental Deficiency, Dallas, TX.*

Froster-Iskenius, U., Bodeker, K., Oepen, T., Matthes, R., Piper, U., Schwinger, E. (1986) 'Folic acid treatment in males and females with fragile X syndrome.' *American Journal of Medical Genetics*, 23, 273–289.

Gillberg, C., Wahlström, J., Johansson, R., Törnblom, M., Albertsson-Wikland, K. (1986) 'Folic acid as an adjunct in the treatment of children with the autism fragile-X syndrome (AFRAX).' *Developmental Medicine and Child Neurology*, 28, 624–627.

Goodwin, M.S., Cowen, M.A., Goodwin, T.C. (1971) 'Malabsorption and cerebral dysfunction: a multivariate and comparative study of autistic children.' *Journal of Autism and Childhood Schizophrenia*, 1, 48–62.

Grüter, W. (1963) *Angeborne Stoffwechselstorungen und Schwachsinn am Beispiel der Phenylketonurie*. Stuttgart: Enke.

Hagerman, R.J., Jackson, A.W., Levitas, A., Braden, M., McBogg, P., Kemper, M., McGavran, L., Barry, R., Matus, I., Hagerman, P.J. (1986) 'Oral folic acid versus placebo in the treatment of males with fragile X syndrome.' *American Journal of Medical Genetics*, 23, 241–262.

Heeley, A.F., Roberts, G.E. (1966) 'A study of tryptophan metabolism in psychotic children.' *Developmental Medicine and Child Neurology*, 8, 708–718.

Hsia, D.Y., Knox, W.E., Quinn, K.V., Paine, R.J. (1958) 'A one-year controlled study of the effect of low phenylalanine diet on phenylketonuria.' *Pediatrics*, 21, 178–185.

Jonas, C., Etienne, T., Barthélémy, C., Jouve, J., Mariotte, N. (1984) 'Intérêt clinique et biochimique de l'association vitamine B$_6$ + magnésium dans le traitement de l'autisme résiduel à l'âge adulte.' *Thérapie*, 39, 661–669.

277

Kleijnen, J., Knipschild, P. (1991) 'Niacin and vitamin B$_6$ in mental functioning: review of controlled trials in humans.' *Biological Psychiatry*, **29**, 931–941.

Koch, R., Shaw, K.N.F., Acosta, P., Fisher, K., Schaeffler, G., Wenz, E., Wohlers, A. (1970) 'An approach to management of phenylketonuria.' *Journal of Pediatrics*, **76**, 815–828.

Lelord, G.,Callaway, E., Muh, J.P., Arlot, J.C., Sauvage, D., Garreau, B., Domenech, J. (1978) 'L'acide homovanilique urinaire et ses modifications par ingestion de vitamine B$_6$: exploration fonctionnelle dans l'autisme de l'enfant?' *Revue Neurologique*, **134**, 797–801.

—— Muh, J.P., Martineau, J., Garreau, B., Roux, S. (1979) 'Electrophysiological and biochemical studies in autistic children treated with vitamin B$_6$.' *In:* Lehmann, D., Callaway, E. (Eds) *Human Evoked Potentials*. New York: Plenum.

—— —— Barthélémy, C., Martineau, J., Garreau, B., Callaway, E. (1981) 'Effects of pyridoxine and magnesium on autistic symptoms: initial observations.' *Journal of Autism and Developmental Disorders*, **11**, 219–230.

—— Callaway, E., Muh, J.P., Martineau, J. (1982) 'Clinical and biological effects of high doses of vitamin B$_6$ and magnesium on autistic children.' *Acta Vitaminologica et Enzymologica*, **4**, 27–44.

Lewis, E. (1959) 'The development of concepts in a girl after dietary treatment for phenylketonuria.' *British Journal of Medical Psychology*, **32**, 282–287.

Lowe, T.L., Tanaka, K., Seashore, M.R., Young, J.G., Cohen, D.J. (1980) 'Detection of phenylketonuria in autistic and psychotic children.' *Journal of the American Medical Association*, **243**, 126–128.

Lowe, T., Cohen, D., Miller, S., Young, J.G. (1981) 'Folic acid and B$_{12}$ in autism and neuropsychiatric disturbances of childhood.' *Journal of the American Academy of Child Psychiatry*, **20**, 104–111.

Martineau, J., Garreau, B., Barthélémy, C., Callaway, E., Lelord, G. (1981) 'Effects of vitamin B$_6$ on averaged evoked potentials in infantile autism.' *Biological Psychiatry*, **16**, 627–641.

—— —— —— Lelord, G. (1982) 'Comparative effects of oral B$_6$, B$_6$-Mg, and Mg administration on evoked potentials conditioning in autistic children.' *In:* Rothenberger, A. (Ed.) *Proceedings: Symposium on Event-Related Potentials in Children, Developments in Neurology, Vol. 6.* Amsterdam: Elsevier, pp. 411–416.

—— Barthélémy, C., Garreau, B., Lelord, G. (1985) 'Vitamin B$_6$, magnesium and combined B$_6$–Mg: therapeutic effects in childhood autism.' *Biological Psychiatry*, **20**, 467–468.

—— —— Lelord, G. (1986) 'Long-term effects of combined vitamin B$_6$-magnesium administration in an autistic child.' *Biological Psychiatry*, **21**, 511–518.

—— —— Cheliakine, C., Lelord, G. (1988) 'Brief report: an open middle-term study of combined vitamin B$_6$-magnesium in a subgroup of autistic children selected for their sensitivity to this treatment.' *Journal of Autism and Developmental Disorders*, **3**, 435–447.

—— —— Roux, S., Garreau, B., Lelord, G. (1989) 'Electrophysiological effects of fenfluramine or combined vitamin B$_6$ and magnesium on children with autistic behaviour.' *Developmental Medicine and Child Neurology*, **31**, 721–727.

McCarthy, D., Coleman, M. (1979) 'Response of intestinal mucosa to gluten challenge in autistic subjects.' *Lancet*, **2**, 877–878.

Rimland, B. (1973) 'High dosage levels of certain vitamins in the treatment of children with severe mental disorders.' *In:* Hawkins, D., Pauling, L. (Eds) *Orthomolecular Psychiatry: Treatment of Schizophrenia.* New York: W.H. Freeman, pp. 513–538.

—— (1974) 'An orthomolecular study of psychotic children.' *Journal of Orthomolecular Psychiatry*, **3**, 371–377.

—— Callaway, E., Dreyfus, P. (1978) 'The effects of high doses of vitamin B$_6$ on autistic children: a double-blind crossover study.' *American Journal of Psychiatry*, **135**, 472–475.

Ritvo, E.R., Yuwiler, A., Geller, E., Kales, A., Rashkis, S., Schicor, A., Plotkin, S., Axelrod, R., Howard, C. (1971) 'Effects of L-DOPA in autism.'*Journal of Autism and Childhood Schizophrenia*, **1**, 190–205.

Sankar, D.V.S. (1979) 'Plasma levels of folates, riboflavin, vitamin B$_6$ and ascorbate in severely disturbed children.' *Journal of Autism and Developmental Disorders*, **9**, 73–82.

Schaumburg, H., Kaplan, J., Windebank, A., Vick, N., Rasmus, S., Pleasure, D., Brown, M.J. (1983) 'Sensory neuropathy from pyridoxine abuse.' *New England Journal of Medicine*, **309**, 445–448.

Segawa, M., Noda, Y., Nezu, A., Uchiyama, A., Soda, M., Nomura, Y. (1987) 'Trials of 5-hydroxytryptophan and low dose L-dopa on early infantile autism.' *Proceedings of the American*

278

Academy of Child and Adolescent Psychiatry, p. 53.

Sepe, J., Levy, H.L., Mount, F.W. (1979) 'An evaluation of routine follow-up blood screening of infants for phenylketonuria.' *New England Journal of Medicine*, **300**, 606–609.

Sverd, J., Kupietz, S.S., Winsberg, B.G., Hurwic, M.J., Becker, L. (1978) 'Effects of L-5-hydroxytyptophan in autistic children.' *Journal of Autism and Childhood Schizophrenia*, **8**, 171–180.

Swaiman, K.F., Milstein, J.M. (1970) 'Pyridoxine dependency and penicillamine.' *Neurology*, **20**, 78–81.

Tada, K., Yokoyama, Y., Nakagawa, H., Ito, H., Wada, Y., Arakawa, T. (1968) 'Vitamin B_6 dependent xanthurenic aciduria (the second report).' *Tohoku Journal of Experimental Medicine*, **95**, 107–114.

PART V

CONCLUSION

24
THEORETICAL CONSIDERATIONS: CNS MECHANISMS UNDERLYING THE AUTISTIC SYNDROMES

Introduction

One of the fascinating challenges of autism is to try to understand the mechanisms in the CNS that underlie autistic symptomatology. In this chapter we review and explore some of the theories regarding the final common pathway that leads to symptoms of autism.

From the foregoing it should be clear that autism is not a homogeneous disease. The attempt to demonstrate a single cause for all cases of autism appears to be futile. Nevertheless, the search for a common denominator, be it at the neuropsychological or neurobiological level or both, might be worthwhile (Frith 1989). The fact that stomach ulcers can be caused by a wide variety of different medical conditions does not mean that a single final factor leading to the development of the ulcer as such cannot be found and reasonably treated. The same might be true of autism.

It should be equally clear that we might have to look for several different pathogenetic pathways when trying to account for the phenomena referred to as autistic behaviours. It has been clearly demonstrated that the disorder known as cerebral palsy—that is, major motor deficits with a presumed CNS origin which show a stable course of development without signs of progressive deterioration —can be brought about by a number of different pathogenetic mechanisms such as bleeding and malformations in the cerebral cortex as well as hereditary developmental abnormalities in the cerebellum and a number of other factors. If we regard autistic behaviours as conceptually similar to cerebral palsy, *i.e.* that they may be a sign of a non-progressive disorder of behaviour with several different aetiologies, we might well end up by having to account for them by demonstrating a number of different CNS dysfunctions impinging on brain areas/neuropsychological faculties subserving empathy functions (Waterhouse and Fein 1989, Gillberg 1991).

Turning to the second possibility first, the systems in the brain which subserve the development of empathy and multifaceted social behaviours are likely to be complex (Waterhouse and Fein 1989). They could be 'located' in the frontal, prefrontal, temporal and diencephalic regions of the human brain—and even in the brainstem and cerebellum. Damage or dysfunction in any one part of these areas could lead to dysfunction in the field of social relationships development, regardless of whether these areas constitute a 'functionally connected system' or not. The multiplicity of brain areas implicated in the study of autism aetiology in research using, for instance, brain imaging techniques could be taken to support the notion that autism can develop on the basis of damage/destruction/dysfunction in any one of these brain regions.

The other possibility, that autism might have a common denominator other than the typical behaviours, now has to be considered from at least two points of view: the neuropsychological and the neurobiological. Let us examine these two levels separately and then go on to see if we can find a common link between the two.

In the last decade, a number of studies have shown that, at least among the relatively high-functioning children with autism (with some communicative speech), there might be a shared deficit in the field of theory of mind development. It appears that most children with autism have severe problems in conceptualizing other people as having separate minds, or indeed as having minds at all (Frith 1989). The inability to conceive of other people as creatures who think and feel could be pathognomonic for autism or at least for autism spectrum disorders/disorders of empathy. Normal young children have been shown repeatedly to have a well-developed theory of mind by the age of 4 years (and there is clear evidence of such a theory of mind emerging at the age of 1 year). Children with classical autism never show obvious signs of such a capacity before age 10 years (Baron-Cohen 1990). This lack of, or extremely delayed development of, a theory of mind in autism is not just a reification of the syndrome of autism as such (which is based on specific behavioural diagnostic criteria). Rather it constitutes an intrapsychic model which can account for the specific development of the behaviours shown by children diagnosed as having autism. Thus it seems, at least at the neuropsychological level, that there could be a denominator common to all cases of autism. Recent research (selectively reviewed by Frith 1989) has shown that other autism spectrum problems could be associated with underlying theory of mind problems as well. This has lead to the development of a new concept in the field of child neuropsychiatry, *disorders of empathy* (Gillberg 1992*a*). Underlying a number of different conditions diagnosed at the behavioural levels as autism, Asperger syndrome, severe obsessive–compulsive disorder, extreme anorexia nervosa, etc., might be a deviant or delayed development of a theory of mind. The theory of mind theory for the emergence of autistic behaviours already has considerable empirical evidence to support it, but only continued research can reveal whether or not it constitutes the major neuropsychological step forward in understanding autism that we believe it to be today. It has certainly opened up a new window on autism spectrum problems through which we can begin to see the coming together of psychology and biology in autism which has long been considered impossible. There might be specific functional systems in the CNS which subserve empathy functions (or the development of a theory of mind). It is now theoretically possible to link the results of empirical psychological studies of theory of mind capacities in individual children, adolescents and adults with and without autism and autism spectrum problems with results of studies using PET and SPECT scanning (see Chapter 13) to visualize regional brain metabolism and the extension/activity of specific neuronal transmitter systems.

It merits mention here that a recent review of the autism literature (Hill and Leary, personal communication) has suggested a very different basic deficit, namely movement disturbance. Akinesia, dyskinesia, stereotypic movement disorders, dyspraxia, and abnormalities of tone and posture have all been reported at very high rates in autism. It is unlikely that classical autism ever occurs without movement disorder. The study of movement/motor disturbance in autism might prove unexpectedly fruitful and shed new light both on underlying brain mechanisms and on potentially useful clinical interventions. Theory of mind and movement disorder hypotheses are not necessarily mutually exclusive.

From the neurobiological point of view, at the time of writing this book, there are still children with autism who do not show signs or histories indicative of neurological disorder, particularly when they are young. Are they brain dysfunctional at all? We submit that indeed they are, but our instruments used in detecting brain dysfunction, in spite of landslide developments in the last few years, are still too crude. The proportion of patients with autism without associated neurological disorder do not differ from the behavioural point of view (Garreau *et al*. 1984, Steffenburg 1991, Gillberg 1992*a*). This is not to say that there may not be symptomatological subgroups which may be separable on the basis of aetiological factors. In fact, there are already a number of studies which have demonstrated quite convincingly that subgrouping at the behavioural level might well match subgrouping according to aetiology (Gillberg 1992*b*). Thus, for instance, Rett syndrome often has a characteristic development of autistic behaviours with extreme aloneness and excessively severe stereotypies in the second to fourth years and amelioration of these symptoms and considerably better gaze contact from about age 5 to 10 years. The fragile X syndrome in boys can show as highly characteristic Kanner-type autism in the very young group, but the emergence of cluttering, partly communicative speech around age 4 to 6 years is usually accompanied by a less characteristic autism phenotype. This in turn, unfortunately, leads some authors to propose that these cases with Rett syndrome and the fragile X syndrome are not associated with 'pure' autism. The fact is that at one age they do indeed show 'classic' autism, but later on they become more atypical. However, this type of developmental course of autistic symptoms is the rule rather than the exception (Wing 1989). Therefore, the observation that in patients older than 6 to 10 years 'all' autism symptoms may no longer be present, should never be taken as evidence that one has not been dealing with autism at all.

When one looks at brain dysfunction in an individual, one asks essentially two primary questions: 'What is the lesion?' and 'Where is the lesion?' The earlier chapters of this book reviewed a number of the aetiologies of autism, so we are beginning to solve the first question. Some possible answers are that it is an abnormally functioning enzyme or a brain infection, or the chronic effects of mildly increased pressure inside the brain.

However, the answer to the question 'Where is the lesion?' or 'Where is the final common pathway that leads a child to have autistic symptoms rather than other types of brain symptoms?' is more elusive. The human brain comprises about 100 billion neurons with a density of approximately 1 trillion synapses per cubic centimetre of cortex. The staggering complexity and multiple redundancies that exist in the brain makes even the boldest investigator hesitant to attempt to explain fully a disease process in the CNS.

What is wrong with the brain of children with autism? Based on current research, a number of tantalizing clues present themselves. Regarding the rate of metabolism in the brain, the PET studies (Rapoport *et al.* 1983) indicate a possibly increased rate of metabolism. The currently most promising drugs, haloperidol and fenfluramine, are drugs that block or dampen down metabolic pathways (see Chapter 22).

Is the brain of the individual with autism immature or advanced? In one autopsy study of an adult, a profound immaturity of the brain was suggested by the retention of the lamina desicans zone which is usually found only in very young children (see Chapter 14). Also, certain REM sleep studies are found to resemble those of very young children, as young as 18 months of age or less (Chapter 12). Endocrine studies demonstrate lack of circadian rhythm for corticosteroids in older patients, such a pattern usually being seen only in children well below 4 years of age (Chapter 11). Yet, on the other hand, there is evidence from studies of cortical auditory and visual evoked potentials that suggest that some of the higher levels of function could be either normal or advanced (Chapter 12). One adult with autism even became a member of a society for geniuses (Sofaer and Emery 1981).

In connection with localization in the brain, patients with autism offer a number of clues to direct our attention toward certain areas. First and foremost, they all appear to have a type of cognitive defect which delays the development of natural, progressive, hierarchic integration of the brain which is so essential for the maturation of the young brain. But, in contrast to many retarded children, children with autism have a profound social immaturity. In addition, they also have sensory processing problems primarily studied in the auditory system, but clearly evident also in the visual and tactile systems if investigated. Relatively spared is the visual spatial system (Shah and Frith 1983); this sparing is related primarily only to the spatial area itself and not to temporal visual processing. Children also have evidence of basal ganglia disease, and there are a number of studies suggesting brainstem dysfunction.

How have past investigators interpreted these symptoms in terms of anatomy? Rimland (1964) hypothesized that the error in these patients lay in the reticular formation of the brainstem, and he propounded a theory suggesting that the cognitive dysfunction was secondary to this brainstem problem. Hutt and Hutt (1970) also suggested that a hyperactive reticular activating system could underlie symptoms of autism with a reactive effort by the brain in an effort to reduce the sensory input. Simon (1975) also suggested a brainstem location, this time in the inferior colliculus. Cohen *et al.* (1976) raised the question of brainstem and midbrain dysfunction involving catecholamine pathways. Damasio and Maurer (1978) related symptoms to the mesolimbic cortex and the anterior and medial nuclear groups of the thalamus. Coleman (1979) suggested that birth injury may affect the thalamus in some cases. There were theorists suggesting that the left side of the brain was damaged (Aarkrog 1968, Hier *et al.* 1979, Prior 1979, Dawson *et al.* 1982), while Myklebust *et al.* (1972) suggested a right-sided lesion and were backed up by some evidence from Baltaxe (1981), Ross (1981) and Weintraub *et al.* (1981).

However, most authorities today agree that a bilateral—not unilateral—brain dysfunction would be required for autism to develop (see Ornitz 1983 for a review). In an attempt to conceptualize the problem, a working hypothesis will be presented which selectively integrates some of the studies and theories of other investigators into a comprehensive theoretical model.

A theory linking brainstem/mesolimbic dysfunction with autistic symptoms
Brainstem dysfunction
There is evidence from several groups and studies that in patients with autism the brainstem has dysfunctional sections. Bonvallet and Allen (1963) noted increased heart-rate variability, failure to habituate to respiratory responses, and enhancement of vascular reaction to visual input. These could be taken as evidence of unusual functioning of the reticular formation in the brainstem.

The UCLA research team has performed a number of studies of vestibular function and have noticed that a large proportion of children with autism have either a decrease or absence of postrotatory nystagmus. They also typically display a lack of dizziness or nausea after spinning and rotation. This too can be interpreted as brainstem dysfunction (see Ornitz 1983 for overview).

Electrophysiological studies have also suggested brainstem dysfunction. Even though baseline EEGs are not specific, the findings on these EEGs are suggestive of centrencephalic rather than circumscribed telencephalic damage (Gladwell *et al.* 1979, Gillberg and Schaumann 1983). Also, auditory brainstem evoked response studies have indicated brainstem dysfunction in a subgroup of children with autism (see Chapter 12). This examination is most sensitive to *structural* brainstem damage, so it is quite possible that even among those with normal results, there are children who have abnormal brainstem *function*.

The autopsy studies of Williams *et al.* (1980), who studied the cortex of four children with autism, also indirectly support this concept since they found no, or minimal, evidence of structural abnormalities in the cortex.

Thus, the evidence of autonomic dysfunction, the vestibular studies, and the electrophysiological studies all point in the direction of brainstem dysfunction in this patient group.

As seen in Figure 24.1, the first part of this comprehensive theory assumes

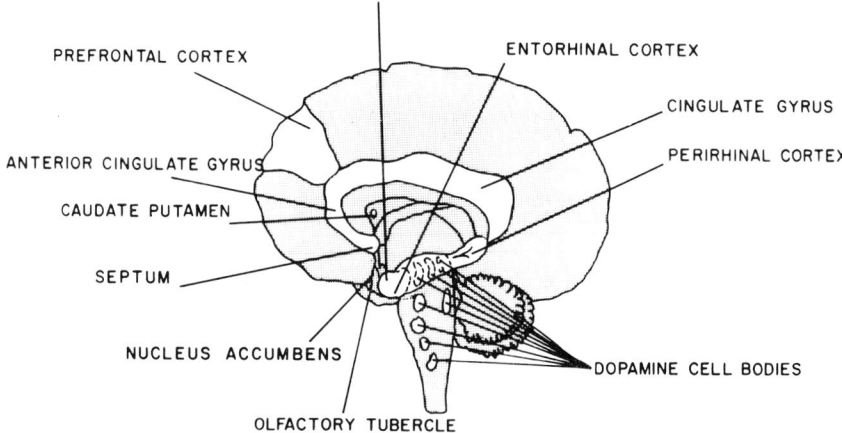

CENTRAL NUCLEUS OF THE AMYGDALA

PREFRONTAL CORTEX

ENTORHINAL CORTEX

CINGULATE GYRUS

PERIRHINAL CORTEX

ANTERIOR CINGULATE GYRUS

CAUDATE PUTAMEN

SEPTUM

NUCLEUS ACCUMBENS

DOPAMINE CELL BODIES

OLFACTORY TUBERCLE

Fig. 24.1. Mesolimbic damage could arise *de novo* or secondary to damage to (or failure of development of?) dopamine cell bodies in the brainstem. Although the dopamine system is pictured here, there is also evidence of dysfunction of related brainstem nuclei, such as the serotonergic and endorphin systems.

brainstem dysfunction or damage. The theory then assumes that one way brainstem dysfunction can present is as an abnormal dopaminergic state that might arise throughout the brain wherever dopaminergic nerve fibres project because of injury to the central neurons in the brainstem through either structural or metabolic injury.

Dopamine dysfunction

The cell bodies for the dopamine neurons are located in the brainstem and diencephalon, and there are studies which indicate a relatively abnormal function of dopamine in patients with autism. Reviewing the evidence that there may be an absolute or relatively excessive amount of dopamine in patients with autism, one finds the following data in support of that hypothesis:

- The enzyme that hydroxylyses (lowers the level of) dopamine-β-hydroxylase (DBH) is depressed in the serum of patients in several studies (Goldstein *et al.* 1976, Lake *et al.* 1977).
- A minor metabolite of dopamine (homoprotocatechuic acid), which is only found in significant amounts when there is a back-up of the dopamine pathway (with excessive dopamine being metabolized into minor pathways), has been demonstrated in 88 per cent of patients with autism in a study by Landgrebe and Landgrebe (1976).
- Dopamine agonists, such as amphetamines, tend to make patients worse, while dopamine antagonists, such as haloperidol, clinically help some children with autism (Campbell *et al.* 1976, 1978).
- The end-product of dopamine is homovanillic acid (HVA) which is elevated in

288

both the CSF (Cohen *et al.* 1977, Winsberg *et al.* 1980, Gillberg *et al.* 1983) and the urine (Lelord *et al.* 1978, Garreau *et al.* 1980).

- The elevated HVA level in children with autism can be lowered by giving them pyridoxine (vitamin B_6)—the co-enzyme of the steps both before and after dopamine (Lelord *et al.* 1978). Since the vitamin lowers HVA, presumably it may be selectively enhancing DBH function, whose job is to lower the level of dopamine. (However, in normal children, the opposite effect is reported. Their normal levels of HVA go up, presumably by enhancing L-AAAD, the enzyme creating more dopamine.) Thus, the catecholamine pathway is affected by pyridoxine differently in patients with autism than in normal children. Double-blind studies show that pyridoxine is helpful clinically to one subgroup of children with autism.

The fact that these dopamine-related results are consistent with each other in different laboratories is encouraging, but it is important to note several limitations at this time. The studies listed above are primarily concerned with measuring from the periphery, and only by analogy from the brain. Even CSF contains a large ultrafiltrate of blood. Also, these are early studies, some of which have not been confirmed independently.

In fact, abnormal functional levels of dopamine could result from a number of factors. As suggested, they could be caused by a relative block in the enzyme DBH, whose job is to catabolize the amine. Alternatively, with normal functioning of the dopamine pathway, they could be due to depressed levels of other neuro-transmitters with which dopamine is in delicate balance. They could be due to denervation of dopamine neurons themselves, making them hypersensitive and hyperfunctional. Or there could be other factors not yet understood.

In contrast, there is also a very small literature which is compatible with depression of dopamine functioning. For example, in PKU patients we know that there is a block in the catecholamine pathway ahead of dopamine which prevents a normal amount of the compound from being formed (see Chapter 17). Also, the gait in some patients with autism has been carefully analysed and described as a childhood equivalent of that seen in Parkinson disease (Vilensky *et al.* 1981). Parkinson disease is a documented dopamine-deficiency disease seen in older age groups.

In our comprehensive model, we therefore postulate that dopamine neurons in the dopamine pathways from the brainstem up into the cortex are functioning abnormally—overdoing or underdoing their job—in many of these patients. Other pathways originating in the brainstem, as yet unexplored, probably are also dysfunctional. This area also contains encephalin substances, so dysfunction of encephalin-containing neurons is also a possibility.

Where do dopaminergic neurons send their axons? The target area of dopaminergic mesencephalic neurons is the mesolimbic cortex, which is architec-tonically and neurochemically distinct and, along with the striatum, constitutes the largest area for those neurons. According to Damasio and Maurer (1978), 'bilateral neural structures that include the ring of mesolimbic cortex located in the mesial frontal and temporal lobes, the neostriatum and the anterior and medial nuclear groups of the thalamus' may be specifically dysfunctional in patients with autism.

Mesolimbic cortex and striatum

With reference to the cerebral cortex, where are the areas that symptoms of autism suggest might be damaged? Several authors have indicated left hemisphere damage and dysfunction, and there are studies of disturbed interhemisphere relationship or relative left hemisphere dysfunction, such as non-right-handedness, special musical skills, special artistic skills and superior visuospatial skills in children with autism. There are also laboratory studies implying a link between autism and left hemisphere dysfunction, *e.g.* left temporal lobe damage evidenced by pneumo-encephalography (Aarkrog 1968, Hauser *et al.* 1975—although Ornitz (1978) and others have criticized the conclusion of the latter study); left parietal occipital reduction of brain parenchyma (Hier *et al.* 1979); and a deficient left hemisphere specialization for language functions (Dawson *et al.* 1982). On the other hand, the dysprosodic characteristics of autistic speech and the failure to convey emotions can be attributed to right, rather than left, hemisphere dysfunction (Baltaxe 1981, Ross 1981, Weintraub *et al.* 1981).

If both sides of the brain are involved, that is, if it is a bilateral problem, which portions of the cortex would one expect to find with abnormal functioning? The mesial portions of the temporal lobe are an obvious choice owing to the nature of autistic symptoms (Hetzler and Griffin 1981). In this and the immediately adjacent areas are the centres for controlling motor language functions, emotion, autonomous functions and auditory processing and the modulation centres for sensory stimuli and voluntary movements. Damage to this region could lead to many of the symptoms typical of autism, while dysfunction in this area might lead to less pronounced problems of a similar kind.

Medial temporal structures are among those most likely to be damaged by reduced optimality in the prenatal period (Griffiths and Laurence 1974). Furthermore, the studies connecting postnatal herpes encephalitis with reversible autistic symptoms also point in the direction of the temporal lobe being affected, since herpes viruses are known to have a predilection for just those areas (Haymaker *et al.* 1958). In the Klüver–Bucy syndrome (Klüver and Bucy 1938, 1939), in which temporal lobe structures are bilaterally destroyed, there is severe incapacity in the fields of recognizing the emotional significance of objects and in social relationships. These symptoms are also typical of autism. Further, in the adult Korsakoff syndrome there is a well-known loss of recall for recent events, which results from bilateral hippocampal lesions in the temporal lobe. This problem, too, can be characteristic of autism (Boucher 1981). The language problem in autism, at one point thought to be similar to that in developmental dysphasia but now shown to be different could be interpreted to favour bilateral temporal lobe damage. Findings by Bryson (1970) suggest the possibility that association fibres connecting the temporal and occipital lobes may be dysfunctional or damaged in autism. The children with autism in that study showed poorer auditory-to-visual and visual-to-vocal performances than visual-to-visual and auditory-to-vocal performances. Psychomotor epilepsy is probably more common in autism than other kinds of epilepsy (Corbett 1982). This, too, would suggest temporal lobe affliction.

What about the mesial frontal lobe area? The mesial frontal cortex has an exceptionally high concentration of dopamine. Originally it was thought to be a silent prefrontal area. Frontal lobes scarcely exist in most animals and are fully developed only in human beings. However, new findings suggest that they have particularly close connections with three deeper brain areas, the thalamus (the site of perception, constant or inconstant), the caudate nucleus (one of the basal ganglia), and the brainstem. Goldman-Rakic and Brown (1982) have shown that, in the frontal lobes, columns of axons from cell bodies in the cortex of one hemisphere alternate with columns of axons from cells of the other hemisphere, and that the silent prefrontal area which was believed to be undifferentiated and diffuse actually has an exquisite and precise organization. Additional evidence for frontal lobe dysfunction in autism has been provided by Rumsay (1984) who found significant deficits in the formulation of rules and also severe perseverative tendencies in nine highly verbal adult males with autism.

With reference to the thalamus, the anterior group of thalamic nuclei are involved in recent memory processing and they are also involved in the balance between stereotypical and exploratory behaviour. The thalamus is the main nucleus for perceptual integration, and the perceptual inconstancy described so graphically by Ornitz and Ritvo (1968) could represent a thalamic (or third neuron up) lesion, rather than primary or secondary deficits seen in disease entities where perception is consistently impaired.

The neostriatal area is involved in the extrapyramidal motor balance system of the body. Dysfunction of this area could conceivably account for the variations of tone that are seen in children with autism, which result in toe-walking or in other minor motor problems (see discussion by Vilensky *et al.* 1981).

Comprehensive model
In Figure 24.1 we summarize a comprehensive model that could possibly account for some autism symptomatology. If the ascending dopaminergic nerve fibres from the brainstem/diencephalon are coming from neurons that are dysfunctional or injured (for whatever reason), then their target cell areas, such as the mesolimbic/striatal/prefrontal cortex, might be dysfunctional and, in a growing child, underdeveloped. It is well established that sensory input is necessary in young children for the development of certain 'end interpretation loci'.

Our model suggests that autism could arise on the basis of brainstem dysfunction or damage—through the mechanism of the dopaminergic pathways (and probably other pathways arising from the brainstem area)—which may cause

291

loss of tropic sensory input necessary for optimal development in the mesolimbic, striatal and prefrontal systems of the CNS. Alternatively, autism symptoms might develop as a result of a disease process in the mesolimbic cortex itself.

One intriguing possibility is that underlying the dysfunction in the dopaminergic pathways might be a primary dysfunction in processes regulating synapse turnover (Ahlsén, personal communication). The finding of a raised level of GFA (glial fibrillary acidic protein) in the CSF of children and young adults with autism is likely to reflect increased glial (astrocyte) breakdown. The astrocytes 'nurture' the nerve cell synapses. In acute brain damage (*e.g.* intracerebral haemorrhage), the GFA in the CSF is raised to about the level found in autism but after the acute stage decreases to normal level. In autism it appears to continue to be at high level regardless of age. Since in most cases autism is clinically not a disorder associated with a downhill course and the impression of ongoing 'acute' brain damage, the high GFA level could not reasonably be accounted for by such recurring damage by external factors. A more appealing model would be that synapse formation in certain systems (such as in the dopamine system) is at a constantly high level, leading to the formation of a large number of non-functional synapses and the consequent breakdown of these synapses. The primary deficit could be an inherited genetic synapse regulation abnormality of the secondary reaction to genomic or brain afflictions of various kinds. Some support for the notion of increased synapse turnover comes from the combined results of studies demonstrating high levels of CSF monoamines and dense cell packing in autism.

Conclusions

Interesting as these theories of biochemical and anatomical localization may be, in the living child whose brain in constantly maturing, specific localization may be misleading. In the young child, dynamic rather than static anatomical approaches often underlie the truest interpretations of symptoms. For example, although autism is thought to be primarily a bilateral phenomenon (as described above), the suggestion has been made by DeLong *et al.* (1981) that there may be both bilateral and unilateral forms, the unilateral being in general milder, more reversible and associated with preserved islands of normal function.

We would like to end by discussing the study of dichotic listening tests by Wetherby *et al.* (1981). A group of subjects with autism ranging from 8 to 24 years of age, who had normal hearing on monaural speech tests, were studied. It was found that only for those subjects displaying echolalia was there an indication of central auditory nervous system dysfunction in the language-dominant hemisphere, as determined from the dichotic tests. Children with autism who were no longer echolalic had normal dichotic test results. One subject who was tested over the course of a year gradually lost echolalia. At the same time, the child showed a normalization in the dichotic test of central auditory function. Thus, in this child with autism, a clinical improvement was documented by an improvement in a functional laboratory test.

It is important to remember that the child's brain is a dynamic, growing organism capable of change. In young children the brain, with maddening ability to switch locations, simply refuses to follow the anatomical rules that were worked out in adult patients. Any theoretical model of brain function in autism based on studies in children needs to keep this fundamental point in mind.

REFERENCES

Aarkrog, T. (1968) 'Organic factors in infantile psychoses and borderline psychoses.' *Danish Medical Bulletin*, **15**, 283–288.

Baltaxe, C.A.M. (1981) 'Autistic characteristics of prosody in autism.' *In:* Mittler, P. (Ed.) *Frontiers of Knowledge in Mental Retardation. Social, Educational and Behavioral Aspects.* Baltimore: Johns Hopkins University Press, pp. 223–233.

Baron-Cohen, S. (1990) 'Autism: a specific cognitive disorder of "mind-blindness".' *International Review of Psychiatry*, **2**, 81–90.

Bonvallet, M., Allen, M.B. (1963) 'Prolonged spontaneous and evoked reticular activation following discreet bulbar lesions.' *Electroencephalography and Clinical Neurophysiology*, **15**, 969–988.

Boucher, J. (1981) 'Memory of recent events in autistic children.' *Journal of Autism and Developmental Disorders*, **11**, 293–302.

Bryson, C.Q. (1970) 'Systematic identification of perceptual disabilities in autistic children.' *Perceptual and Motor Skills*, **31**, 239–246.

Campbell, M., Small, A.M., Collins, P.J., Friedman, E., David, R., Genieser, N. (1976) 'Levodopa and levoamphetamine: a crossover study in young schizophrenic children.' *Current Therapeutic Research*, **19**, 70–86.

—— Anderson, L.T., Meier, M., Cohen, I.L., Small, A.M., Samit, C., Sachar, E.J. (1978) 'A comparison of haloperidol, behavior therapy and their interaction in autistic children.' *Journal of the American Academy of Child Psychiatry*, **17**, 640–655.

Cohen, D.J., Johnson, W.T., Caparulo, B.K. (1976) 'Pica and elevated blood lead level in autistic and atypical children.' *American Journal of Diseases of Children*, **130**, 47–48.

—— Caparulo, B.K., Shaywitz, B.A., Bowers, M.B. (1977) 'Dopamine and serotonin metabolism in neuropsychiatrically disturbed children: CSF homovanillic acid and 5-hydroxyindoleacetic acid.' *Archives of General Psychiatry*, **34**, 545–550.

Coleman, M. (1979) 'Studies of the autistic syndromes.' *In:* Katzman, R. (Ed.) *Congenital and Acquired Cognitive Disorders.* New York: Raven Press, pp. 265–275.

Corbett, J. (1982) 'Epilepsy and the electroencephalogram in early childhood psychoses.' *In:* Wing, J.K., Wing, L. (Eds) *Psychoses of Uncertain Aetiology. Handbook of Psychiatry, Vol. 13.* London: Cambridge University Press, pp. 198–202.

Damasio, A.R., Maurer, R.G. (1978) 'A neurological model for childhood autism.' *Archives of Neurology*, **35**, 777–786.

Dawson, G., Warrenburg, S., Fuller, P. (1982) 'Cerebral lateralization in individuals diagnosed as autistic in early childhood.' *Brain and Language*, **15**, 353–368.

DeLong, G.R., Bean, S.C., Brown, F.R. (1981) 'Acquired reversible autistic syndrome in acute encephalopathic illness in children.' *Archives of Neurology*, **38**, 191–194.

Frith, U. (1989) *Autism: Explaining the Enigma.* Oxford: Basil Blackwell.

Garreau, B., Barthélémy, C., Sauvage, D., Muh, J.P., Lelord, G., Callaway, E. (1980) 'Troubles du metabolisme de la dopamine chez des enfants ayant un comportement autistique. Résultats des examens cliniques et des dosages urinaires de l'acide homovanilique.' *Acta Psychiatrica Belgica*, **80**, 249–265.

Gillberg, C. (1992*a*) 'The Emanuel Miller Lecture 1991: Autism and autistic-like conditions—subgroup of disorders of empathy.' *Journal of Child Psychology and Psychiatry*, **33**, 813–842.

—— (1992*b*) 'Subgroups in autism. Are there behavioural phenotypes typical of underlying medical conditions?' *Journal of Intellectual Disability Research*, **36**, 201–214.

—— Schaumann, H. (1983) 'Epilepsy presenting as infantile autism? Two case studies.' *Neuropediatrics*, **14**, 206–212.

293

—— Svennerholm, L., Hamilton-Hellberg, C. (1983) 'Childhood psychosis and monoamine metabolites in spinal fluid.' *Journal of Autism and Developmental Disorders*, **13**, 383–396.

Gladwell, S.R.F., Kaufman, K.R., Driver, M.V. (1979) 'Psychosis or epilepsy? Differentiation in a complex case.' *Developmental Medicine and Child Neurology*, **21**, 95–100.

Goldman-Rakic, P.S., Brown, R.M. (1982) 'Postnatal development of monoamine content and synthesis in the cerebral cortex of rhesus monkeys.' *Brain Research*, **256**, 339–349.

Goldstein, M., Mahanand, D., Lee, J., Coleman, M. (1976) 'Dopamine-beta-hydroxylase and endogenous total 5-hydroxyindole levels in autistic patients and controls.' *In:* Coleman, M. (Ed.) *The Autistic Syndromes*. Amsterdam: North Holland; New York: Elsevier, pp. 57–63.

Griffiths, A.D., Laurence, K.M. (1974) 'The effects of hypoxia or hypoglycemia on the brain of the newborn human infant.' *Developmental Medicine and Child Neurology*, **16**, 308–319.

Hauser, S., DeLong, G., Rosman, N. (1975) 'Pneumographic findings in the infantile autism syndrome: a correlation with temporal lobe disease.' *Brain*, **98**, 667–688.

Haymaker, W., Pentschew, A., Margoles, C., Bingham, W.G. (1958) 'Occurrence of lesions in the temporal lobe in the absence of convulsive seizures.' *In:* Baldwin M., Bailey, P. (Eds) *Temporal Lobe Epilepsy*. Springfield, IL: C.C. Thomas, pp. 166–202.

Hetzler, B.E., Griffin, L. (1981) 'Infantile autism and the temporal lobe of the brain.' *Journal of Autism and Developmental Disorders*, **11**, 317–330.

Hier, D.B., LeMay, M., Rosenberger, P.B. (1979) 'Autism and unfavorable left-right asymmetries of the brain.' *Journal of Autism and Developmental Disorders*, **9**, 153–159.

Hutt, S., Hutt, C. (1970) *Behavior Studies in Psychiatry*. Oxford: Pergamon Press.

Klüver, H., Bucy, P.C. (1938) 'An analysis of certain effects of bilateral temporal lobectomy in the rhesus monkey with special reference to psychic blindness.' *Journal of Psychology*, **5**, 33–54.

—— —— (1939) 'Preliminary analysis of functions of the temporal lobes in monkeys.' *Archives of Neurology and Psychiatry*, **42**, 979–1000.

Lake, C.R., Ziegler, M.G., Murphy, D.L. (1977) 'Increased norepinephrine levels and decreased dopamine-beta-hydroxylase activity in primary autism.' *Archives of General Psychiatry*, **34**, 553–556.

Landgrebe, A.R., Landgrebe, M.A. (1976) 'Urinary catecholamine studies in autistic children.' *In:* Coleman, M. (Ed.) *The Autistic Syndromes*. Amsterdam: North Holland; New York: Elsevier, pp. 65–72.

Lelord, G., Callaway, E., Muh, J.P., Arlot, J.C., Sauvage, D., Garreau, B., Domenech, J. (1978) 'L'acide homovanilique urinaire et ses modifications par ingestion de vitamine B$_6$: exploration fonctionnelle dans l'autisme de l'enfant?' *Revue Neurologique*, **134**, 797–801.

Myklebust, H., Killen, J., Bannochie, M. (1972) 'Emotional characteristics of learning disability.' *Journal of Autism and Childhood Schizophrenia*, **2**, 151–159.

Ornitz, E.M. (1978) 'Neurophysiologic studies.' *In:* Rutter, M., Schopler, E. (Eds) *Autism: A Reappraisal of Concepts and Treatment*. New York: Plenum, pp. 117–139.

—— (1983) 'The functional neuroanatomy of infantile autism.' *International Journal of Neuroscience*, **19**, 85–124.

—— Ritvo, E.R. (1968) 'Neurophysiologic mechanism underlying perceptual inconstancy in autistic and schizophrenic children.' *Archives of General Psychiatry*, **19**, 22–27.

Prior, M.R. (1979) 'Cognitive abilities and disabilities in infantile autism: a review.' *Journal of Abnormal Child Psychology*, **7**, 357–380.

Rapoport, J.L., Rumsey, J., Duavas, R., Schwartz, M., Kessler, R., Culten, N.,Rapoport, S.I. (1983) 'Cerebral metabolic rate for glucose in adult autism as measured by positron emission tomography.' *Journal of Cerebral Blood Flow and Metabolism*, **3** (Suppl. 1), 264–265.

Rimland, B. (1964) *Infantile Autism*. Englewood Cliffs, NJ: Prentice-Hall.

Ross, E.D. (1981) 'The aprosodias: functional-anatomic organization of the affective components of language in the right hemisphere.' *Archives of Neurology*, **38**, 561–569.

Rumsey, J.M., Grimes, A.M., Pikus, A.M., Duara, R., Ismond, D.R. (1984) 'Auditory brainstem responses in pervasive developmental disorders.' *Biological Psychiatry*, **19**, 1403–1418.

Shah, A., Frith, U. (1983) 'An islet of ability in autistic children: a research note.' *Journal of Child Psychology and Psychiatry*, **24**, 613–620.

Simon, N. (1975) 'Echolalic speech in childhood autism: consideration of possible underlying loci of brain damage.' *Archives of General Psychiatry*, **32**, 1439–1446.

294

Sofaer, J.A., Emery, A.E.H. (1981) 'Genes for super-intelligence?' *Journal of Medical Genetics*, **18**, 410–413.

Steffenburg, S. (1991) 'Neuropsychiatric assessment of children with autism: a population-based study.' *Developmental Medicine and Child Neurology*, **33**, 495–511.

Vilensky, J.A., Damasio, A.R., Maurer, R.G. (1981) 'Gait disturbances in patients with autistic behavior.' *Archives of Neurology*, **38**, 646–649.

Waterhouse, L., Fein, D. (1989) 'Social or cognitive or both? Crucial dysfunctions in autism.' *In:* Gillberg, C. (Ed.) *Diagnosis and Treatment of Autism.* New York: Plenum, pp. 53–61.

Weintraub, S., Mesulam, M.M., Kramer, L. (1981) 'Disturbances in prosody: a right-hemisphere contribution to language.' *Archives of Neurology*, **38**, 742–744.

Wetherby, A.M., Koegel, R.L., Mendel, M. (1981) 'Central auditory nervous system dysfunction in echolalic autistic individuals.' *Journal of Speech and Hearing Research*, **24**, 420–429.

Williams, R.S., Hauser, S.L., Purpura, D.P., DeLong, G.R., Swisher, C.N. (1980) 'Autism and mental retardation. Neuropathologic studies performed in four retarded persons with autistic behavior.' *Archives of Neurology*, **37**, 749–753.

Wing, L. (1989) 'The diagnosis of autism.' *In:* Gillberg, C. (Ed.) *Diagnosis and Treatment of Autism.* New York: Plenum, pp. 5–22.

Winsberg, B.G., Sverd, J., Castells, S. Hurwic, M., Perel, J.M. (1980) 'Estimation of monoamine and cyclic-AMP turnover and aminoacid concentrations of spinal fluid in autistic children.' *Neuropediatrics*, **11**, 250–255.

25
THE FIRST NEUROPSYCHIATRIC ASSESSMENT OF PATIENTS WITH AUTISM, AUTISTIC-LIKE CONDITIONS OR ASPERGER SYNDROME

This book is background for taking the history and conducting the physical, neuropsychological and laboratory evaluations of a child with autism. Nevertheless, both because of the difficulties of even touching some of these children with their severe haptic defensiveness and because of other unusual aspects of the examination, a few additional comments (based on the experiences of the authors of this book) are included with the examination checklist presented at the end of this chapter (Table 25.1). We claim no uniqueness; there are other fine approaches to this evaluation (*e.g.* Adrien *et al.* 1989).

First of all, it is important to realize that the neuropsychiatric diagnosis of a child with autism is often a long and complicated task without short cuts. The work-up should progress through the full assessment until a diagnosis is established and detailed information about the child's level of cognitive functioning, seeing and hearing is available for the educators who will be working with the child.

The likelihood that a medical diagnosis can be made for a child with autism is no longer remote. In a recent study by Steffenburg (1991) 37 per cent of a population-based series of carefully defined autism cases—conforming to DSM-III-R (American Psychiatric Association 1987), and Rutter (1978) criteria—were diagnosed after intensive neurobiological investigation as having at least one of the medical conditions described in this book. (Moreover, this percentage does not include the epilepsy/infantile spasms cases in this group.) One important finding of the Steffenburg study was that in at least half of these cases the diagnosis would not have been made had the medical investigation not been exhaustive.

In addition to the 37 per cent of children who had a definite medical diagnosis, 50 per cent had clear signs of major brain dysfunction not seen in normal children. Another 6 per cent had a close relative with Asperger syndrome/autism, providing the only clue to a possible aetiology. A few more also had a positive family history combined with clear evidence of brain damage. Of the total study group, in only about 5 per cent was there no clue at all as to the underlying aetiology of their autistic symptoms.

These figures could be taken to mean that at least 35 per cent of all autism cases are causally related to an underlying known medical condition, 5 to 10 per cent are clearly related to other hereditary factors (autism/Asperger syndrome or some other autistic-like condition), 50 per cent have unspecified major signs of brain dysfunction which could be brought about by medical conditions (hitherto undiscovered), hereditary factors or a combination of the two, and only 5 per cent have no strong or clear-cut clue as to the underlying aetiology. The Steffenburg study was presaged long ago in the 1970s when Lorna Wing and Judith Gould presented evidence that about 60 per cent of all children with 'classic' autism had major signs of associated brain damage/dysfunction (Wing and Gould 1979).

Optimally, a child with autism should receive his/her work-up and diagnosis in early childhood. In the assessment outlined below most emphasis is placed on the young age-group. The reader should keep in mind that modifications are appropriate for older children and adults. No major study has been published of adults with autism systematically evaluated and diagnosed as adults; their work-ups may have to be tailored for them as immunization and screening programmes often were not available when present-day adults were young. An example from Chapter 16 is the recent diagnosis of deletion of the short arm of chromosome 5 (the cri-du-chat syndrome) made in two adult men who were studied because they were in a chromosomal survey of adults with autism (Cantu *et al.* 1990).

The examination needs preparation, such as getting the medical records of the child and mother in advance. If possible, the examination room should be large with stairs available.

In these haptically defensive children, observation is an important skill to cultivate.

When the physical examination is started, one of the very first items may be one of the most difficult, since placing a cranial circumference tape around the head of a child with autism can be most difficult. Their haptic defensiveness is often most severe in the head area making measurements there hard to achieve. Auricle length may be a diagnostic indication for fragile X testing so this measurement is important to achieve.

Examination for minor physical anomalies is part of the work-up for a child with autistic symptoms: several studies have shown these to be more frequent in children with autism than in controls (Walker 1976, Campbell *et al.* 1978, Links *et al.* 1980).

Evaluation of the skin for the possibility of one of the three known (or other) neuroectodermal disease entities is often neglected (Fig. 25.1). A Woods lamp should be available if there are areas of depigmented skin, and the iris should be examined for Lisch nodules (Lubs *et al.* 1991). If any signs are found, the parent accompanying the child should also have the skin examined immediately, since these disease entities are almost always autosomal dominant.

Motor function in children with autism is often gauged by observation of posture, gait and ability to imitate motions. For examples, the Imitation of Gestures test of Bergès, with sensory and developmental components, may also reveal motor dyspraxia (Jones and Prior 1985). Spontaneous adventitious movements should be recorded (*e.g.* hand flapping, clapping, clasping or posturing; hands over the ears, eyes or in the mouth; jumping; rocking; whirling; facial grimacing).

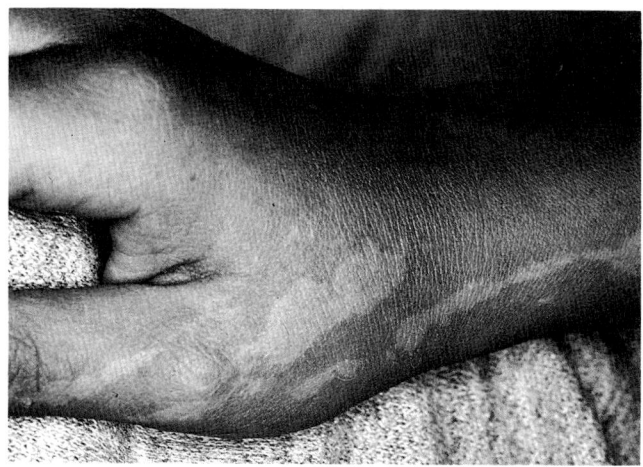

Fig. 25.1. Right hand of an 8-year-old boy with hypomelanosis of Ito and autism. Note hypomelanotic areas.

Regarding extrapyramidal function, investigators have noted that choreic posturing and hypotonia may be found in children with autism well past infancy (Walker and Coleman 1976).

The cranial nerve examination requires a great deal of cooperation; often it can be done only by inspection and a brief twist of cotton to the eye. It is an important examination in autism.

The reflex examination is relevant in this patient group because hyperactive or pathological reflexes can be an indication of brain damage later seen in EEG or imaging studies. It is interesting theoretically that infantile reflexes, such as the snout and visual rooting reflexes (see table), may be found in older children with autism; they may have developmental implications for the patient with autism (Minderaa *et al.* 1985).

Higher-functioning and older children with autism/Asperger syndrome may have speech, and some direct communication may be possible during the examination. It is relevant to observe whether the speech is flat, monotonous or improperly modulated; errors in stress, pitch, phrasing, intonation and inflection should be noted.

With respect to CSF examinations, current practice tends to vary considerably. In the Scandinavian countries, a lumbar puncture with CSF protein-electrophoresis is considered one of the basic procedures in the work-up of severe developmental disorders without a clear cause; some other countries have a more conservative attitude. We recommend this procedure as part of the work-up.

The importance of the ophthalmological (Fig. 25.2) and auditory examinations cannot be overstressed; these must be thorough (Rosehall *et al.* 1988). Not only are they of value in some cases diagnostically, but they help define the child's

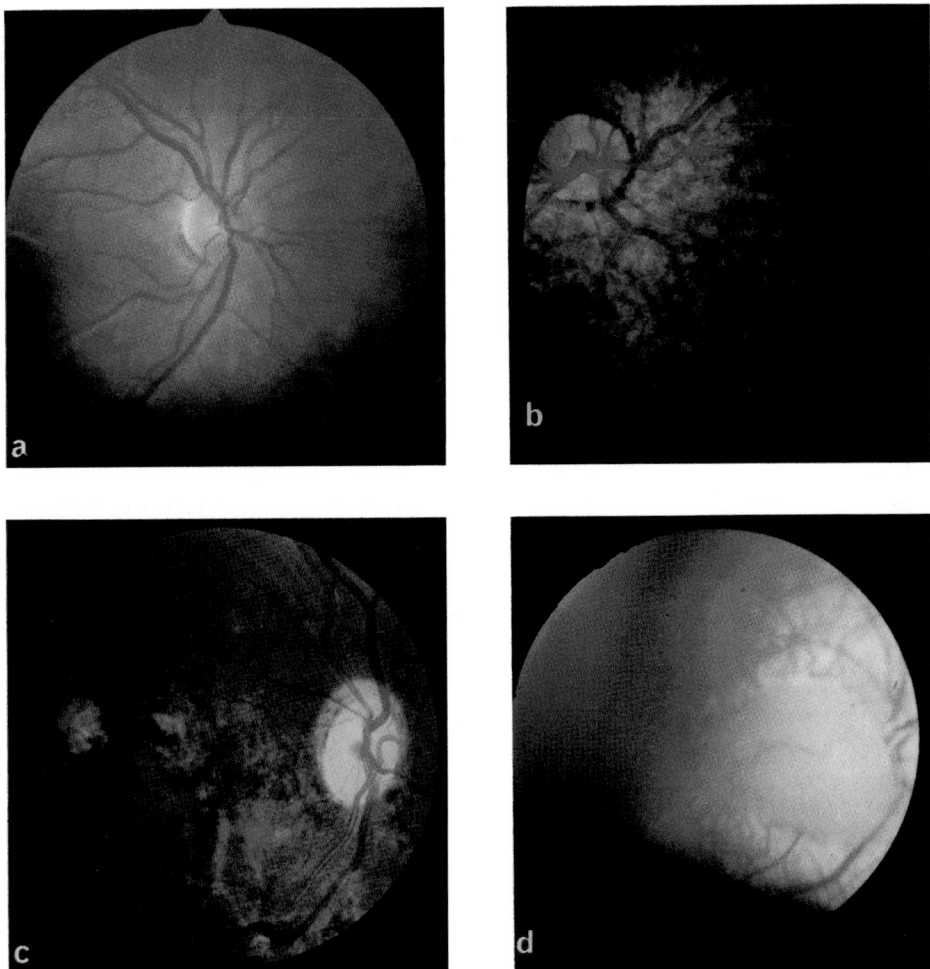

Fig. 25.2. Examination of the fundi can be helpful in patients with autism. (*a*) Normal fundus. (*b*) Rubella pigmentary retinopathy. (*c*) Herpes simplex type II choroidoretinitis. (*d*) Lucid white mass is a phakoma, a retinal tumour seen in tuberous sclerosis.

capacities and limitations regarding educational intervention.

We would now recommend magnetic resonance imaging (MRI) in preference to CT scanning as recommended in the first edition of this book. Because there is no radiation with MRI, more areas of the cranium can be scanned, increasing the likelihood of detecting any abnormality. In fact, there are a number of new studies showing that the MRI may be highly relevant to diagnosis (see Chapter 19).

These examinations are often limited by non-compliant and haptically defensive children. Skill, patience and sufficient time are ingredients likely to lead to success.

TABLE 25.1

Neuropsychiatric assessment checklist for autism

Materials needed

1—Autism assessment questionnaire: use validated questionnaire such as HBS (Wing 1980) or CARS (Schopler 1980)

2—Medical records of patient (gestational, birth, neonatal, paediatric)

3—Cranial circumference tape

4—Small ruler to measure auricle length and interpupillary distance

5—Woods lamp (to look for diagnostic skin changes)

6—Standard equipment for neurological examination

7—(optional) Video equipment for making a permanent recording of child's behaviour for your records

Special space requirements

1—Room for child to run

2—Stairs for child to climb

History and clinical assessment

Before seeing the patient and family

Review of medical records:

- ?maternal infections, bleeding, etc. during gestation
- ?optimality in pre-, peri- and neonatal periods
- ?postnatal potentially brain-damaging events
- ?medical illnesses of infancy
- ?growth patterns normal

Parent(s) present only

1—Detailed structured assessment in respect to autism using validated questionnaire

2—Detailed psychiatric history:

- family factors and psychosocial milieu
- temperament, attention span, sleep patterns, food fads of child
- family history for heredity (especially autism, Asperger syndrome, learning disorders, language delay, mental retardation, childhood psychosis, childhood schizophrenia, tuberous sclerosis, neurofibromatosis, phenylketonuria, uric acid disorders including gout, fragile X syndrome or other chromosomal disorders, geniuses, psychiatric disorders—especially affective disorders, anorexia nervosa, adult schizophrenia). Note kinship and make family pedigree chart

Child joins parent(s) and examiners

General physical examination

Non-intrusive observation throughout the examination. Observe posture, gait and what the child is grasping in his/her hand. Is child rocking or whirling? Or catatonic? Observe any adventitious movements, such as self-biting, hands over ears, hand flapping, clasping, wringing, clapping. Fingers or other objects in the mouth? Is there facial grimacing? Is child performing visual self-stimulation on a pattern in your office? Note and record any myoclonic jerks. If possible, observe spontaneous handedness. Record spoken language by child, if any

Measurements

- height, weight, cranial circumference, auricle length, interpupillary distance

Inspections

- look for minor physical anomalies (particularly ear anomalies and seating of ear, mouth anomalies, syndactyly in toes)

- look carefully at the skin for evidence of neuroectodermal diseases (use Woods lamp in any possible depigmented area, check for café-au-lait spots, adenoma sebaceum, etc.) and self-induced abrasions; check if freckles in armpits. Look at iris for Lisch nodules
- inspection of external genitalia (prepuce, penile and testicular size and volume) Examination of heart-beat variation if child is adequately cooperative

Age-appropriate neurodevelopmental/neurological examination
Cranial nerves—assess by inspection if child uncooperative

Reflexes—check standard deep tendon reflexes; also plantar flexion and clonus. Test for snout reflex[1] and visual rooting reflex[2]

Sensory examination—usually impossible; make a try at praxis testing at least

Extrapyramidal examination—assess muscle tone, observe child on stairs. If child runs, look for dystonic, choreic and/or athetoid posturing. Check milkmaid sign[3]

Neuropsychological evaluation
Should be performed by a clinical psychologist experienced at testing children with autism. The psychologist must know how to do cognitive testing of children with autism, which includes tests appropriate to age, developmental level, amount of language and degree of cooperation (WISC-R, Leiter, Raven and Griffiths may all be appropriate)

Laboratory examinations
1—Blood tests:
- whole blood
  —serotonin
  —chromosomal culture (standard and folate-deficient)
- serum
  —phenylalanine
  —pyruvic acid, lactic acid
  —herpes, cytomegalovirus titres
- red blood cells
  —magnesium
2—24-hour urine:
- uric acid
- calcium and phosphorus
- magnesium
- HVA
- creatinine (to check adequacy of 24-hour urine and for calculation of ratios)
3—CSF: protein electrophoresis (to rule out progressive encephalopathy)
4—Other essential laboratory tests:
- Ophthalmological examination
- Auditory examination, include brainstem AEP if child is language delayed
- EEG
- MRI

---

[1]*Snout reflex*—primitive reflex in infants, an involuntary pouting elicited by tapping the centre of the closed lips.
[2]*Visual routing reflex*—another primitive reflex, an involuntary rooting in response to the sight of food.
[3]*Milkmaid sign*—a sign of underlying basal ganglia disease; the examiner 'milks' the finger of the patient as if milking a cow: the sign is positive if the finger tremors.

REFERENCES

Adrien, J.L., Barthélémy, C., Lelord, G., Muh, J.P. (1989) 'Use of bioclinical markers for the assessment and treatment of children with pervasive developmental disorders.' *Neuropsychobiology*, **22**, 117–124.

American Psychiatric Association (1987) *Psychiatric and Statistical Manual of Mental Disorders. DSM-III-R (3rd Revised Edn)*. Washington, DC: APA.

Campbell, M., Geller, B., Small, A.M., Petti, T., Ferris, S. (1978) 'Minor physical anomalies in young psychotic children.' *American Journal of Psychiatry*, **135**, 573–575.

Cantu, E.S., Stone, J.W., Wing, A.A., Langee, H.R., Williams, C.A. (1990) 'Cytogenetic survey for autistic fragile X carriers in a mental retardation center.' *American Journal of Mental Retardation*, **94**, 442–447.

Jones, V., Prior, M. (1985) 'Motor imitation abilities and neurological signs in autistic children.' *Journal of Autism and Developmental Disorders*, **15**, 37–46.

Links, P.S., Stockwell, M., Abichandi, F., Simeon, J. (1980) 'Minor physical anomalies in childhood autism.' Part I: Their relationship to pre- and perinatal complications.' *Journal of Autism and Developmental Disorders*, **10**, 273–285.

Lubs, M-L., Bauer, M.S., Formas, M.E., Djokic, B. (1991) 'Lisch nodules in neurofibromatosis type 1.' *New England Journal of Medicine*, **324**, 1264–1266.

Minderaa, R., Volkmar, F., Hansen, C.R., Harcherik, D., Akkerhuis, G., Cohen, D.J. (1985) 'Brief report: snout and visual rooting reflexes in infantile autism.' *Journal of Autism and Developmental Disorders*, **15**, 409–416.

Rosenhall, U., Johansson, E., Gillberg, C. (1988) 'Oculomotor findings in autistic children.' *Journal of Laryngology and Otology*, **102**, 435–439.

Rutter, M. (1978) 'Diagnosis and definition of childhood autism.' *Journal of Autism and Childhood Schizophrenia*, **8**, 139–161.

Schopler, E., Reichler, R.J., Devellis, R.F., Daly, K. (1980) 'Toward objective classification of childhood autism: Childhood Autism Rating Scale (CARS).' *Journal of Autism and Developmental Disorders*, **10**, 91–103.

Steffenburg, S. (1991) 'Neuropsychiatric assessment of children with autism: a population-based study.' *Developmental Medicine and Child Neurology*, **33**, 495–511.

Walker, H.A. (1976) 'The incidence of minor physical anomalies in autistic patients.' *In:* Coleman, M. (Ed.) *The Autistic Syndromes*. Amsterdam: North Holland; New York: Elsevier, pp. 95–116.

—— Coleman, M. (1976) 'Characteristics of adventitious movements in autistic children.' *In:* Coleman, M. (Ed.) *The Autistic Syndromes*. Amsterdam: North Holland; New York: Elsevier, pp. 135–144.

Wing, L., Gould, J. (1978) 'Systemic recording of behaviors and skills of retarded and psychotic children.' *Journal of Autism and Childhood Schizophrenia*, **8**, 79–97.

—— —— (1979) 'Severe impairments of social interaction and associated abnormalities in children: epidemiology and classification.' *Journal of Autism and Developmental Disorders*, **9**, 11–29.

302

26
CONCLUSION

We have reviewed a great deal of information now available about the biology of the autistic syndromes. We end by discussing an interesting hypothesis whose cloth comes from the threads of many different coloured studies.

Autism is a behavioural disorder; its symptoms may reveal both the timing and the type of noxious agent that has affected the young child's brain. It now appears that an argument can be made that for some patients, autism may be a mid-trimester syndrome; that is the hypothesis that emerges from information of highly disparate disciplines as reviewed throughout this book.

No one piece of evidence can prove an hypothesis about as complicated a problem as 'what causes autism?' But there is a play and replay of the same mid-trimester theme in many different studies from a variety of disciplines. Using the framework of this hypothesis, one can find that a number of puzzling findings in autism may appear less enigmatic.

Chapter 9, which discusses the medical literature on preconception and prenatal factors, introduces the first critical piece of information. The only prospective study ever done of prenatal factors in autism was the Collaborative Perinatal Study of the National Institutes of Health (Niswander and Gordon 1972). 14 patients with autism were identified in a prospective study of 55,908 pregnancies (Torrey *et al.* 1975). Comparing the mothers of these children to those of both normal and mentally retarded controls, the study looked at 15 factors and identified a single prenatal event that appeared to be significantly associated with the subsequent development of autism—maternal uterine bleeding during gestation. Among the mothers of the children with autism there was significant mid-trimester bleeding, whereas in the two control groups, mid-trimester bleeding was extremely rare ($p < 0.01$).

Chapters 11 and 18, concerning immunology and infectious diseases, add information of a most interesting kind. One surprising finding is the monthly distribution of the births of children with autism. This distribution is so skewed that four well controlled studies (in three different countries) all found an excess of births in the same months of the year. Three studies found the excess in the summer months and the month of March (Bartlick 1981, Konstantareas *et al.* 1986, Burd 1988), the fourth in March alone (Gillberg 1990). Thus every study performed, without exception, found an excess of March births. Could this result be due to some unbelievable coincidence or could there be another explanation? Chapter 18 struggles with several possible reasons; a likely one is the fact that the early winter months (the season of virus epidemics) are the mid-trimester for March births. Late winter and early spring are the mid-trimester times of summer births.

Moreover, the type of infections which appear to be aetiologically linked to autism—almost without exception—are viral infections (see Chapter 18). That rarity, accurate documentation of the timing of a maternal infection in the case of a congenital infection of the infant, has been reported in a child with autism with congenital cytomegalovirus infection (Ivarsson *et al.* 1990). The primary infection of the mother occurred shortly before the twentieth week of gestation, *i.e.* mid-trimester. In addition, there are the new, provocative C4B null allele data (Warren *et al.* 1991), which could be interpreted as indicating that some women, known to have given birth to a child with autism, may not clear viral infections in an immuno-competent manner (Chapter 11).

Chapter 19, which discusses clinical results related to imaging studies, also has information pointing toward the mid-trimester of pregnancy. In a recent (MRI) study focused on the cerebral cortexes of 13 high-functioning subjects with autism, seven were found to have cortical malformations related to neuronal migration abnormalities (Piven *et al.* 1990). Similar MRI findings were reported in two Asperger syndrome patients (Berthier *et al.* 1990). These findings may have stunned the investigators because of the high level of functioning of the individuals being studied.

How can the patients with the highest level of functioning be the ones who have grossly visible malformations in the cortex? The answer may lie in what happens in the human brain during the second trimester: most neurons migrate to their final places (a few groups are still moving later than this), and the patterns and interrelationships among neuronal networks are set in place. It is a period of enormous brain growth and development of spatial formations. The cortical malformations described in the high-functioning patients with autism/Asperger syndrome were due to errors, misplacements and failures of neuronal migration.

The theory would assume that the higher-functioning children with autistic symptoms, those often diagnosed as having classical infantile autism or Kanner autism, go through the first trimester intact; the disease entity which causes their autistic symptoms does not effect their CNS until the second trimester. By then, the face and body are fully formed, and much of the fetal brain is beginning to function. There are already known to be a number of different noxious agents (viruses, trauma, genetically triggered metabolic failure not adequately compensated for by the placenta, etc.) that can interfere with the normal developmental process, probably very selectively, in the parts of the CNS outlined in Chapter 24. (As an example, it is known that herpes virus has a predilection for the temporal lobe; congenital herpes virus infection has now been described in childen with autism —see Chapter 18.)

The high-functioning infant with autism/Asperger syndrome is born, appearing normal, with symptoms only gradually surfacing as development unfolds. Because the injury was a second trimester event, the child appears relatively intact, not usually retarded, and even with areas of superior intelligence in some cases. It is likely that some sections of the brain have already developed normally, so it is too late for the pattern of migration to be changed by the damaging agent. This could explain how a child with Asperger syndrome who would have a good normal intelligence might also be found to have polymicrogyria (Chapter 19). It all depends upon the second trimester timing.

On the other hand, those children who suffer from both mental retardation and autism apparently have a disease entity that has a noxious effect throughout all the trimesters of the pregnancy. They have the mental retardation seen from first trimester injury, possibly adding autistic symptoms from continuing second trimester damage and so on. These children are those with chromosomal abnormalities, first trimester infectious diseases, overwhelming genetic metabolic disorders and so on.

In discussing the mental and emotional development of any young child, it is essential to recognize the developmental processes involved and the timing of how they unfold. One does not see all layers of brain function in a baby; even a severely cerebral-palsied child appears virtually normal at birth. In the case of mental retardation, one can never assess the extent of the intrauterine damage until a child is 3 years old. Intelligence tests are not fully predictive before that age. In the case of the autistic syndromes, 30 months or 36 months has been selected as the age of cut-off of onset of symptoms for diagnostic purposes. This is basically the same time-frame as in mental retardation when predictions and diagnoses can be made. For developmental reasons, it is hard to be sure of the effect of any prenatal damage until a child is several years old—this is true of the cognitive system, motor system and the emotional/social system.

However, perhaps the strongest argument of all for autism to begin in many children after the first trimester is the beautiful, non-stigmatized faces of so many children with autism, as seen in figures throughout this book. In many children, certainly nothing affected their facial development—a process which is completed by the end of the first trimester.

Finally, there are the children who undeniably have an insult to the CNS after birth, not just intrauterine damage showing itself as development matures, but a true postpartum noxious attack on the CNS. Such a patient is the previously normal 14-year-old girl with herpes simplex virus encephalitis that left her with permanent autistic-like symptoms the rest of her life (Gillberg 1986). In these cases, the noxious agent must selectively affect that section of the CNS which is the final common pathway of autistic symptoms (Chapter 24).

Thus, if this hypothesis is correct, in many cases the autistic syndrome may be a timing syndrome—a second trimester syndrome. Can it be that whatever causes the disorders of empathy—those characteristics that make children so appealing, so attractive, so huggable, so connected to us—has already done its damage long before the child even has its first hug?

REFERENCES

Bartlick, B.D. (1981) 'Monthly variation in births of autistic children in North America.' *Journal of the American Medical Women's Association*, **36**, 363–368.

Berthier, M.L., Starkstein, S.E., Leiguarda, R. (1990) 'Developmental anomalies in Asperger's syndrome: neuroradiological findings in two patients.' *Journal of Neuropsychiatry*, **2**, 197–201.

Burd, L. (1988) 'Month of birth of non-speaking children.' *Developmental Medicine and Child Neurology*, **30**, 685–686. *(Letter.)*

Gillberg, C. (1986) 'Brief report: onset at age of 14 of a typical autistic syndrome. A case report of a girl with herpes simplex encephalitis.' *Journal of Autism and Developmental Disorders*, **16**, 369–375.

—— (1990) 'Do children with autism have March birthdays?' *Acta Psychiatrica Scandinavica*, **82**, 152–156.

Ivarsson, S.A., Bjerre, I., Vegfors, P., Ahlfors, K. (1990) 'Autism as one of several disabilities in two children with congenital cytomegalovirus infection.' *Neuropediatrics*, **21**, 102–103.

Konstantareas, M.W., Hauser, P., Lennox, C., Homatidis, S. (1986) 'Season of birth in infantile autism.' *Child Psychiatry and Human Development*, **17**, 53–65.

Niswander, K.R., Gordon, M. (1972) *The Women and their Pregnancies (DHEW pub. no. 73-379.)* Washington, DC: U.S. Government Printing Office.

Piven, J., Berthier, M.L., Starkstein, S.E., Nehme, E., Pearlson, G., Folstein, S. (1990) 'Magnetic resonance imaging evidence for a defect of cerebral cortical development in autism.' *American Journal of Psychiatry*, **147**, 734–739.

Torrey, E.F., Hersh, S.P., McCabe, K.D. (1975) 'Early childhood psychosis and bleeding during pregnancy: a prospective study of gravid women and their offspring.' *Journal of Autism and Childhood Schizophrenia*, **5**, 287–297.

Warren, R.P., Singh, V.K., Cole, P., Odell, J.D., Pingree, C.B., Warren, W.L., White, E. (1991) 'Increased frequency of the null allele at the complement C4B locus in autism.' *Clinical and Experimental Immunology*, **83**, 438–440.

APPENDIX
GLOSSARY OF GENETIC TERMS

Autosomes. Chromosome pairs numbers to 1 to 22, in contrast to the gonosomes (q.v.)

Centromere. Constricted portion of the chromosome which divides it into long and short arms.

Deletion. Part of a chromosome arm broken off. The symbol for a deletion from the short arm of a chromosome is p– (from the French *'petit'*, meaning small) and that for a deletion from the long arm is q–.

DNA. Deoxyribonucleic acid: a sequence of nucleotides, usually double-stranded.

Dominant trait. One expressed in the phenotype in the heterozygous condition.

Duplication. Presence of a segment of a chromosome in a double dose on the same chromosome.

Exons. Coding parts of genes for structural proteins (non-coding parts are called *introns*).

Gamete. Mature germ-cell of either sex (ovum or sperm) with a haploid set of 23 chromosomes in normal circumstances.

Genes. Units of genetic information consisting of DNA.

Genetic mutation. Error in the exact sequence of the constituent DNA. (It is like a misspelling of the DNA sequence.)

Genome. All the chromosomal DNA (in humans, about 3×10^9 base pairs of DNA).

Genomic imprinting. Gene expression is modified by whether it is the father or the mother who passes on the chromosome to the child.

Gonosomes. The sex chromosomes X and Y, also called the 23rd pair of chromosomes.

Haplotypes. Sets of RFLPs (q.v.).

Histones. Basic proteins with 50 to 200 amino acids, notably arginine, lysine and histidine. Chromosomes are composed of DNA on a framework of histones.

Inversion. A fragment of a chromosome may break off, become inverted, and fuse again with the same chromosome so that a distorted sequence of genes results.

Isochromosome.   Chromosome with two identical halves (sometimes two identical short arms, sometimes two identical long arms).

Isodicentric.   Chromosome complexes with two centromeres.

Karyotyping.   Chromosomes in a cell arranged and analysed according to size and banding patterns.

Marker chromosome.   Chromosome material (from the regular chromosomal set-up) which appears as a separate chromosome not part of the normal karyotype.

Mosaicism (mixoploidy).   Two or more cell populations (clones), each with a different karyotype, in the same individual.

Recessive trait.   One expressed in the phenotype in the homozygous condition.

RFLPs.   Restriction fragment length polymorphisms, or suite of DNA markers; they are inherited.

Ring chromosome.   A chromosome in the form of a ring. There is deletion in the long and short arms and fusion of the two break-points, forming a ring.

RNA.   Ribonucleic acid: a sequence of nucleotides, usually single-stranded.

Satellite.   Small mass of chromatin separated from the short arm of the acrocentric autosomes by a small stalk (secondary constriction).

Transgenes.   Foreign genes introduced directly into the nucleus of a fertilized egg, integrated into nuclear DNA, and expressed in the phenotype. These are genetic chimera.

Translocation.   Transfer of a piece of one chromosome to another chromosome. If two non-homologous chromosomes exchange pieces, the translocation is balanced.

Trisomy.   Two haploid sets of 23 chromosomes plus one extra chromosome. The total number of chromosomes is 47 (rather than the usual 46).

Uniparental disomy.   An individual carries two copies of a chromosome, both inherited from the same parent.

ACKNOWLEDGEMENTS

The authors thank the following people who shared manuscripts in press or gave of their time and thought in the preparation of this book:

Ann Barnet, M.D.
Simon Baron-Cohen, Ph.D.
Magda Campbell, M.D.
Carina Gillberg, M.D.
Randi J. Hagerman, M.D.
Raffaele Ferri, M.D.
Uta Frith, Ph.D.
Gilbert Lelord, M.D.
Michele M.M. Mazzocco, Ph.D.
Maria Råstam, M.D.
Susan L. Smalley, Ph.D.
Suzanne Steffenburg, M.D.
Peter Tanguay, M.D.
Lorna Wing, M.D.

Mary Coleman wishes to thank her husband, Jay Y. Gonen, for his selfless support during the preparation of this book.

We also thank Helen Gravås at the Göteborg University Library and the staff of the Crearer Medical Library of the University of Chicago, in particular James Vaughan.

Carina Löf and Gun Jakobsson both contributed in the everyday work with this volume in many important ways, too numerous to mention.

We are indebted to Dr Pamela Davies and, in particular, to Pat Chappelle for excellent editorial work.

INDEX